Dementia

PERSPECTIVES ON INDIVIDUAL DIFFERENCES

CECIL R. REYNOLDS, *Texas A&M University, College Station*
ROBERT T. BROWN, *University of North Carolina, Wilmington*

Current volumes in the series

COGNITIVE ASSESSMENT
A Multidisciplinary Perspective
Edited by Cecil R. Reynolds

DEMENTIA
Allen Jack Edwards

EXPLORATIONS IN TEMPERAMENT
International Perspectives on Theory and Measurement
Edited by Jan Strelau and Alois Angleitner

FIFTY YEARS OF PERSONALITY PSYCHOLOGY
Edited by Kenneth H. Craik, Robert Hogan, and Raymond N. Wolfe

HANDBOOK OF CREATIVITY
Assessment, Research, and Theory
Edited by John A. Glover, Royce R. Ronning, and Cecil R. Reynolds

HANDBOOK OF MULTIVARIATE EXPERIMENTAL PSYCHOLOGY
Second Edition
Edited John R. Nesselroade and Raymond B. Cattell

INDIVIDUAL DIFFERENCES IN CARDIOVASCULAR
RESPONSE TO STRESS
Edited by J. Rick Turner, Andrew Sherwood, and Kathleen C. Light

LEARNING STRATEGIES AND LEARNING STYLES
Edited by Ronald R. Schmeck

PERSONALITY DIMENSIONS AND AROUSAL
Edited by Jan Strelau and Hans J. Eysenck

PERSONALITY, SOCIAL SKILLS, AND PSYCHOPATHOLOGY
An Individual Differences Approach
Edited by David G. Gilbert and James J. Connolly

SCHIZOPHRENIC DISORDERS
Sense and Nonsense in Conceptualization, Assessment, and Treatment
Leighton C. Whitaker

THEORETICAL FOUNDATIONS OF BEHAVIOR THERAPY
Edited by Hans J. Eysenck and Irene Martin

A Continuation Order Plan is available for this series. A continuation order will bring delivery of each new volume immediately upon publication. Volumes are billed only upon actual shipment. For further information please contact the publisher.

Dementia

Allen Jack Edwards

Southwest Missouri State University
Springfield, Missouri

Plenum Press • New York and London

Library of Congress Cataloging-in-Publication Data

Edwards, Allen Jack, 1926-
    Dementia / Allen Jack Edwards.
        p.   cm. -- (Perspectives on indvidual differences)
    Includes bibliographical references and index.
    ISBN 0-306-44286-8
    1. Dementia.   2. Dementia--therapy.   I. Title. II. Series.
    [DNLM: 1. Dementia--diagnosis.   2. Dementia--psychology.   WM 220
E26d]
RC521.E4   1992
616.8'3--dc20
DNLM/DLC
for Library of Congress   92-49161
                                                                    CIP

ISBN 0-306-44286-8

© 1993 Plenum Press, New York
A Division of Plenum Publishing Corporation
233 Spring Street, New York, N.Y. 10013

For Joel,
who still makes good things happen

Preface

Dementia is a state that has implications for several groups. There are, first, those who wish to assess its nature and impact in an objective and scientific fashion, using tools of research to uncover dementia's causes, effects, and parameters. The result has been a rapidly expanding literature in diverse disciplines: physiology, chemistry, neurology, psychology, and sociology, among others.

Second, there are those professionals and caregivers who work directly with patients and other caregivers and who must assess and apply interventions. Third, physicians are involved in diagnosis and treatment (so far as possible) and are responsible for communicating the ominous meanings of the destructive disease process. Fourth, there are the caregivers, who accept accountability for the future of a human who increasingly shows a "robbing of the mind" in his or her behaviors. The needs and stresses of those who care for and about those with progressive dementia are among the most intense imaginable. They need support of many kinds, frequently without knowing what to ask or of whom to ask it. Finally, there are the patients, who increasingly become dependent as their mental competencies decline. They need empathic care—including answers to questions about cause, stabilization, or reversal of the dementing process. Even more, they need cure. Further, present and future generations need the assurance of prevention.

This volume surveys present "knowledge" about dementia and its consequences. As a result, no one discipline is emphasized; indeed, there is a frank intent to reflect the interests, needs, and resources of each of the groups just described. It is hoped that the selectivity that had to be used with the resulting copious (if not always enlightening) literature does not damage the intent seriously.

To accomplish the goal of appealing to disparate audiences, topics were selected that have specific but unrestricted interest. Accurate diagnosis, including differentiating criteria, of the various conditions that may lead to dementia is a major concern. The diagnostic procedures used medically, buttressed by psychological tests and brain scans, are the subject of the text. Description of a number of instruments, both standardized and nonstandardized, is included to assist the reader in appreciating the problems involved. The cause, prognosis, course, and outcome of each precursor of a dementing state are assessed by loooking at representative studies of these processes.

The meanings and effects of dementia for both patients and caregivers are a second focus of the book. Psychological and social ramifications for both groups have been heavily researched and reported. As a result, the literature explores outcomes of dementia in considerable depth. Unfortunately, what might be done to rectify the many negative effects has not been investigated as thoroughly, and the results of those studies that have been conducted are less than compelling. As disciplines (such as psychology and sociology) and sub-disciplines, in particular (such as verbal learning and neuropsychology in psychology), communicate and cooperate in model building and in research efforts, the outcomes should be rewarding for the well-being of patients and caregivers.

Although only a portion of the available literature has been surveyed, the focus of this volume is, admittedly, *research*. After reading well over 1,000 published papers, I believe that what is included is reasonably representative—while it is doubtless that significant studies have been left out. My apologies both to researchers and to readers of this volume for any important omissions.

Humankind faces a major challenge in the twenty-first century. Unless there is continuing, sponsored research, future generations of a steadily aging world population will face increasing peril from the devastating effects of a variety of syndromes. This book represents a look at where we stand at this moment. Although that is sufficient reason for its publication, whatever positive effects this effort has on future events will be a bonus. It is my hope that a prospective volume (and I wouldn't object were it by me) can report significant medical, psychological, and social progress.

Several people must be acknowledged for their assistance in making the manuscript a reality. Foremost is my colleague and friend, Elissa M. Lewis, who patiently critiqued, questioned, encouraged, and challenged the content to help produce a better manuscript. Whatever merits the book has are due largely to her efforts. My thanks, as well, to Carol and Bob, who always unselfishly and unquestioningly took in an author who needed access to the Health Sciences Library at the University of

Missouri. My gratitude to Jean for support and encouragement. To any others I have not mentioned directly, I offer my sincere gratitude.

ALLEN JACK EDWARDS

Springfield, Missouri

Contents

3. Identifying Dementia

4. Technology and Diagnosis

5. Dementia and Psychological Testing

6. Dementia and Psychiatric Disorders

7. Dementia and the Patient—I

8. Dementia and the Patient—II

9. Dementia and the Family

10. Intervention Techniques

11. Dementia and the Future

CHAPTER ONE

The Nature of Dementia

The last half of the twentieth century has seen the growth of a remarkable awareness of health care, both in terms of needs and research. Many conditions that resulted in slow and painful death in past generations are now made more tolerable by drugs or surgery, whereas some are treatable to the extent that their progress is halted or slowed, and a few are now curable. These last conditions, however, are restricted almost exclusively to diseases with known causes and/or major research efforts.

With an aging population worldwide, there is an increasingly recognized condition that has received far too little research and for which causes are not yet clear. These are the syndromes that affect the nerve cells of the brain, altering their structures in such a way that they no longer perform in the normal fashion. Because damaged neurons do not regenerate, the alterations are permanent, and any effects they create, including behaviors, are usually permanent.[1] Usually there is no way to stop the progression of the disease, because there is no treatment. Thus the process may progress to other nerve cells—gradually but inevitably leading to the behavioral deficits, excesses, and/or inaccuracies known as *dementia*. The consequences may well be described as a "systematic robbing of the mind" whereby the person becomes increasingly dependent, unsure, demanding, unaware, and incompetent. With an aging population that is growing in size, there is the probability that dementia will reach epidemic proportions in the twenty-first century.

DEFINING "DEMENTIA"

Despite the rather common use of the word by physicians and lay persons, there is little evidence that the term *dementia* is being used to mean the same thing in all cases. One may even make a case for the position that it is a scrapbasket diagnosis that refers to a variety of different conditions with similar outcomes in their behavioral effects. After all, the Latin term *mens* means only "mind," whereas *de* signifies "from." In the less literal sense, then, dementia must mean a loss of mental competence, without reference to causation or consequences. It seems clear that this is really too broad a meaning to have much practical application, and so there is a need to be more specific.

The *International Dictionary of Psychology* (Sutherland, 1989) defines the syndrome as

> an impairment or loss of mental ability, particularly of the capacity to remember, but also including impaired thought, speech, judgment, and personality. It occurs in *senile dementia*, and in conditions involving widespread damage to the brain (such as *Korsakoff's Psychosis*) or narrowing of the blood vessels. (p. 112)

This clearly refers to observable, and seemingly measurable, behaviors. The principal effect is a loss of memory, though the particular forms of memory so affected are not specified. Further, thought and judgment are adversely influenced, in large part because the memory of the patient does not function adequately. There is even the extension to speech and to personality, indicating the broader effects of a devastating syndrome. Finally, there is reference to certain physical problems that may produce such effects.

Sutherland further introduces a slightly different term, *senile dementia*, which deserves its own definition. "Senile" comes from the Latin adverb "senilis," derived from "senex" (pertaining to age or growing old). Some dementias, then, must occur only or largely in the aged, for unspecified reasons. The *International Dictionary of Psychology* defines senile dementia as

> a progressive syndrome *starting in old age* with no clear cause, in which intellect, memory, and judgment are impaired; it is often accompanied by apathy or irritability. (Sutherland, 1989, p. 397; italics added)

This definition is quite close to that of dementia, with the addition of some loss in intellect to accompany deficiencies in memory and judgment. In addition, responses to be expected in the patient are apathy or irritability although this is not universal.

These definitions provide us with some "signs" or "symptoms" that should alert us to a problem in ourselves or other persons. That problem *may be* dementia (or senile dementia if we are old enough) but not necessarily so. It is possible to show signs of memory loss or poor judgment, yet not be demented. For example, one may suffer depression (a treatable disorder) and behave in a manner that indicates poor memory and poor judgment. If the depression is treated, there will be relief with memory and judgment restored to the level they had before the depressive episode.

A more precise definition of dementia may be found by referring to those who have studied the syndrome and should know its salient characteristics. Miller (1977, pp. 4–5) points out that dementia has been used in two different ways. This complicates our understanding. First, there is a general meaning that reflects changes in the individual resulting in deterioration in behaviors over what would normally be expected for this person. Miller illustrates this usage with the example of a localized brain tumor that lowers cognitive competence despite educational and social advantages that the individual has had. If there are psychological deficiencies—such as apathy and withdrawal—that accompany these changes, then the patient may be classified as "demented." However, the physical and behavioral changes are so common to so many causes that the term signifies little or nothing uniquely and fails to provide a dis-criminative pattern for psychological diagnosis or treatment.

This brings us to Miller's second meaning. The label *dementia* may be restricted to a group of conditions, related in describable ways, or to a specific syndrome. This is the more practical use of the term and the one recommended by Miller. He points out that its principal application should be for a group of related conditions, dichotomized on the basis of age of onset. Those states that occur after a certain age (he mentions age 65 as the dividing line, but only as a convenience) will be dementias of the senium, labeled *senile dementias*. Those that more commonly occur before that arbitrary age cutoff will be labeled *presenile dementias*. The distinction is more apparent than real, as Miller has clearly indicated, not only because there simply are no syndromes that can be shown to occur only after or before a given age but also because a basis for making a diagnosis is unclear. Behaviorally, the effects of dementias due to any one of several causes are similar, perhaps even indistinguishable. "Tests" to assure accuracy of diagnosis are lacking; many will be decided only by exclusion of treatable conditions. Nevertheless, if there is agreement on the syndromes to be included (Miller designates those he believes are appropriate), then there is better understanding of what "dementia" means.

Reference to other sources demonstrates that agreement and under-standing are far from complete. Spar (1982), for example, has discussed the diagnostic evaluation of persons who complain of symptoms that may reflect a dementia. Assessing the reality of the symptoms expressed and the condition suffered, in order to make an accurate diagnosis, re-quires evaluation for pseudodementias (such as depression). If these, and other treatable syndromes, are excluded, the decision may be made that the only remaining possibility is a diagnosis of a syndrome leading to dementia. The next step is to consider if intervention is possible to relieve some of the symptomatology. Spar suggests that some of the difficulties suffered by the patient as a result of the dementia may be alleviated by psychopharmacology or psychotherapy. The patient diagnosed as having Alzheimer's disease, for example, may experience depression because there is awareness of the disorder's effects. Depression should not only be recognized but can be treated also. One can see the "ripple effect" that is involved even when demarcation of the disease process occurs.

Wolanin (1983) provides much the same opinion as Spar, but with even broader description of influencing factors and confusing events. Her discussion includes the difficulties of discrimination of symptoms for diagnosis, the possible confusion and overlap among many conditions both treatable and untreatable, and even social and cultural diffences between the elderly and those who are younger. These differences, in a climate where people are alerted to look for problem behaviors in the aged, may lead to unwarranted concern and even the belief that there is a dementia where none actually exists. If this attitude is found in a diagnostician as well, the older person may be in danger of being misclassified and treated inappropriately.

Yet another recognized figure in the field is A. E. Slaby. He has presented a quite straightforward definition for dementia as "a chronic impairment of cognitive ability secondary to cerebral cortical or subcortical cellular dysfunction" (Slaby & Cullen, 1987, p. 135). The emphasis here is on the loss in cognitive ability, a decrement that is chronic and therefore probably irreversible, perhaps even progressive. This intellectual deficit is the result of some neuronal dysfunction in the cortex of the brain or the area below the cortex. There could be a variety of conditions leading to such dysfunction, but regardless of the cause the result will be found in the cognitive deterioration. Slaby adds that not only is prevalence unknown, but dementia itself is not a diagnosis (p. 135).

This approach opens new possibilities. In the attempt to define, one must distinguish effects from cause and label from disease. Commonly, emphasis is placed on describing the "effects" that are found with dementia. Slaby and Cullen (1987, pp. 135–136), for example, describe signs found early in the developmental period. The principal one is increasing incompetence for recent memory events. As this change occurs, those associating with the patient in the vocational setting or at home may note that repetition of routine instructions may be required beyond that normally needed for this person. With increased dementia, more and more situations will require this need for repetition. It is important not to "explain away" or ignore such events but to recognize them and to have the person seek a mental evaluation from a qualified professional. If identified early, the chances for effective intervention, perhaps even reversal, are greater.

There are other noteworthy signs as well. A loss of initiative, for example, may indicate that the individual is having trouble coping with routine life events. By refusing to act, the demented person may cover the disturbing reality that something is wrong. A personality change may accompany a decrease in effective coping. For example, the person may become increasingly irritable and thereby cut off routine challenges in order to avoid confrontation. These and similar signs (Slaby and Cullen cite loss of interest in life activities, problems coping with circumstances requiring original thinking, increasing difficulties with activities of daily living) are cues to the observant family members and colleagues of a significant problem. The use of mental-status screening devices can be helpful in determining the extent of the problem so that more thorough diagnostic procedures may follow.

Differential diagnosis[2] must occur next. This process will permit the clinician to distinguish the reversible from the irreversible and the treatable from the untreatable. Some 20% of dementia cases may be reversed, and perhaps another 25% or so may be partially treatable (Slaby & Cullen, 1987, pp. 135–136). Some differential diagnosis focuses on identifying drug or other toxic causes and metabolic disturbances. Such a distinction, as early in the process as possible, offers hope if individuals will admit to having cognitive malfunction. Ignored and avoided, the time may come when intervention is not successful. This process allows one to delineate two "types" of dementia based upon signs of mental incompetence: One results from a disease process with its medical implications; the other from toxicity, due to purposeful or accidental ingestion by the individual. Diagnosis is important principally for deciding which "type" is pertinent and deciding subsequent intervention. The distinction is meaningful, but there remains the problem of describing the more traditional diagnoses of dementia, their courses and consequences.

A Definition Used in This Book

Though other authorities might be cited and other sources used as illustrations, there would be little advantage in so doing. The point should be clear that there is no single nor perfect definition. Rather, all are of the "working hypothesis" type and must be accepted as such.

The definition used in this text is something of an amalgam derived from Miller and from Slaby. Dementia is defined, then, as *a result of a set of conditions, medically diagnosed, and leading to recognized and measurable behavior changes in an individual.* The "set of conditions" referred to will include the following so-called "diseases": Pick's, Alzheimer's, Creutzfeldt–Jakob, Huntington's, and Parkinson's, although all will not receive equal consideration in this book. In addition to these syndromes, there will be discussion of multiinfarct dementia and normal pressure hydrocephalus. Identifying characteristics and diagnosis will be described for each syndrome. All of these conditions are diagnosed and labeled by a physician, though psychologists may contribute to the final decision. Greater attention will be paid to their effects, that is, the behavioral changes that may be recognized and measured. The changes will be described, and the methods for recognition and measurement will be surveyed. The "result" alluded to at the beginning of the definition will be focused on the patient and other persons affected by the condition, such as family members, primary caregivers, and secondary (institutional) caregivers.

CONDITIONS LEADING TO DEMENTIA

The conditions that lead to the outcome of dementia are best described in terms of medical diagnoses. There are currently several syndromes, which are understood at various levels and to various degrees, that meet this criterion. The following descriptions are provided in order to permit a rudimentary understanding and will be more fully elaborated in a subsequent chapter. The order of presentation should not be construed as reflecting relative importance, degree of severity, level of knowledge, nor amount of physical and mental involvement.

Pick's Disease

This syndrome was first described by the Czechoslovakian psychiatrist and neurologist, Arnold Pick (1851–1924). He published his descriptions in 1892, detailing an atrophy of the cerebral cortex leading to dementia. In this syndrome there is a progressive impairment of intellect and judgment (necessary to fit the definition for dementia) with transitory aphasia. This latter condition, reflected in an inability to understand or produce either spoken or written language, may be the major sign used to diagnose the state. With the extent of brain damage resulting from the atrophy, in most cases both of the expressive forms of communication will be lost. There are a variety of aphasias, but they do not necessarily lead to dementia; that is, even with one of the aphasias, dementia is not a foregone conclusion. Pick's, then, is a case with a special outcome, due to the general atrophy of the brain. Such degeneration may be disclosed by use of a scan (such as computerized axial tomography), but all atrophy that may be found is not the result of Pick's. The combination of total aphasia and demonstration of atrophy is central to this diagnosis. Sutherland (1989, p. 326) points out that the diagnosis is more common in females than in males, although why this occurs is not known. He also notes that the symptoms include incoherent thinking, stereotyped behavior, and eventual loss of all mental faculties. Most commonly, the disease expresses itself in middle age. In the traditional scheme, then, Pick's leads to "presenile dementia."

Creutzfeldt–Jakob Disease

This syndrome bears the names of two physicians who described it at about the same time. Hans Gerhard Creutzfeldt was a German psychiatrist (1885–1964) who, in 1920, published his description of the condition. This was followed in 1921 by Alfons Maria Jakob's (1884–1931) article in the same journal. The disease has a known cause: a slow virus[3] that results in infection affecting the nerve cells of the brain. Cohen (1988, p. 120) notes that communicability is unconventional because it is not transmitted in the usual ways, with the possibility of a genetic connection that is exercised only in the presence of the virus.

The course of the disease is progressive and fatal, with presenile dementia usually occurring in middle age (Webster's *Medical Desk Dictionary*, 1986), but Cohen notes that it may occur also in young adulthood or old age if the conditions of transmission are met. The course of the disorder is usually rapid, with death commonly occurring within 1 year of onset (Cohen, 1988, p. 120). A distinguishing feature of Creutzfeldt–Jakob disease is the presence of muscular incoordination, particularly ataxia. The condition is rare and has been diagnosed in only a few hundred cases per year in this country.

Alzheimer's Disease

This syndrome was first described by the German neurologist, Alois Alzheimer (1864–1915) in 1907, although it is currently the condition that most Americans are afraid and aware of. He had noted behavioral changes in two of his female patients who were in their fifties. He felt these changes reflected premature aging, as their mental abilities deteriorated in a fashion to be expected only in very old persons. He described the memory losses and confusion these females experienced and labeled them *presenile dementia.* Today, the disease process is still believed to occur in the presenium, though the majority of diagnoses are in persons over the age of 65. In fact, the evidence indicates that there will be a significant increase in the frequency of diagnosis of Alzheimer's in persons over age 75 as we have more persons living longer lives.

Currently the syndrome is considered a degenerative disease of the central nervous system. Sutherland (1989, p. 19) describes it as "a form of presenile dementia caused by atrophy of brain cells, usually starting at about 55, and producing severe intellectual, sensory, and motor deterioration, and ultimately death." Cohen (1988, pp. 116–117) more precisely details memory loss as the dominant feature, with a subsequent decrement in other intellectual functions. Thus those behaviors that depend upon adequate memory function will change for the worse. The onset is gradual and insidious, showing an irregular course that eventually produces deterioration of mental competence so that the patient is unable to respond appropriately to normal tasks. At some point, then, care and supervision must be provided with eventual total dependence occurring before death. The course of the syndrome varies, with patients living from a few years to as many as 20 or more years. Unexpectedly, those showing the effects prior to the senium usually have the shorter life course, though very aged persons (over age 85) will have shorter prognoses as well.

The cause of Alzheimer's is not yet known, so that diagnosis is imprecise. Probable diagnosis is possible, if brain tissue is examined microscopically. Because biopsies of brain material are rare, diagnosis usually is by exclusion. After considering and eliminating all other possible causes of behavior changes, either reversible or irreversible, the diagnosis may be made. This procedure allows for the possibility of error in diagnosis, an issue that has been investigated in postmortems. Unfortunately, the availability of viable brain tissue from corpses is small, and the issue of diagnostic accuracy remains an open one.

Huntington's Disease (Chorea)

This syndrome was described by a family physician in a single medical publication and subsequently named for him even though he was not the first to write about the condition. George Huntington (1850–1916) was an American who published his paper in 1872 (Webster's *Medical Desk Dictionary*). He gave a detailed account of the symptoms found in the chorea, especially of the regression that brings on dementia (Webster's *Medical Desk Dictionary*, 1986). A chorea is any of a number of disorders that have an infectious or organic origin. The results behaviorally are involuntary, uncontrollable, and purposeless movements of the body. There is, in particular, incoordination of the limbs, and the condition historically has been called "St. Vitus' dance."

Huntington's disease is hereditary, with onset usually in one's 30s or 40s. At first, it expresses itself with abrupt movements of the joints and progresses to severely distorted movements of the body. As the motor dysfunction increases, so may the presence of signs and symptoms of dementia. Guyton (1991, p. 631) says that the abnormal movements may result from the loss of cell bodies that produce certain inhibitory neurotransmitters such as Gamma-aminobutyric acid (GABA). Without inhibition, the movements are spontaneous and uncontrollable.

However, the dementia associated with Huntington's disease is more likely the result of loss of neurons that produce acetylcholine (Guyton, 1991, p. 631). The result will be a decrement in mental competencies, including severe memory loss.

Parkinson's Disease

James Parkinson (1755–1824), a British surgeon, in 1817 published a monograph on *paralysis agitans* and proposed a clinical entity. The syndrome, caused by degeneration of the nervous system, is insidious and progressive. It is most noticeable in the individual's poor motor coordination, with tremor and an inability to initiate voluntary actions. The cause is unknown, but it is suspected that the function of the neurotransmitter dopamine, produced in the basal ganglia, is impaired. In fact, the symptoms may be better controlled through the use of a substitute for dopamine, a chemical called L-dopa, which the brain apparently uses to create a balance between inhibition and excitation in portions of its structure. However, the effect is cosmetic and is not a treatment for the condition itself. Guyton (1991, pp. 630–631) reports that in research conditions, surgical destruction of parts of the basal ganglia or the thalamus or perhaps even portions of the motor cortex, causing feedback to be blocked, may help control the syndrome. At present, such surgical procedures are not accepted as an appropriate intervention with patients. Dementia is not a certainty with the Parkinson's patient, but it does result in enough cases to warrant its inclusion here.

Multiinfarct Dementia

The term infarct refers to the death of an area of living tissue because of an obstruction in the circulatory system. It may be due to a blood clot in a blood vessel that prevents proper circulation of the blood or by some particle, like an air bubble, not normally found in the tissue but brought to it by blood circulation. Infarcts may occur anywhere in the body, of course, but they assume a special relationship to dementia when they occur in the brain. In effect, the infarcts produce strokes.

Whenever neurons are destroyed, the loss is permanent because brain cells do not regenerate. With sufficient destruction of certain portions of brain tissue, there will be increasing behavioral disruption so that the individual demonstrates a dementia. Multiinfarct dementia is the result of a series of strokes, often slight or subtle so that they may not be diagnosed individually but in the aggregate contribute to a decline in competency. In this case, the initial pathology is commonly outside the brain itself (for example, heart disease) but produces the behavioral effects through a clot formed elsewhere that goes to the small blood vessels in the brain. The resulting clogging brings about a stroke of greater or lesser magnitude. Those who receive a diagnosis of multiinfarct dementia usually have a history of heart disease or hypertension. Whether or not dementia occurs depends on the areas of the brain affected by the strokes (Guyton, 1991, p. 209).

Because the progress of dementia depends upon the destruction of brain tissue by a series of strokes, the deterioration assumes a stepwise appearance. There may be months between strokes in some instances and only weeks or perhaps days in others. The result is that the steps may not be regular in either a horizontal or vertical direction. This is a distinctive feature of the dementia, resulting from multiple infarcts, that differs from the course found with other causes, such as Alzheimer's disease. However, when it does occur, the result is as inevitable and as destructive as with any other condition leading to the loss of mental competence and the same behaviors occur.

Normal Pressure Hydrocephalus

Within the cranium, the brain tissue is surrounded with cerebrospinal fluid. The balance between the two may alter with age as tissue shrinks and fluid increases, although the ratio is normally maintained, at least into old age. Sometimes, however, for unknown reasons, cerebrospinal fluid pressure increases and produces in adults the effects of hydrocephalus. In this case, the brain has not atrophied, but the ventricles[4] have enlarged due to the pressure of the fluid and have forced the compression of the brain tissue into a smaller than normal size. When the condition occurs, it is believed that a dementia will begin and proceed rapidly. There will also be incontinence and ataxia. Miller (1977, p. 123) points out that these symptoms are not very reliable for diagnostic purposes and that, although scans will disclose ventricular enlargement, beyond that fact there is still little agreement on diagnosis. Miller (1977, p. 123) states that better definition of the syndrome is needed to permit more effective treatment for patients who will develop dementia from the condition. At this point, then, there is a case for some small number of individuals who may show demented behavior apparently because of the change in pressure levels of cerebrospinal fluid in the brain. More definitive study is being conducted and should provide a basis for accurate and reliable description and discussion in the future.

As this survey would indicate, there are at least a half dozen identified syndromes producing the results that are labeled dementia. However, perhaps the direct antecedent is not so important as the behavioral consequences, especially if intervention does not occur. The outcomes, then, must be considered next.

THE EXPRESSIONS OF DEMENTIA

The behavioral expressions of dementia have been well described, particularly for the loss of memory, but a more meaningful discussion may result if there is first a review of certain functions of the brain. Our actions and thoughts seem so natural to us that we may be in danger of oversimplifying a most complicated system. The brain is a complex organ, so complex that it is still only partially understood. Our understanding does include an awareness of the several functions that allow us to live our lives in reasonable accord with the environment.

In the cortex, there are three "association areas" that receive signals from the sensory sites. One of these associative areas carries on a constant interpretation of our body in its spatial orientation, both for the various parts of the body and for its position in the environment. Guyton (1991) points out that "to control the body movements, the brain must know at all times where each part of [the] body is located and also its relation to its surroundings" (p. 637). This means that each of our functions is a kind of small universe in the midst of many such universes. We must be aware of our own identity and its place in reference to other identities if we are to function. If that awareness is not present, we will not be able to relate to those other "universes" or to the environment, and our actions will not be those necessary to success.

Essentially, then, each of us must be oriented in time and space constantly if we are to be independent as well as interdependent. Loss of this orientation will leave us with all kinds of capabilities that we cannot employ because we are a universe with inaccurate reference points or without contact altogether. Imagine, if you will, that you leave the room you are now in. As you exit the doorway, you find a world different from that you expected, at variance with the one about which you are aware and with which you deal confidently. Instead, everything is strange: There are no familiar landmarks, sounds are incomprehensible, and persons seem unconcerned and distant. Such an event would leave one confused, unsure of how to proceed or to react, probably frightened rather than challenged, and almost certainly without confidence. As alien as this other world might seem, that might well be the result if the cells in the brain's association area responsible for orientation were to become diseased or damaged. You could still hear, you could still see, you could still be aware, but you would no longer be able to interact effectively. Terry and Parker (1990, p. 69) describe this state by pointing out that *consciousness is not altered.* This is one of the outcomes of dementia and is the result of degeneration of nerve cells in the association area.

If one is disoriented, the possibilities of problem solving, judgment, decision making, or any of the other so-called "higher-order-thinking" processes will be impossible. What especially complicates the picture is that there may be certain times when one is disoriented and other times when one is not, or, just as likely, some types of behaviors show disorientation, whereas other types do not. Consider the frustration of the individual suffering such unpredictable interaction with the environment and empathize with the family that observes what seems to be erratic or obstinate behavior in a person who has previously been competent in dealing with the world.

In short, the behaviors that will be adversely affected by dementia depend upon the neurons that are diseased. Miller (1977, p. 7) notes the similarity in such a disease process to "normal aging." In both cases, there will be atrophy (shrinkage) of the brain due to degeneration and death of neurons. In both cases, there will be plaques and neurofibrillary tangles. There is a difference in the extremes to which each of these proceed, however, and one should not assume that the occurrence of dementia is inevitable if one lives long enough. More to the point here is the fact that in dementia the most affected areas are the frontal and temporal lobes and the hippocampus (Miller, 1977, p. 7), precisely those areas that include the association areas and memory functions.

Memory Loss

Memory loss is the most commonly described effect of dementia. Of course, without memory every stimulus is a new one, and every response would have to be developed from scratch, leading to such disruption that orderly, predictable actions would be impossible. The more complete the memory and the more extensive it is, the easier we may adapt to constant and to changing conditions. Rapidity of correct response is an increasing probability for constant conditions, whereas change in the environment may be adapted to through the use of prior experiences and responses.

There are several "kinds" of memories that are currently recognized. Though the authors' labels for these may vary, the functions are similar from one model to another, and all the descriptions deal with how we may encode experience to use in the immediate present or in the future. In all, there is an assumption of some form of storage that will then permit retrieval of experiences, and it is this process that is most interrupted by dementia. First, we must consider how memory may be developed.

Sensory Register

There are many experiences in our lives that we do not need to preserve beyond the immediate. For example, if you are driving down a street and approach an intersection with a traffic light, you must be concerned as to whether it is green, yellow, or red. If you observe that the light is red or yellow, you will slow down preparatory to stopping. If it is green, you must decide whether or not you will proceed, and this decision likely will be based on how long it has been green. Once an action has been carried out, you no longer need to preserve for future use the particular conditions prevailing at the time. The "memory" of color will not be stored in any form because it has no relevance to future behavior. True, you used past experience that *had* been stored in order to make a reasonable decision, but this particular incident would no longer be needed. This example represents what we know of the type of memory we call "sensory register." As the title indicates, we normally register experiences related to sensations that require an immediate response, but that are largely or solely independent of future actions.

Sensory register should not be dismissed as unimportant. In fact, it may be our most widely used form of memory. Certainly it does represent the first step in memory storage, for without it other forms would have nothing upon which to base storage. Somehow the "mind" makes a decision about storing or not storing a particular experience. Further, that decision has some reference to the length of time that storage is necessary. Included in this must be some habituation based upon the repetition of certain experiences or the intensity of experience, but even here there is surely some limit. How many repetitions of "green means go, red means stop" do we need before we discontinue the storage? The question does not have an answer at present, though we are sure that repetition does facilitate neural patterns to permit accurate and rapid responding. When that point is reached, we no longer need to store that particular example.

Short-Term Memory

The immediacy of sensory register will not satisfy all needs for memory. We must store some events for a period of time, even though that period of time may be only for minutes or hours. This second stage provides the basis for such experiences. Here, the event cannot be responded to immediately and/or requires a greater use of stored experiences. Through some mechanism as yet not clear, there must be a "consolidation" (Guyton, 1991, pp. 645–646) involving chemical, physical, and anatomical changes in synapses involved in memory. This process may take from a few minutes (perhaps 5 to 10) up to an hour or more. Once accomplished, however, the event is stored for future use. Perhaps the process involves "rehearsal"—a capability accorded to the brain for certain types of information. In addition, as the consolidation proceeds, the memories will be classified into different categories.

However the process works, there seems to be a need to accept this level of memory storage in order to act efficiently. As an example of short-term memory, we can consider a task commonly used to test it. I may say to you that I am going to say some numbers and that I want you to repeat them when I have finished. I may begin with a span of four digits, presented in a random order, then go to five digits, and continue until I reach a span that you can no longer retain long enough to repeat exactly. To perform on this task, you must encode the numbers and retain them in the order I present them for a period long enough to "pass" the span. It has already been demonstrated that the "magic number" of such units is 7, plus or minus 2. This means that most persons can recall some span between 5 and 9. Longer spans are rarely attempted because an effective ceiling has already been reached.

The "short-term" nature of this memory task is demonstrated in another way. If, 10 minutes after the task is completed and unless you were warned that a test would follow, the chances that you will remember the span of six digits would be so low as to assume no probability. There simply was no perceived need to encode beyond the time of testing, and so the transfer to a level requiring such memory did not occur. The experience of that span "washed out" from lack of relevance.

The distinction between short-term and long-term memory is not always so clear. Certainly, if there is a temporal restriction on experience limiting it to the immediate present, short-term memory is all that is required. However, there is the possibility for some overlap. For example, you may need to store some material for use at a later time; in effect, there will be a "test." You may study the material and rehearse it by attempting recall without looking back at the material. If your recall is good, you may assume that you have now "learned" adequately and that storage in long-term memory is assured. When the "test" occurs, however, you may find that you had insufficient rehearsal so that you accomplished short-term status but not long-term. The experience did not receive enough habituation and/or consolidation and/or classification.

Long-Term Memory

Now we have reached the ultimate—stored experiences available to us for long periods of time, perhaps for a lifetime. It would seem reasonable that we store in long-term memory only the events that will be needed over and over or that are so significant that they should be permanently available. Practically, however, we're all aware that we maintain a variety of thoughts that are so trivial in fact that we call them "trivia."

The process of long-term memory involves a decision about the importance of the event so that it may or may not be enhanced as a memory trace. The way this decision is "made" in the brain is not known, but the limbic system is involved to a significant degree (Guyton, 1991, p. 643). The procedure is the same for all persons, but there is certainly a unique dimension from one individual to another. Each of us may have the same experience, but it may not assume the same status for memory storage. Indeed, even when two of us agree on the importance of the event, what is stored in long-term memory may vary greatly.

Within this context, we build a lifetime of experiences, stored so that we may use them to act with purpose and rationality. What is stored will be modified by new experiences so that we cannot assume the validity of every event reported to us by others. But, by and large, our past assists us in dealing with the environment and interacting with it to our benefit. What we record and report is our identity. With neurons intact, we are functional; with neurons lost or damaged, we are dysfunctional.

These levels of retention apply to dementia in some clear ways. As a dementia progresses, the patient will have greater and greater difficulty in responding effectively to the environment. Earlier in the process, there will be evidence of inability to utilize short-term memory. Events occurring that require encoding with minimum dependence on already-stored recall will be responded to poorly. In this regard, the patient will have difficulty with a memory span test, a frequently used measure to determine the possible presence of a dementia. Beyond this superficial example are more important ones. For example, the dementia patient may be presented with a clear instruction that normally would be responded to effectively. One may say to the person, "Your lunch is on the kitchen table. Do you want to get it for yourself?" The answer may well be "yes," but the message is not encoded and the patient may do nothing. Later, the patient may be upset and ask, "Why didn't I have any lunch?"

Decrements in memory function eventually will affect all three levels, though when and to what degree cannot be predicted. The long-term memories are the most likely to be maintained so that remote events, often rehearsed, may persist for years in the development of the dementia. Because there is an irregular pattern, appearances to those unfamiliar with the individual may be deceiving. The patient will continue to respond to such superficial questions as how one feels today, statements about weather conditions, polite notations about seeing one another, and the like. If questions are used that require encoding and the use of "new" material, however, the patient will be increasingly at risk of failing to respond accurately and effectively. With sufficient progression of the disease, some stored memories will no longer be available.

The dementia expresses itself in memory loss in two ways (though not necessarily at the same time or in the same degree). First, the person is less and less able to used stored experiences to assist in meeting the demands of daily life. The bookkeeper can no longer add a column of figures accurately, the farmer can no longer be trusted with the tractor, the restaurant employee is unable to carry out a dishwashing task, and so on. Such expressions are critical indeed because they disrupt normal, routine functioning that cannot be disguised. Such incidents more often than not are the "sign" to the caregiver and the patient that something is so wrong that it can no longer be ignored. By this time, the dementia has progressed to such a point that intervention may be impossible.

Coexisting with such major interruption in memory will be the inability to respond effectively to current stimuli. The cues are present, but the patient cannot interpret and/or react appropriately to them. Increasingly, the individual may have to depend on "crutches" to cover inadequacies. Professionals who have dealt with dementia patients know of the skill developed in utilizing the caregiver as such a crutch. When something is asked, for example, to which the person cannot effectively respond, she or he may turn to the caregiver and say, "Oh, yes, now how does that work?", or so "condition" the caregiver that the answer comes from that source almost automatically.

In an alien world where memory is impaired or lost, confusion seems a reasonable reaction and result. The confused state also is frequent in the patient and represents a manifestation of memory loss. The individual may be "lost" in his or her own home where she or he has lived for many years. Needing to urinate, the location of the bathroom is not known or, being in the bathroom, whether to use the tub, commode, or lavatory is not clear to the patient. Such examples are legion and represent major difficulties for those faced with dementia in either role.

We have what appears to be a normal person. Certainly there is no physical problem evident (because dementia is a robbing of mind and not obviously of physical systems), and there may be seemingly lucid use of language. However, this individual is not whole, and it requires some awareness and patience to distinguish the functional behaviors from the dysfunctional.

SUMMARY

Dementia is a term with a central focus—loss of mental competence expressed in observable and measurable ways—but not always used to reflect only that focus. In some instances, the label is reserved to these outcomes, but at other times it is used to signify the syndrome that causes the behavioral outcomes. In this book, the two are separated in order to preserve clarity. Both are important; thus the apparent causes are described as well as the symptoms and signs. This introductory survey will lead to more extensive treatment in succeeding chapters.

CHAPTER TWO

The Brain and Dementia

Dementia is the result of certain syndromes that alter the status of nerve cells in the brain. This alteration expresses itself in several observable behaviors, principally memory loss but also confusion and disorientation, and the effect is one of systematically "robbing" the mind. This means that there are two related but discrete elements involved: the structural integrity of the brain on the one hand and the loss of competencies deemed possible because of a mind on the other. The two need to be described separately as well as in terms of their relationships. In this chapter, there is an attempt at this task with the restriction that only the most essential elements will be highlighted.

A brief review of the evolution of the brain should be the first step. In some respects, the human brain does not differ greatly from that of other animals. This not only means that certain behavioral tendencies are shared (such as involuntary activities of the tongue or muscles, co-ordination of motor activity, and maintenance of balance) but also that study of the brains of lower animals may reveal some evidence about human behavior. The principal difference between humans and other animals is in the evolution of the cerebral cortex that gives us the capabilities that make us particularly human.

Indeed, the cerebrum, made up of the cerebral cortex, the underlying white matter, and the basal ganglia, is the most highly developed and multifunctional part of the human brain. The *cerebral cortex* is a grayish outer layer that is made up of densely packed cells called neurons. There are so many of these cells that they are in layers, with the ability to interact with one another, greatly expanding the utility and potential of the brain. Each of these nerve cells is unmyelinated, that is, they lack a substance that increases the speed of conduction of nerve impulses.

The "*white matter*" mentioned above consists of fibers that appear white and are myelinated, that is, they have a white, fatty substance around them that acts as insulation. As a result, they are capable of a higher velocity in the conduction of nerve impulses than are the un-myelinated neurons of the cortex.

The *basal ganglia* also consist of gray matter and are involved in the control of posture and movement. Of these three, though all three are important, our major interest for purposes of this text is in the cortex.

The cerebral cortex is a dull shade of gray, appears to have large wrinkles, and seems to have segments or compartments due to deeper fissures. Its very design is one of its strengths because the multiple folds permit inclusion of many millions of cells in a limited space. If the human cortex were to be flattened out, it would be only about an eighth of an inch thick, but it would be 3 feet long and 2 feet wide. Because it is folded in on itself, it is possible to have about three times as much tissue within the cranium as appears on the surface area.

Given this design, the human brain has evolved to permit behaviors both unique and profound. Humans can interpret the environment in ways unknown to other species and as a result can rearrange the environment to suit individual needs and desires (admittedly a talent with outcomes of mixed value). Humans have an ability for language that exceeds that of all other animals because it goes beyond the immediate and concrete to deal with the abstract and creative. Our species devises symbols such as the alphabet to serve purposes not inherent in the symbols themselves.

Indeed, we are so adept at developing these that we take it for granted. Our children model their language expression on our own and by age 2 or so possess a vocabulary sufficient to communicate at complex levels. Despite physical immaturity, they can begin to substitute the written symbol for the spoken one within the first decade of life. Once they have acquired that skill, there are virtually no limits to which they can take their talents. Written documents allow us to preserve history, to document change, to foster allegiances and causes, to create and invent, to challenge and stimulate. All of these can occur in the absence of direct contact with other persons or events, once we have achieved literacy.

We expect all adults to have some basic functioning in such skills, and their absence is a signal that we must provide in special ways for the few who do not. Having demonstrated competence in oral and written language in adulthood, we expect that skill to be maintained and expanded throughout the rest of life. An interruption or reversal is not only unexpected but is felt to indicate a significant abnormality. However, we are living in an era when such cases are increasing, to our surprise and dismay. The culprit is dementia—effects that first arrest then deteriorate the ability of the individual to continue functioning as an active member of society. The change affects not only the afflicted person but others as well. Immediate family members must assume support roles that they neither expected nor prepared for; social and governmental agencies may be solicited for assistance with the "costs" attached to a variety of deficits; and society is faced with the privations accrued due to the individual's inability to contribute any longer. To translate these deficits and losses into merely financial terms would depreciate their importance. Indeed, what we must be most concerned about is the loss of an important human being—a loss that results from some physical condition, not yet understood, that destroys the quality of the most significantly human organ and causes deterioration from maturity to dependence. As dramatic as this sounds, it is not possible to overemphasize the importance of the cortex and its healthy functioning.

THE STRUCTURE OF THE CORTEX

The brain consists of two hemispheres that cooperate with each other through the corpus callosum that joins them and that also perform somewhat different functions. In most humans, the left hemisphere is dominant. Sometimes characterized as the "logical and rational" side, the left half is the site of predominance of language function (plus other skills, of course). Disease or damage in this hemisphere, then, may have particularly adverse effects on the ability of the person to use and understand those symbols that are uniquely human. The right hemisphere may be described as the more "subjective and creative." Damage to cells in this half may have more detrimental effects on the ability to deal with novel stimuli and to be artistic in one's expression. If disease processes affect both halves, the person will be less likely to demonstrate the variety of competencies normally expected of the individual. Figure 2.1a shows the left hemisphere in a surface view, whereas Figure 2.1b is the right hemisphere shown in a section cut to disclose components within the brain.

Both hemispheres are divided into areas called "lobes." These areas are roughly designated according to the way fissures occur. Though largely a convenience, such divisions do make it possible to describe where major sites for particular competencies are located.

The Lobes of the Brain

There are four of the areas designated as "lobes."[1] The frontal lobe is, of course, in the front part of the brain; the parietal lobe runs across

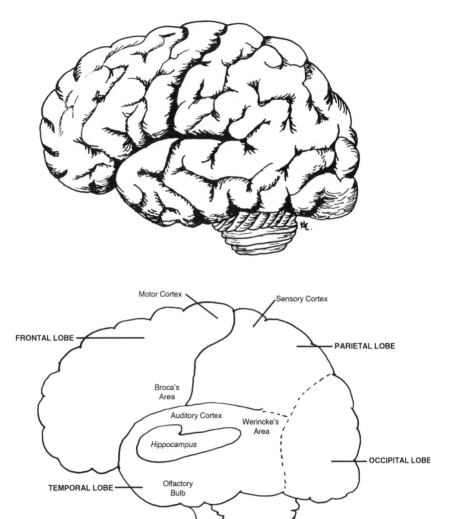

FIGURE 2.1. (a) Left hemisphere of brain in surface view; (b) right hemisphere of brain in center view.

the top central area; the temporal lobe is on both sides; and the occipital lobe is in the rear.

Each of the lobes contains nerve cells that have evolved to perform certain functions or to assist in those functions. The frontal lobe, for example, contains "Broca's area," which has been identified as the place where word formation occurs. Within the frontal lobes generally there is also the "association area"[2] that is used in planning complex movements. It appears that any elaboration of thought, a higher intellectual process, is carried out primarily in this lobe as well.

The parietal lobe contains the motor and sensory cortexes. Additionally, it is involved with the occipital lobe in an association area that keeps our bodies coordinated and helps us stay aware of our bodies in space (orientation). In conjunction with the temporal lobe, the association area includes "Wernicke's area," the most significant portion of the brain so far as our intellectual abilities are concerned because Wernicke's is responsible for language comprehension.

The temporal lobe contains the auditory cortex and the olfactory bulb. Below Wernicke's area and slightly behind it is the portion of the brain involved in naming of objects. Finally, the occipital lobe is the center for the visual cortex. One of the functions served here is the visual processing of words.

Most of the capacities described are essential to one's functioning as a competent adult. Damage in the cells of one portion of the brain may have deleterious effects in another portion that is responsible for higher-order thought. For example, if we are unable to visually process words, we will not be able to read even though we understand the word when presented orally. Because the visual cortex may have other healthy cells except in the processing area, we may even be able to recognize that there is something written, but what that "something" is becomes incomprehensible no matter how well practiced in the past.

There is one other structure that needs to be identified and described. The *hippocampus* is a bit of gray matter just a little more than an inch long. Located beneath the temporal lobe on both hemispheres, it is believed to be the site where long-term memory begins. Its involvement in *why* some memories are stored and others are not is unknown. Much of the knowledge of the role of the hippocampus is based on cases in which damage to the hippocampus has resulted in disruption of long-term memory.

There are many other capabilities and functions for the brain than those cited. The preceding presentation is meant only to be a limited representation of the abilities most central to the adequate functioning of the intellect.

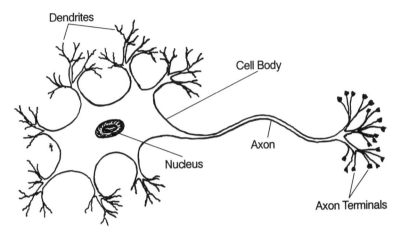

FIGURE 2.2. Drawing of typical neuron.

THE WORKING UNIT OF THE BRAIN: THE NEURON

Throughout the human body there are billions of nerve cells that serve the systems of the body so that we may function efficiently and effectively. There are estimates of as many as 100 billion such cells (100,000,000,000), each capable of interacting with several thousand other cells. The potential is staggering in its implications *if* all such cells are healthy. However, damage to these cells occurs during our lives, and destruction of a neuron is permanent, so that whatever functions it may be responsible for or whatever memories it may have stored will be lost permanently. Such massive numbers, then, may be an evolutionary precaution against too great a loss.

Cohen (1988, pp. 170–173) has discussed the possibilities of compensation in dendritic sprouting and axonal formation for a damaged cell where the cell body is healthy. The use of mentally stimulating environments in such cases would be of great benefit. Unfortunately, the conditions leading to dementia do not attack only the dendrites and axons. Inevitably, the cell body will be diseased, greatly decreasing the efficacy of many interventions though not completely eliminating their usefulness.

Though all neurons do not have the same shape (varying with the function of that cell), they do share certain features. (See Figure 2.2 for a typical neuron.) In each, there is a *cell body* with a nucleus. The latter contains the deoxyribonucleic acid (DNA) responsible for the programming of that cell's functioning. All neuronal cells also have *dendrites*, extensions from the cell body that are designed to receive signals (electrical impulses) from other nerve cells. The more dendrites the better because this increases the possibility that the cell will receive information upon which the brain can act. There is an increase in the number and length of dendrites from birth until only age 10 or so. Admittedly, we have the potential for many more behaviors than we will ever develop or use under present circumstances, but the fact that cell loss accumulates as we live our lives should cause us some concern. In fact, as we grow older, dendrites begin to shrivel, leading to less likely communication between cells. Recently, de Ruiter and Uylings (1987) compared cellular morphology in five patients (four Alzheimer's and one multiinfarct dementia) with five postmortem controls. All cases were age 65 or older. They reported clear differences, with significant dendritic degeneration more pronounced in the dementia cases than in the controls.

Virtually all neurons also have an *axon* extending from the cell body. The axonal end is involved in transmitting the electrical signal to the dendrites of adjacent cells. The axons vary widely in length from a fraction of an inch to as much as 3 feet, depending upon the function of the cell.

Associated with the neurons are the *glial cells*. They serve various roles, from myelinization to removal of dead cells. The myelin is deposited on the dendrites, and so the glia assume the responsible function of myelinization during the period when proliferation of dendrites continues.

Between the axon of one cell and the dendrite of another is a very small space called the *synapse*. The electrical signal must jump across this space in order to continue its journey. Assisting in this task are various *neurotransmitters*, chemicals that may be discharged across the synapse in order to allow binding with a receptor site on the dendrite of the next neuron. There are a number of these neurotransmitters with the possibility either to excite the neuron to "fire" or to inhibit it. Thus these chemicals are of extreme importance to the functioning of the person. Several of them have been implicated in the processes that lead to dementia. For example, *dopamine* has been identified as insufficient in Parkinson's patients, whereas *acetylcholine* is lacking in the Alzheimer's victim. A number of studies have been reported in recent years that describe such relationships (e.g., Winblad, Hardy, Backman, & Nilsson, 1985; Gottfries, 1985; Goodnick & Gershon, 1984). Because this issue and its meaning are important to our understanding of dementia and its expressions, it will be addressed again in Chapter 7.

THE INTELLECT

To this point, we have described a few of the physical properties of the human brain. In some cases, there is empirical evidence of direct brain–behavior relationships. For example, it is clear that stimulation of a particular portion of the brain will lead to a physical expression. Most of these demonstrated outcomes are muscular, but there is also evidence about other systems. The results of dementia, even though eventually influencing physical actions (such as changes in gait or development of incontinence), are of primary importance for their changes in mental functioning and in their effects on the adaptability of the individual. We need, then, to develop an understanding of the intellectual nature of humans, allowed but not explained by an understanding of the complex structure of the brain.

For this purpose, we will examine part of the efforts to define intelligence and to measure adult intellectual functioning, describe what we know of its attributes, and discuss its relation to dementing conditions.

The Nature of Intelligence

The importance of intellect to our ability to respond to the world and its demands is obvious. In fact, we have a variety of terms that pay homage to our efforts. Words like "dumb," "clever," and "original" are everyday expressions, and each says something about the way we have dealt with a problem. Implicitly, then, we not only acknowledge the presence and use of intelligence, we imply as well that we recognize and understand it.

However, the fact is that our observations of the effects of what we believe intellect to be are based on behaviors allowed by the quality, not on an understanding of its nature. Indeed, the two principal sources of evidence about intelligence consist of results from tests designed to measure the amount of ability on the one hand (the so-called "intelligence tests") and laboratory experiments requiring participants to demonstrate the ability to grasp and solve problems of various kinds on the other.

The dilemma revolves around the relationships of cause and effect. Scientifically, if we can describe and measure a "cause," we may be able to demonstrate empirically the variety and contexts of its effects. In the case of intelligence, however, we are able to observe effects without knowing the true nature of their causes. We are left then with the necessity of *inferring* what the true nature of the cause may be, not only a less scientific mode of proof but one that is fraught with a strong probability of error in unknown ways.

Nevertheless, the construct is too important to ignore. We must be particularly concerned because dementia has such an adverse effect on the outcome variables resulting from intellect. A good beginning point will be to examine the possible definition of intelligence and survey measures and outcomes based on such a definition.

Sutherland (1989) defines intelligence as "in general, the aptitude for solving those problems that can be solved by thought." We recognize, then, the quality by its effects. There is the implication that the quality permits more than limited recognition of stimulation, interpretation of that stimulation, and responding to it. "Higher-order" faculties or thinking is a common expression, without saying specifically how much higher or in what ways.

The most influential figure in the adult intelligence test movement has been David Wechsler (1896–1984). As a soldier during World War I he had been introduced to group tests developed by a number of outstanding psychologists and used for classification purposes. He also had the opportunity to meet Carl Spearman and was greatly intrigued and influenced by Spearman's concept of a "general" nature of intellect with a large number of "specific" abilities influenced by that general quality. During the 1930s Wechsler developed his own definition, based on the Spearman model. This definition was to remain unchanged (though expanded in certain limited ways) throughout the rest of his life (Edwards, 1974, pp. 5–6).

To Wechsler, intelligence in its nature is a global capacity that occurs in some amount in all of us. Although there will be differences in the amount of this capacity, these need not be particularly large. The capacity each of us possesses is supposedly present at birth, remains unchanged by experience, and allows us to deal with the everyday encounters of which life is comprised. He proposed three general expressions of our global capacity that he did not mean to be inclusive or restrictive—merely representative. What we can *do* with our capacity results in the ability to think in a rational way (thus objectively dealing with experience), act with purpose (thus defining goals and means of reaching those goals), and deal in an effective manner with environmental stimulation (Edwards, 1974, pp. 5–6). His often-quoted definition is:

> Intelligence is the aggregate or global capacity to act purposefully, to think rationally and to deal effectively with the environment. (Wechsler, 1944, p. 3)

During the 1930s, Wechsler became chief psychologist at Bellevue Hospital in New York City (Edwards, 1974, p. 10). One of his chief duties was to serve as a member of a psychiatric team that was responsible for a recommendation for disposal of psychological cases (say for treatment with or without commitment or for discharge). His particular charge was to evaluate the educational and intellectual status of each case so that this information could be a part of the data upon which the recommendation was based. There were several adequate measures of educational achievement (the ability to read and write, numerical facility, and the like). However, the only individually administered intelligence test available (and the principal one used in other settings) was the Stanford Revision of the Binet Scale, a test designed for use with children and normed on the assumption that mental growth was completed by age 16 (Terman & Merrill, 1937, p. 29). To Wechsler, it seemed inappropriate to use such a measure on adults in a decision-making process that could influence their lives for better or worse. The alternative was to design and norm a test intended for adults and to include content appropriate to the target population and purpose (Edwards, 1974, pp. 11–14).

Earlier, he had decided that the most pertinent approach was to use a series of tests (called subtests), each containing a set of items representing a designated ability and graded from easiest to most difficult. This tactic, called a *point scale*, would allow the use of the same items and the same subtests across a wide age range. In this case, the test was to be constructed so that all adults could be tested and compared using the same test. Originally called the Wechsler-Bellevue, the test had two scales. One was the Verbal Scale, consisting of five subtests (later enlarged to six), all of which allowed the individual to display the abilities possessed in the use of verbal symbols. The other (also with five subtests) was called the Performance Scale. Each of these permitted the expression of an ability to perceive and manipulate concrete objects under a time limit. He made this Verbal–Performance division on the basis of a belief that intellect may express itself in more than one way. However, for expediency, it was necessary to limit the content of the test. As a result, he decided that these two modes of expression would be adequate for his purposes and would allow the person to show strengths in either or both directions (Wechsler, 1944, pp. 136–138).

Wechsler borrowed freely from test ideas already available (Wechsler, 1944, p. 76) and adapted them to his needs and purposes. Although it may not be original, this approach showed the pragmatic good sense of assuring a reasonable probability that the test would "work"—as it certainly did and has continued to do. Essentially, performance on the scale should reflect the outcomes of the individual's capacity: purposeful action, rational thinking, effective dealing with the environment. In addition, each of the subtest's content may be related to some specific ability that may be important to a decision about the individual. There is even the potential for the examiner to observe the way the examinee approaches tasks and reacts to the different kinds of subtest content. Inferentially, then, some predictions may be made beyond the precise test behavior, though such inferences always demand external validation.

The results of an individual's performance on the Wechsler-Bellevue (or one of its progeny such as the current Wechsler Adult Intelligence Scale—Revised) yield a score that ranks the individual in his or her age group. This "score" is a derived quotient (called the intelligence quotient or IQ) that is compared to a normal distribution of such scores. The mean is 100, so this particular score signifies an individual who performed at the average of the age group. A score of 130 exceeds 95% of the age group, one of 70 is exceeded by 95%, and so on. Other conclusions that may be drawn from this test are inferential and subject to error. Wechsler, educated as an experimental psychologist, believed that some inferences must be made, but he cautioned against unverifiable conclusions. Much of the antipathy about this test is due to the *interpretations made by test users*, not to the design, scoring, or quotients in and of themselves.

As mentioned, the point scale allows testing across a wide age range with all items being administered to all individuals for comparative purposes. This is a strength that has diminishing returns in some ways. The WAIS–R, for example, is standardized for use with persons between ages 16 and 75 (Wechsler, 1981, p. 51) so that norms end with age 74. Although Wechsler (1981, p. 51) maintains that the test may be used for those older than 74, he also recognizes certain problems are involved because the norms will not be representative. There is the further problem that the age range of the scale may be too broad anyway, so that there needs to be a separate test devised for persons over age 55 or 60, and certainly for those over age 75. It is interesting that in the last years of his life, Wechsler was considering the possibility of a scale to be devised for use with and normed on older persons. Richard van Frank, at the time the senior editor for the behavioral sciences at Academic Press, Inc., even suggested what seemed a most appropriate title: The Wechsler Intelligence Scale for the Elderly, that is, the WISE. At his age and with the expense involved in developing and norming a test, the idea was not implemented. There would seem to be a need for such a test, albeit not necessarily in the same structure as the WAIS–R and certainly not containing only content similar to that test. Such an instrument would not only overcome some of the limitations of the current WAIS–R but would permit more appropriate scores and consequent inferences for the increasing numbers of aging individuals in our society.

In any event, much of what we know about adult ability is based on the use of the Wechsler adult scales. There has been research done both with those aging successfully and those not, including some comparisons of persons with dementia. Generally, the results have been disappointing. For example, Wechsler (Levi, Oppenheim, & Wechsler, 1945, pp. 405–407) had proposed that certain subtests would be more influenced by any form of brain impairment than would other subtests. He identified four subtests (Digit Span, Digit Symbol, Similarities, and Block Design) as ones where neurological damage would be particularly detrimental to the individual's performance. On the other hand, he said, four others (Information, Object Assembly, Picture Completion, and Vocabulary) should not alter greatly in the presence of such brain changes.

Some studies offer support for Wechsler's position. Jarvik (1988), for example, has reported longitudinal data that low Digit Symbol scores were predictive of a later diagnosis of dementia in two-thirds of her sample. At the same time, low scores on Vocabulary and Similarities were even more predictive. As a result, she stated that "it may be possible to utilize standardized cognitive tests to distinguish older persons who will subsequently develop dementia from those who will not" (Jarvik, 1988, p. 742).

Other results have not been so supportive (e.g., Lezak, 1983; Aram & Ekelman, 1986). This is not to say that such conditions as dementia do not affect the abilities of the patient, including specific tested ones like those demonstrated on Similarities or Digit Symbol. Indeed, it seems reasonable to believe that there are such deleterious effects and that they are identifiable—but that may not help in the sense of *diagnostic* capability. In this sense, Loring and Largen (1985) found that patients receiving a diagnosis of presenile dementia (a sample only of three persons) had lower IQs on the WAIS than did patients with a diagnosis of senile dementia (a sample of 24). As we would expect, the presenile group was significantly younger than the senile one. The young group also showed significant impairment on the Performance Scale of the WAIS, leading the authors to suggest that dementia developed prior to the senium will show greater impairment on age-adjusted tests that require concentration and mental tracking.

Similarly, Schultz, Schmitt, Logue, and Rubin (1986) compared several different diagnostic categories, including Alzheimer's and Multiinfarct Dementia, on memory tests. The poorest performance was found for the dementias, whereas normal persons and those with affective disorders had the best recall scores. Groth-Marnat (1990) has made the cogent point that an attempt to predict or relate mental abilities with dementia "is based primarily on the presence and extent of subtest deviation from other subtests. Much of this interpretation is an art, based on integrating knowledge about the person, brain function, Wechsler subtests, and past clinical experience" (p. 145). The degree to which the procedure is "art" rather than "science" is a matter for concern and some doubt.

But if the Wechsler Scales are not sufficient to predict dementia, perhaps the problem lies in the test itself, or even in the definition of intelligence used by the test author. Certainly, there have been other definitions of intelligence (e.g., Guilford, 1959) and other dimensions of its expression (e.g., Horn, 1968), but these have provided little for the understanding of normal intellectual changes occurring during the senium, and nothing of value in determining the effects of dementia on the coping behaviors that require intellect.

The second approach to the understanding of intelligence includes a large number of laboratory studies that provided excellent controls over conditions so as to permit analysis of the intellectual process. Among the many possibilities for investigation, the one that seems most pertinent to our purpose is the study of problem solving. In the demented person, the ability to realize the components of a problem and to utilize stored experience to solve it diminishes progressively. Unfortunately, the research efforts have focused more on the strategies used by the subject than in developmental changes that occur under conditions associated with aging. Thus the usual experimental procedure involves establishing the rules used in solution to report the process of problem solving. Two general approaches have been described. One may solve a problem using a set of rules that, when applied correctly, will guarantee a solution (called an algorithm), or one may try various strategies based on personal experience until a solution is achieved (called an heuristic). In other words, the research has not been designed to try to relate intellectual change in dementia to the ability to solve problems.

The issue of intellectual deterioration in dementia is a very practical one, nevertheless, and efforts must continue to identify and relate mental decline with accepted tests of competence. Certainly, measures such as the WAIS–R will continue to be a part of the screening process even if not used directly for diagnosis. Fogel and Faust (1987, p. 62) propose that assessment of intellectual and cognitive functions is a potentially useful *part* of neuropsychological assessment. It can provide information on the "higher-order" thinking processes as well as memory retrieval. In concert with other screening devices and measures, a more complete and helpful picture of the current functioning of the individual is possible. Certainly, inclusion of a measure of intelligence is common practice as part of the diagnostic procedure (Miller, 1977, pp. 105–110). As such, it must be accorded some attention until a more definitive or helpful approach is developed.

There are several reasons for including intelligence test scores in the diagnostic process. One is that the Wechsler scale has been carefully developed, with a history of over 50 years use, and has been extensively and systematically renormed on several occasions. Regardless of its limitations, the test remains the single best estimate of adult ability available to us. Second, there has been a large body of research collected wherein the results on the scale have been used as one of the dependent variables for predictive purposes. Despite the fact that research results are not as helpful as one might wish, the data are still necessary and useful. Third, the decision about the future of an individual should include a variety of types of information, each making some contribution to the decision itself. One of these kinds of information is general ability. Fourth, and perhaps most important, the content of the test includes material related to functional abilities involved in dealing with life. The foremost of these is memory, principally because memory is an essential component to efficient problem solution. As described in Chapter One, there is general agreement that memory is of several types, depending on the needs of the individual. Basically, memory storage seems to be a function of the synapses (Guyton, 1991, p. 480). When signals pass through synapses a number of times, the process of transmission is facilitated. With practice, then, the impulse need not occur at all; we may have the *perception* of the sensation in the sense of a *memory* even though the sensation in fact is not physically present.

Upon storage, the brain can compare experiences with extant memories to select what information is already stored, what needs to be stored, and where the storage should occur. The cerebral cortex is an extensive compendium for memories, and it works with other parts of the nervous system to assure more efficient operations by us (Guyton, 1991, p. 481). This permits many applications to daily life, particularly all those we ascribe to "learning." The development of the cortex in the human expands the possibilities for stored experience, to be used by us in an intelligent fashion, so that we may function in an increasingly complex environment (made more complex, of course, because of our superior abilities). It is true that all of us may not be equally adept in the tasks of life (though it is not clear whether this is due to true differences in intelligence or brain structure, or to opportunity, or to some interaction of both). What does seem clear is that the human who has reached maturity and is functioning at some reasonable level with the demands of life should be expected to continue to do so throughout the adult span. If there is a breakdown in the structure of the brain, there will be adverse consequences on the functioning previously demonstrated by the person. Dementia does not discriminate; the nuclear physicist, the janitor, the homemaker, the banker, the teacher are equally at risk. If the destructive condition altering the status of the cortex is present, the result is certain. The individual will show decline in mental competence.

To this point, there is no answer to the cause of most dementias and no medical interventions that will reverse or even stabilize the course. For this reason, there is a greater attention to the outcomes: the behavioral effects and the consequences to patient and caregiver. Though research is underway to determine cause, there seems no reason to believe that an answer will be forthcoming for some years.

This brings us to the fact that the complex structure of the brain permits the human to develop and use capacities of almost unlimited potential. We possess what might be called a "mind," dependent upon the *quality* of the brain but certainly different from the *structure* of the brain itself. How may we reconcile the distinctions?

THE QUALITY OF MIND

To try to describe the nature of "mind" would seem to be less a scientific problem than a philosophical one. Yet the fact that the brain permits behavioral expressions and talents far greater than are found in other species requires some explanation for humankind. Von Bonin (1963, p. 80) concluded:

> Man is born with a very immature cortex and . . . most of what is in it later in life is added after the second to fourth years of his life. How the cortex does things is the only element in the operation of the brain that is laid down before birth; what the cortex does and what man thinks about are elements that develop only during the life of the individual.

As he points out, the physical structure is largely set at birth, with some genetic plan that permits the cortex to serve its many functions given appropriate experiences. Most of life is invested in benefitting from the multitude of events we encounter. Perhaps, as von Bonin notes (1963, p. 80), distinguishing process from outcome is not possible at present; we do not know the evolution of *mind*. However, recent study does permit analyses that help to delimit the problem.

Jerison (1985, pp. 2–4) proposes that mind is reflected in the personal world that is constructed by the brain. This personal world is what each of us sees as the "real" world, but it is not the same as the external world. It is our contact, our experience with the external world that must be assigned a reality in order to achieve meaning. Yet each of us will have somewhat different "real worlds" because we have somewhat different experiences to be transformed and processed. Even in the face of the same external world, we may differ somewhat in the constructed reality we derive.

One of the major dimensions of mind is the use of language. Language has developed as a medium for sharing experiences (Jerison, 1985, p. 5) so that there is a reduction of the limits imposed by the boundaries of our bodies. Even subtle experiences (feelings and emotions, for example) may be shared through the medium of language (Jerison, 1985, p. 6). Ultimately, the world that each of us considers "real" is a creation of the brain and is dependent upon its capacity to perceive the world (Jerison, 1985, p. 10). Although that capacity is, in fact, enormous, it is realized only as the mind of the person puts the potential to work. Experience, as cited from von Bonin, is the agent permitting the interactive effects that allow us to move from what might be to what is. The principal reason for the differences between humans and other animals in behavioral potential is the development of language (Jerison, 1985, p. 22).

LeDoux (1985, p. 198) says that language is crucial in human consciousness. With it, we are able to accomplish a common categorization of many different experiences and to construct a sense of self and reality. If there is specific damage to human brain cells, there are deficits reflecting the change. In some cases, these deficits adversely affect the ability to interpret stimulation; in others, they lead to the inability to retrieve stored memories; in still others, they interfere with the ability to attend, and so on. Whether this means that mental events are equivalent to brain states or that the brain is the necessary element for mental events to be expressed is not certain (LeDoux, 1985, p. 198). Scientifically, much more evidence is needed to clarify the relationships.

LeDoux (1985, pp. 210–211) concurs with Jerison in the position that reality is a personal state, subjectively constructed through the use of language. Our reality is what we believe we are and can be.

> The behavior of all primates, including man, is minimally dictated by invarient stimuli outside the organism; man, however, possessing nature's most sophisticated mechanism (natural language) for coding, storing, analyzing and retrieving past experience, individually constructs a subjective reality to an extent unmatched by other creatures. (LeDoux, 1985, p. 211)

This idea is repeated and reinforced by Oakley and Eames (1985, pp. 219–220). That is, as we collect and store representations of experience, we establish a backlog permitting rerepresentation in terms of priorities. Being able to rerepresent may be labeled self-awareness (Oakley & Eames, 1985, p. 220), permitting us to perceive ourselves in terms of the outside world or to perceive our inner world of thoughts, feelings, and emotions.

This position leaves us with the proposition that mind is predicated upon a cortex that structurally has evolved to permit a world of experience including but greater than that of the sensorimotor one. Much of our experience is like that of other animals in its importance (for example, reaction to heat and cold), but the *human* cortex allows for a subjective evaluation that constructs a unique reality. This reality may be shared to some extent with other persons but is probably never exactly the same. We are conscious of ourselves in this unique world, and our actions are undertaken to be congruent with and to protect us in the external world. So long as we can maintain a sufficiently intact brain, we benefit from experience to make more personal and "real" the world we have subjectively built.

The reality of dementia is a destructive change in this ability to continue to function in and expand the personal world that permitted interaction with others. Certainly, the patient must still have some subjective reality, but it is less and less communicable to others, and it is eventually altered to the point that it appears to the outside view as an impersonal one. Understanding this change, appreciating its meaning, and learning to deal with its effects is the primary task of the professional and the caregiver.

There is no magic formula, whether it be behavioral or medical, that will make this task easier. Perhaps too much emphasis has been placed on the attempts to operationalize effects through diagnosis and treatment, and too little on the effects of the victim's subjective reality within which she or he must operate. Rather, both forms of contingencies must be accepted and explored to gain an understanding of the nature and meaning of dementia.

Research efforts have focused on the behavioral consequences developing with a dementia. This is both necessary and worthwhile; the results have given us a clearer picture of what happens to the patient and how adaptation is altered. But the approach also implies that what is happening to the mind of the patient is largely a void. If the person cannot perform in the real world as we perceive it, then that individual must be incompetent in the sense that there is little or no mind left. Perhaps it is time to question such an assumption; perhaps what is happening is that the reality of the dementia patient's world is slowly but systematically changed toward new directions. This would call for research that would attempt to discover what reality the patient establishes as the disease process continues. Instead of comparing the responses of the individual to *our* reality, present the reality we see to the patient for interpretation and report.

For many professionals and caregivers, this idea will not seem pertinent nor helpful. They will point out that the patient must still be taken care of and that task is more burdensome than can be helped by "understanding" some alternate reality. The point is well taken and will influence the content of the remainder of this book.

SUMMARY

There are two components to consider in understanding the ability of humans to deal with the complexities of life. One of these is the structure of the brain, similar in many regards to other animals but differing in one major aspect—the cerebral cortex. Some of the important components of the cortex are described in this chapter. Particular attention was given to the lobes with their relatively compartmentalized functions, the structure and functions of neurons, and associated cells such as the glia.

The possibilities provided by the evolution of the human brain include a superior intellect. The work of David Wechsler in defining and measuring adult intelligence was surveyed, with reference to some of the findings provided in the research. Problem solving as it is investigated in psychological laboratories was described.

The distinction between brain and mind concludes the chapter. Despite our limitations in understanding and demonstrating the evolution and nature of mind, the construct must be appreciated because so much that is human goes beyond the possibilities provided in the subcortical areas of the brain. The cortex would seem to be the "seat" of mind, and its outcomes need investigation as much as its structure and function do.

The meanings of these dimensions to our knowledge of the course and consequences of dementia were described.

CHAPTER THREE

Identifying Dementia

Dementia expresses itself in so many adverse ways that it would be worthwhile if a definite diagnosis, proposed early in the progression, were available. Unfortunately, diagnosis usually comes only after some accumulation of problems has occurred and, sometimes, only when some incident has happened that is so bizarre that it cannot be explained away. It is true that, after diagnosis, caregivers can frequently cite a number of events, which occurred over several years, that were "warning signs" that something was wrong. However, as mentioned in the preceding chapter, we expect the mature adult to be able to continue functioning in a normal manner. Deviations, particularly if not extreme and if occurring only occasionally and in restricted behavioral areas, will be ignored, denied, or explained away—by both the eventual patient and caregiver. Retrospective data, of course, is not very trustworthy, although it may be sought; even when trustworthy, it is obviously too late for the case at hand. Better education of the public about behavioral changes and their meanings is needed and should be a central part of medical examination and treatment, particularly with aging persons.

Even if greater awareness and willingness to admit to apparent changes in one's competencies were present, the scientific basis for an accurate diagnosis is limited. First, it would be necessary to be able to recognize relatively quickly the nature of the specific condition that will lead to expressions of dementia (e.g., Alzheimer's disease, Pick's disease, strokes leading to Multiinfarct Dementia, etc.). This task is feasible with some diseases but not with others. In addition, many of the necessary tests that might assist in diagnosis are not routinely performed. For example, unless the patient presents some symptoms that suggest the need for neurological examination, most primary care physicians will not request a brain scan (say, computerized tomography) or other tests. The cost and the intrusions involved seem not to warrant such measures when the patient appears to be living a normal life and has no complaints.

The education of professionals (psychiatric, psychological, and neurological) is a continuing effort. Perhaps the best evidence is in the publication provided by the American Psychiatric Association, detailing the features, expression, course, and differential diagnosis of a variety of syndromes. This *Diagnostic and Statistical Manual of Mental Disorders* (3rd ed. rev.) (DSM-III-R) (American Psychiatric Association, 1987) is a helpful source for recognition of the signs and symptoms of dementia.

DEMENTIA IN THE DSM-III-R

Dementia is a general term, denoting certain effects resulting from a variety of organic causes (see Chapter 1). Though each of the causes may be medically described and diagnosed, the DSM-III-R is not concerned with that function. Instead, the emphasis is on the nature of the *mental* disorders that result. The following discussion is based on that presentation (pp. 103–107).

Features of Dementia

The essential feature of any dementia is memory loss. There is a certain inability to recall facts and details at any point in a normal adult's life, though it is certainly perceived more negatively for the older person. If the 70-year-old does not remember whether she or he locked the house before leaving, there often is more concern about the meaning of that lack than will be true for the 20-year-old. In fact, the young adult will be chastised for being careless; the 70-year-old may be judged as becoming senile. Such normal events, of course, seldom have any adverse affect on the ability to maintain oneself independently and fruitfully. The difficulty is in the eye of the beholder in such cases.

Memory loss as it is reflected in dementia is much more serious and comprehensive. At first, short-term memory will be most affected, but, at some point in time, portions of long-term memory also will be lost. Associated with this element of memory loss, there are increasing difficulties in carrying on abstract thinking and in showing sound judgment. Of course, one may expect such higher abilities to be altered if the individual manifests increasing inability to recall experience and apply it correctly. The DSM-III-R also includes as a criterion for dementia "disturbances of higher cortical functions." These include language disorders (aphasia), inability to perform motor activities in spite of adequate comprehension and motor function (apraxia), inability to recognize or identify objects even though sensory functions are adequate (agnosia), and difficulties in perceiving the construction of certain tasks (assembling blocks, copying three-dimensional figures, and the like).

Further, the DSM-III-R points to the possibility of personality change. The person may become more subdued than formerly or more volatile. Traits formerly possessed may be accentuated or reversed. There is no single pattern for all cases, but change of some kind is more likely than not.

The consequences of whatever changes occur express themselves in interference with the ability to function at work, in social activities, or in interpersonal relationships. The artisan may find it increasingly difficult to perform tasks once easily accomplished, so that there may begin to be damaged products. The surgeon may be unable to recall the procedure just performed so that surgical notes are not dictated and patient complications are not recorded. The bookkeeper may have increasing problems with basic calculations, making errors or simply not carrying out the necessary computations for accurate reporting. The homemaker may begin to hide dirty dishes rather than wash them and deny any such action.

In such instances, there is the assumption that the behaviors displayed are the result of an organic factor, though it may not be possible to identify that cause specifically. As an example, the DSM-III-R lists a disorder labeled "Primary Degenerative Dementia of the Alzheimer Type." The *cause* is not known, but it is classified psychiatrically as a dementia because:

There is demonstrable memory loss (plus poor judgment or lack in abstract thinking, or disturbance in higher-order faculties, or personality change) that is significant enough to interfere with normal functioning.

Medically, there has been an attempt to find some specific organic factor that would account for the behaviors observed. This search, however, has not disclosed a possible cause even though all available tests have been performed.

The kinds of conditions that are not due to changes in the brain (and thus are nonorganic) have been assessed with negative results. Whether the cause is *truly* Alzheimer's disease will not yet be known, although that may be determined if an autopsy is performed upon the death of the patient. What remains, then, are the observed positive symptoms, that is, the various deleterious behavioral changes that interfere with functioning and that are accepted as reflecting dementia.

In the DSM-III-R, the definition of dementia is based on clinical symptoms only. Reference to prognosis is neither given nor intended. Under such circumstances, it is possible that some dementias may be stabilized, even reversed, if the pathological state is treatable. In other instances of dementia, no such possibility exists.

Once the DSM's description of dementia is accepted, it is possible to consider several ways in which it may be expressed.

Degrees of Impairment

DSM-III-R proposes three different levels of severity. First, the condition will express itself in a *mild* form where there is impairment vocationally or socially but with the ability to live independently still present. Judgment will remain generally unimpaired, and personal hygiene is maintained. These criteria may be used to infer specific behavioral outcomes. As observed in patients, there will be moderate memory loss, more typically for recent events that can no longer be encoded accurately or completely. Specifically, the patient will have problems with the names of other persons or will be unable to remember directions or the content of events. For example, the individual may still be able to drive safely, observing traffic signals and rules of courtesy, but not be able to remember how to get to the destination desired. She or he may drive aimlessly or become frustrated or return to the starting point and deny that any problem existed. As another example, some event may be partially remembered but reconstructed with elements that are incorrect (a behavior called "confabulation"). Again, the patient may deny any change and resist any correction.

In the *moderate* degree, there is less likelihood of independent living, and where continued, the dangers inherent in situations will be greater. As a result, the patient will need supervision to some degree. Beyond this criterion, there are other behavioral changes that have been noted among patients. There is further memory loss, which may be illustrated behaviorally in several ways. Now, only material that has been rehearsed a large number of times will be retained. (This conforms, of course, to the idea in the previous chapter that highly practiced behaviors may bring about synaptic perception even in the absence of the stimulus itself.) While the person is in this level, new material and information will be forgotten rapidly. Though the individual will seem to comprehend what is presented, there is little or no encoding of the experience so that it will not be stored and available after only a few moments. For example, a family may obtain a new videocassette recorder (VCR). All members are instructed on where and how to insert the cassette, the proper channel setting on the television, the use of the "play" button to start the tape. One with dementia at this level may even repeat the instructions accurately, yet in just a few minutes be unable to remember part or all of the steps.

The moderate level is also shown when a task is being performed correctly but then is interrupted. Under these circumstances, the individual will not remember to return to the task and complete it. The mechanic may remain competent to do repairs, but if the telephone rings and she or he answers it, the person may not remember to go back and complete the task being worked on once the call is completed. Instead, a different repair task may be started, without awareness of what has not been done completely.

In its *severe* form, the DSM specifies the interference that now is found in carrying on activities of daily living. Impairment has reached a level that requires continued supervision. This criterion is illustrated by the massive forgetting of even heavily rehearsed information. The name of one's spouse may be gone, and there may even be a denial that this is the spouse. Caregivers report instances, often heartbreaking to them, where the wife or husband asks where the spouse is. Upon being told that he or she *is* the spouse, there may be not only emphatic denial but strong rejection as well. The caregiver will be accused of lying, of keeping the true spouse away, of taking advantage.

It is not unknown for the patient to forget his or her own name. The inability to recall so intimate a fact as that clearly and amply illustrates how profound the dementia has become. The person has now lost at least part of the orientation that allows connection with others. Consequently, the reality that constitutes her or his world must be very different from that which the rest of us recognize.

The severity of dementia is progressive, but there is no particular schedule. The mild form may exist for several months or years, perhaps even allowing the individual to function adequately in a number of ways before deteriorating to the moderate degree. Eventually, because the condition is usually progressive, there will be a time period when the losses are more crucial. People tend to expect severe dysfunction to be reflected in some physical changes. Thus because there is nothing visible in the individual's physical condition to indicate malfunction, the changes become increasingly difficult to accept and deal with for both patient and caregiver. When there has been progression to the severe level, the person becomes totally dependent on the caregiver. No longer is it appropriate to expect the patient to carry out unsupervised normal activities of daily living.

Deficits in Abstract Thought

Perhaps the most direct way in which these changes express themselves is in the inability to solve novel tasks, and this is particularly true when there are time constraints. In the preceding chapter, there was a description of the Wechsler adult scale that is often used as one part of the evaluation if dementia is suspected. On the Verbal Scale, some kinds of abilities may remain constant for years; a good example is vocabulary. Even as the dementia progresses, the person usually continues to be able to define the words on the Vocabulary subtest. However, many more difficulties will be experienced on the subtests of the Performance Scale, in part because these are timed. On one of the subtests, called Digit Symbol, the person being tested must substitute a symbol (such as a caret:^) for a given number. The numbers 1 through 9 are represented, each with a different symbol as its substitute. Because the model is left exposed, the examinee does not have to learn and remember any symbols. There is, in addition, a practice section to assure that the examinee understands the task. Dementia patients have considerable difficulty in performing well on this task, in part because there is a time limit and because the patient cannot accommodate to the novelty. As mentioned in Chapter 2, Jarvik (1988) found performance on this task to be a predictor of later possible diagnosis of Alzheimer's disease. Other studies have concurred with the position that solution of novel tasks is deficient in the demented patient, using subtests either from the Wechsler scale or other sources.

The difficulties in abstract thinking may become so uncomfortable for the person that she or he may try to avoid any situation that requires that new information be processed or complex material be dealt with. This suggests the interesting possibility that the world of reality experienced by the mind of the Alzheimer's patient still recognizes the emotional discomfort even if (or perhaps because) the intellectual task cannot be accommodated.

Impaired Judgment and Impulse Control

Although there are wide differences, many caregivers report the occurrence of behaviors atypical of the past and incongruent with social norms. The person may begin to use foul language, for the first time in her or his life or in inappropriate social situations such as church meetings. This is embarrassing and difficult to explain, and even then the explanation of dementia may not be accepted as a sufficient excuse by many who will be offended by the behavior. Not infrequently, the individual becomes unconcerned about hygiene and grooming. She or he may even refuse to change clothes or to bathe. Logical arguments are wasted, and sometimes the patient is stronger than the caregiver, so that force is not possible. Yet caregivers do learn to cope. An incident reported by one husband is pertinent. He found it increasingly difficult, even impossible, to persuade his wife to bathe. Using physical force exhausted him and caused his wife to be more of a behavior problem. One day, he turned on the shower, undressed, and suggested to his wife that they shower together. She was intrigued, and the problem was solved. Unfortunately, this gimmick will not work for every case, so there is a constant search for new and different solutions.

Beyond the intimate, there can be other examples of poor judgment that are devastating to the family. The businessman who has been successful for many years and is still trusted to make the right decisions may invest heavily in a venture that is unsafe but legal. Recovery of the investment may be difficult or impossible if some medical diagnosis and legal adjustments have not already been made. In the same sense, a respectable citizen may act illegally without intent or knowledge. There is the documented case of the man who walked into a store and picked up a box of cigars. He left the store without paying, was stopped by the proprietor, and arrested for shoplifting. Though there was a satisfactory resolution in this case (and he was diagnosed then by a physician), the discomfort to him and his family was marked.

The DSM-III-R reports that such impaired judgment and/or loss of impulse control occur most commonly in dementias that primarily affect the frontal lobe of the brain.

Disturbances of Higher Cortical Function

The most commonly recognized instances in this case involve alterations in language. The individual who has been competent in language expression may begin to show some vagueness and imprecision in the use of language. With time, the expressions may become more and more stereotypic, consisting of superficial or irrelevant phrases. There may even be increasing aphasia, with the person unable to remember even common terms and expressions. Apraxia and agnosia are more likely. Particularly troubling to the patient and caregiver is the intensity of nominal aphasia (anomia). Though the inability to recall the correct word, or to understand it in listening, may be found in many of us as we age, the degree of anomia is more severe in the dementia patient. In assessing the competencies of an Alzheimer's patient with the Mental Status Questionnaire (a set of 10 reality questions), the writer recalls that a patient was unable to answer any of the questions. At the end of the test administration, the patient reacted that he knew the answers but he "just couldn't get them out." Eventually, over a number of years, there may be babbling sounds like those of a baby, followed by mutism.

Another type of disturbance in this area is "constructional" apraxia. On the Wechsler scale, for example, the Block Design subtest would be useful. Here, the examinee is presented with a drawing that must be duplicated using several 1 in. cubes with different colors on the various sides. Because this task is also timed, the dementia patient will encounter difficulty on more than one dimension.

Personality Change

The principal changes that occur in personality, *if* they occur, will be some alteration of traits already present. In one direction, for example, the shy individual may become more and more outspoken, eventually becoming aggressive and abusive perhaps. By contrast, the more ebullient person may become withdrawn and quiet, conforming without question to demands placed upon him or her. Sometimes, traits may be accentuated so that they are more extreme than formerly. A hostile individual may show increased hostility, including using verbal abuse not displayed before. In still other instances, the personality of the patient may be relatively unchanged over the course of the progression of the syndrome.

Associated Features

One can appreciate that the inability to recall some segment of one's life, brief though it may be, can be frightening. Initially, perhaps, because it may be for only a short period and does not reoccur, it would be easy to explain it away as a temporary and unimportant aberration. If, however, there is some syndrome insidiously leading to dementia, the incidents will occur again and within a shorter time span. There will be some imbalance in one's life, an awareness that one is functioning inappropriately at times and no explanation of what it may be. If a physician is consulted, there is the chance that monitoring may begin in order to document the incidents that would allow for more complete examination and diagnosis. But even this, if it happens, will not reduce the stress. The result is, perhaps, increasing fear, confusion, and/or anxiety: What is wrong, how serious is it, what does it mean, what will treatment require, will recovery be possible? If the anxiety persists, the individual may become depressed, perhaps even to a clinical level. Depression is not uncommon in patients during the early stages of dementia. It is, however, identifiable and treatable in its own right. Again, if medical advice has been sought, the physician should be alert to these psychological expressions and refer the client to a specialist for appropriate intervention. With the progression of dementia, the ability of the person to assess personal fears and meanings will decline, and depression will be less likely.

Being aware that one's life is in some degree of disarray and hoping to cope well enough to disguise the fact from others may lead to the adoption of techniques that compensate. The patient may resort to behaviors such as excessive orderliness, thereby making it less likely that there will be some incident that requires quick adaptation. In another version of this technique, there may be an effort to set up rigid schedules and allow no deviation by anyone. There will probably be some social disengagement, expressed in a self-protecting way such as the complaint that some events and meetings are no longer appealing. Infinite variety can be introduced into this approach, depending on the person, but such efforts are an attempt to minimize or deny what eventually becomes too apparent to conceal any longer. Often, not only does the individual refuse to admit to and accept the deterioration but also hopes that things won't get worse if they are disguised.

Often, patients also begin to use remaining language abilities as a means to cover the deficits. They may tell stories from the past in great and minute detail to suggest that their recall is unchanged, thereby avoiding confrontation. One dementia patient would recount the way in which he became a pilot. During World War I as an enlisted man in France, he was given instruction by the pilots in his unit and became proficient enough to later pass the examination in this country. The tortuous detail was repeated to the extent that he would drag out the story for over 15 minutes! Interruption was resented, and he would return to the *beginning* of the story as soon as possible. Of course, listeners were aware of what he was doing if they knew of his dementia, but it is surprising how often he succeeded in persuading casual acquaintances of the clarity of his mind and the depth of his memory.

In some cases, the individual may express delusional ideation, thereby fixing the cause of any problems on some other source. The DSM-III-R delimits the concept of "paranoid ideation" to such delusional states and specifies that the delusion may be expressed in different forms, including grandiosity or persecution. Other clinicians see paranoia in the elderly as more often focusing on persecution with or without delusions (Kermis, 1986, p. 186). Where a brain syndrome is present, disorientation and even hallucinations may be found. Where delusions occur, they are more apt to reflect influence by others or passivity, seen by some clinicians as an exaggeration of normal personality traits (Kermis, 1986, p. 186). The paranoia, in this less restricted sense, is most commonly expressed toward one who is close and dear, such as the spouse or another family member. The behavior may distract the relative who does not understand what is happening and interfere with a realization of what exactly is occurring. Because the patient has been competent in the past, the delusion also enables the relative to believe that perhaps there has been some contribution to the present state by others. The force with which the delusion is expressed is another factor leading to feelings of guilt and shame in the relative that she or he may have been a part of the problem. However, this attribution of blame to external events also enables relatives to minimize or deny the other evidence of brain dysfunction.

Whether or not such behaviors occur, and in what manner or degree, the patient must be recognized as a person who is vulnerable. This means that the behaviors that reflect dementia achieve the level of stressors and may well be disruptive. The cumulative effects of such stressors are easy to describe in the more extreme cases. For example, the person with dementia may need some minor surgery. Normally, this could be adapted to with only minor trauma, but with a loss in competence and the resulting feeling of insecurity, the effects may be major. Tager (1980, pp. 177–178) has discussed the induction of stress from loss in old age (such as death of a spouse or decrease in functional capabilities) that may lead to prolonged stress responses (such as muscle tightness or hypertension). Sometimes these disorders may lead to more serious consequences. Additionally, in old age, there may be temporary disability as an aftereffect of major surgery. With the dementia patient, there might be a drop in the competence of the individual immediately after the surgery is performed, and there is a possibility that the former mental status will not be regained. Less obvious incidents can also have their adverse effects. A loss of some kind—say of a friend who dies—can have more extreme effects than the bereavement process would predict. Even a change in routine that seems minor can be devastating. If the patient is still competent to walk around the block (despite being unable to remember where the kitchen is in his or her own home) and there is a disruption such as the closing of the street for repairs, the effects can be major. The person cannot understand, may react with anger, confusion, and disorientation, and be less competent from that point on than was true just the day before. Predicting that such outcomes will occur is much easier than predicting precisely *what* will be especially stressful, in what way the patient will be affected, or to what degree.

Age at Onset

In Chapter One, a distinction was made between presenile and senile dementia; such a distinction bows to convention and is for convenience only. If dementia is considered in the general case, it is clear that an aging population will show increasing numbers of cases. The DSM-III-R points out that the condition is found largely in the elderly, but it is possible at any age. In fact, the DSM states that a diagnosis of dementia may be possible at any age *after the intelligence quotient has estabilized (around the age of 3 or 4)*. But the major danger remains with older persons, though dementia is not directly due to aging and the reason for higher incidence is not clear.

In the past, estimates (statistics in such areas are seldom available) suggested that from 7% to 10% of the population suffered some form of dementia, with the large majority of those being Alzheimer's patients. More recently, an estimate of 4 million having Alzheimer's was proposed, and prognostications go as high as 14 million for Alzheimer's by the year 2040. The increases, if they occur, will be due to more people living longer lives and thereby becoming more at risk for age-related diseases. If research identifies a cause and develops means of intervention (hopefully, prevention), then the prospects for successful aging will be substantially increased.

Course

Dementia in the aging population may be progressive and degenerative in most cases. The outcomes are dependent on *cause*. However, even knowing cause does not assure reversibility. For instance, it is known that a slow virus is responsible for Creutzfeldt–Jakob disease, but it is nonetheless fatal because there is no treatment for the viral condition. This is not an unusual state of medical affairs.

For different causes of dementia, there are different effects. Multiinfarct dementia (MID) progresses in a stepwise fashion, depending on the times at which strokes occur and their severity. The length and depth of the steps will be irregular (see Figure 3.1), and as a result the course may run over a period from a few weeks or months to several years. In contrast, Alzheimer's disease (AD) presents in a more irregular but steadily progressive fashion (see Figure 3.2). There may even be the appearance of "recovery" by the patient, but inevitably the course will turn downward again until its course is completed.

Several dementias are slow in presentation (as in MID and AD), whereas others are of rapid onset (a brain injury from a bullet wound,

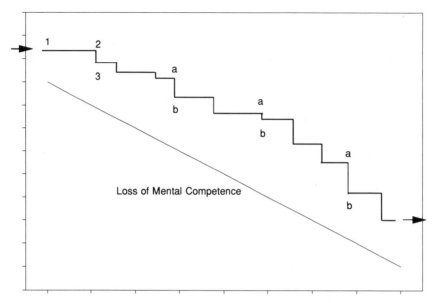

FIGURE 3.1. Progression in multiinfarct dementia. (1) = Period of life without strokes; (2) = occurrence of a "silent" stroke; (3) = degree of losl of competence; (a) = recurrent strokes; and (b) = loss of mental competence.

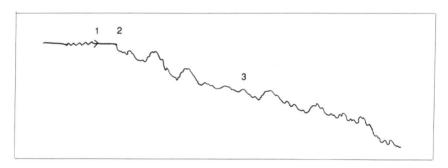

FIGURE 3.2. Progression in Alzheimer's disease. (1) = Period of life when disease not expressed; (2) = onset of decline in mental competence; and (3) = irregular nature of decline in mental competence.

for example). There are a few that can be arrested, so that they stabilize or may even be treatable or reversible (such as those due to operable tumors or to normal pressure hydrocephalus). For most dementias, however, there is little or no hope at the present time even for intervention, much less for control or reversibility. In certain instances, the current research is investigating only stopgap methods. An example is the project evaluating the use of physostigmine with Alzheimer's patients. This drug inhibits an enzyme that breaks down acetylcholine, one of the neurotransmitters involved in transmission of the signal across the synapse between neurons. If the acetylcholine is not present in sufficient quantity and quality, the "message" cannot be transmitted. This acetylcholine deficit has been associated with AD in research on Alzheimer's patients.

If there were a means of *increasing* the presence of acetylcholine in the cells of an AD patient, there might be better neuronal functioning. Already, some study has been done that indicates that for *some* patients, physostigmine increases memory abilities for a period of time. Currently, this study is being conducted with a form of the drug that will remain in the bloodstream for a greater period of time. Will it benefit more patients in memory retrieval for longer periods of time? The question is legitimate, and this particular study is appropriately designed to find an answer.

The research examined 300 individuals, all of whom were diagnosed as having AD. The drug was administered at one of 16 medical centers (see Table 3.1) with the patient carefully monitored for side effects. For those who had no side effects, the drug was administered for an additional nine months. The study did not include any individuals who could no longer care for themselves ("severe" degree of dementia) or who had other major medical problems (say, hypertension).

The study has generated excitement, particularly among caregivers, because they welcome any drug that promises positive changes for behavioral losses. Often, however, they misconstrue or fail to understand what may result. Even under the most ideal circumstances, physostigmine will not be a cure for Alzheimer's; in fact, it will not have an effect on the general course of the condition at all. At best, it will be a means of intervening so that patients will be able to function more adequately than expected and for a longer period of time. There is the possibility that, as in the previously mentioned study, only some individuals will benefit and only for a limited time period. There is the assurance that the intervention will be effective only in the earlier period of the course of the disease and then only with those who have no other health problems. For successful use of physostigmine, certain criteria must be met. First, there must be early (and accurate) identification of the disorder so that the drug is used during the period when it is most effective. This criterion may not be met because victims and family members tend to minimize symptoms and even deny the presence of problems as they become more evident. Second, the patient must not have other "major

TABLE 3.1.
Medical Centers Investigating Role of Physostigmine
in Alzheimer's Disease

University of California, San Diego, Alzheimer's Disease
  Research Center, San Diego, CA
University of Southern California, Los Angeles
Neuromedical Research Associates, Miami Beach
University of Minnesota Hospital, Minneapolis, MN
Kansas University Medical Center, Kansas City, KS
Massachusetts General Hospital, Boston
Albert Einstein College of Medicine, The Bronx, Bronx, NY
University of Alabama at Birmingham, Birmingham
Francis Scott Key Medical Center, Johns Hopkins Medical
  Institution, Baltimore
University of Washington, Seattle, WA
Baylor College of Medicine, Houston, TX
Southwestern Medical Center, University of Texas, Dallas TX
Michael Reese Hospital, Chicago
Maimonides Medical Center, Brooklyn, NY
Neurological Institute, New York City
The Graduate Hospital, Philadelphia

medical problems." Though there are Alzheimer's patients who will meet this criterion, others will not. The prevalence of several medical disorders in the same elderly individual has not been documented. However, data from the Baltimore Longitudinal Study of Aging (Shock, 1984, p. 58) disclosed that, of 336 subjects excluded from the "normal group," there were 531 individual exclusions, so that some subjects had more than one disease sufficiently serious to preclude their participation in the study. It seems apparent that, even if study results with physostigmine are successful, the drug will have only limited utility. Only a fraction of AD patients will receive even temporary benefits, as important for those individuals as that outcome would be.

Differential Diagnosis

The DSM-III-R points out that a diagnosis of dementia is possible only if there is demonstrable evidence of memory loss, with its associated features, that interferes with the social or occupational functioning of the individual. Further, it must be possible to rule out disorders with similar features, such as amnestic disorder or major depression. Only when these conditions are met should the diagnostic label "dementia" be assigned.

MEDICAL PROCEDURES

Once a patient and/or caregiver has recognized and admitted to the patient's behavioral problem, there usually will be consultation with a physician. This step is necessary to consider the possible causes for the problem and to determine a diagnosis. Because the diagnosis will establish the potential for and types of interventions and treatment the medical examination should be comprehensive and thorough.

If there is no result that identifies a definite cause for behavioral changes, a referral to another physician may follow. Although most primary care physicians will be competent to evaluate the routine medical test results, they probably are not prepared to perform a detailed assessment of neurological involvement. Thus the patient will be referred to a neurologist or psychiatrist. A different, more specialized set of tests will then be administered, including sophisticated mechanical procedures to be described in the next chapter. These tests may be diagnostic but more frequently are used to exclude identifiable, and perhaps treatable, conditions that the prior, routine tests may have missed (e.g., a brain tumor). Once this procedure is complete, a diagnosis may or may not be given, depending upon the breadth and adequacy of the evidence collected. In most cases, a specific diagnosis will be based on an *absence* of an identifiable cause. Alzheimer's disease, for example, can be identified with some accuracy by examining neuronal tissue for the presence of neurofibrillary tangles and neuritic plaques (plus some other signs), but the neuron can only be examined microscopically. The usual medical tests, including even the newest of the scans, cannot disclose the nature of the cell. Biopsy of brain tissue is a rarity because of the potential destruction of cells to acquire tissue from the areas likely to be involved (the frontal lobe, the hippocampus, etc.). Under these circumstances, the diagnosis of Alzheimer's is an "educated" or "best" guess. It may also be in error. No one wants to be exposed to such a mistake because the diagnosis includes the assumption that progressive degeneration of neurons will occur with no possibility of intervention or treatment. Essentially, the diagnosis commits the patient to futility. In addition, there is the maxim that "absence of evidence is not evidence of absence." How do you explain these things to a patient and caregiver?

Given the lack of evidence of validity in diagnosis and the desire to offer positive outcome possibilities, the physician may opt for some less precise, definitive, or distressing label. This brings us to the issue of categorization, both in the layperson's and the professional's languages.

The Meaning of the Diagnostic Label

There are some recognized and diagnosable syndromes that lead to dementia in some form and degree, as they were described in Chapter One. However, the identification of these is obscured by a vocabulary that has developed out of historical events and has been amended by personal preferences and attempts to avoid concepts that have acquired pejorative value. Nowhere is this more evident than with Alzheimer's disease.

Alois Alzheimer described premature aging in two female patients, both of whom were in their 50s. They showed severe memory loss and confusion, behaviors he felt were more representative of the very old than of their age group. The term he used to describe these patients was *presenile dementia*, by which he meant that they showed evidence of senility at a time in their lives prior to the senium. For 1907, his position was typical and acceptable. However, it also established certain historical precedents. First, it was *atypical* for persons in their 50s to be senile (but expected in much older ones). The characteristics that were shown in analyses of their brain tissue (neurofibrillary tangles and neuritic plaques) must, he believed, be typical of old age. If these changes occurred prior to old age, they were not only unusual but pathological as well. Thus the attitude was accepted that patients who present structural changes like those of Alzheimer's cases must suffer from presenile dementia. Further, when Kraepelin later suggested the disorder be named for Alzheimer, the attitudes simply transferred to the new title: Alzheimer's patients should be middle-aged rather than elderly. In addition, there remains some of the belief that when one is very old, the adverse outcomes due to senility, if not the physical evidences, must be present. This position has received credibility by the fact that older individuals who are not demented may show neurofibrillary tangles and senile plaques upon postmortem examination. The web may be tangled, but it is also logical.

This generated the possibility that elderly persons will not suffer from Alzheimer's disease but from senile dementia *like* Alzheimer's. Today, one will find in the literature the designation "senile dementia of the Alzheimer's type" (SDAT). Unfortunately, the user may or may not mean to infer the difference that seems implicit in the terminology, that is, that SDAT is similar to presenile dementia in its effects but different in its cause. If the cause is the same, why not use the label *presenile dementia of the Alzheimer's type?* Obviously, because it has been understood that *all* cases in the presenium are considered to be Alzheimer's.

The medical diagnosis should succinctly describe the syndrome that alters the status of the brain cells. By this reasoning, there should be no reference to dementia at all. As in the case of the DSM-III-R, the label used is "Primary Degenerative Dementia of the Alzheimer Type," and it is a psychiatric label. Does this mean that neurologists should or should not use the term? If the internist or family physician is communicating with the patient and caregiver, is this the appropriate diagnosis? It certainly does provide some mixture of all that has been described heretofore. There is the term *dementia*, and there is the allusion to the presenium with *Alzheimer Type*. However, there are additional terms as well. The course is inferred from the descriptor *degenerative*. That is, one should expect things only to get worse. Further, it is "primary" in its focus, proceding directly from the causative condition and dominating the clinical picture. Are we better or worse off? More to the point, should a physician prefer this label over others?

The point should be well made by now. One may find a variety of labels used, as well as cases where a diagnosis is avoided altogether. To some degree, the diagnosis communicated to the patient and caregiver must remain an individual preference. Still, the major need is for the physician to be able to describe to the caregiver and patient what is wrong, what caused it, what it means for the future, and what may be done about it.

It is essential, however, that consistency be maintained and the reality of the syndrome addressed so that the fears and lack of knowledge experienced by patient and caregiver can be reduced to the minimum. Normally, neither will know what questions to ask. Their needs must be anticipated and dealt with as frankly and completely, at their level of understanding, as possible. Some organization (the American Medical Association and/or the Alzheimer's Association) needs to focus on this issue in order to serve the best interests of a public ill-educated and confused.

It would be unfair to ignore the educational efforts of such units as the Alzheimer's Association (Alzheimer's Disease and Related Disorders of Aging). There are bulletins, articles, brochures, and other materials produced and distributed by them, particularly through local chapters in the United States. But, the efforts are relatively recent and seem to locate and serve only a portion of the cases. There is the other problem, as well, that the "related disorders of aging" receive much less attention than does Alzheimer's.

Physicians in all specialties (but particularly in internal medicine, family practice, neurology, and psychiatry) seem to need a much more thorough education. With the size of the problem at present and the portending major increase in prevalence of dementia, some curriculum that is current and complete and includes effective skills of communication to patients and caregivers is sorely needed. Undoubtedly, some medical schools and some continuing medical education programs are attempting to meet these requirements. If the commonly expressed experiences of caregivers with medical personnel is at all accurate, however, the education of many physicians is insufficient.

SUMMARY

In this chapter, there has been a discussion of the elements involved in the diagnosis of the several conditions leading to a possible dementia. All such diagnosis is medical and needs to remain so because that profession is best equipped to measure the status of the individual physically. Medical evaluation will identify a variety of conditions whether associated with the potential occurrence of dementia. In some cases, a reversible cause will be found that, with treatment, will allow avoidance of mental incompetence. In other cases, no treatable cause is found, but an untreatable condition will be discovered that has been related to dementia as an outcome. In most cases, neither alternative will exist, and there must be a diagnosis by exclusion.

In addition to the conventional medical exam, it may be necessary to utilize neurological or psychiatric personnel to make a final diagnosis. Again, some brain condition may be discovered, either treatable or untreatable. If none is found, then there will probably be the diagnosis of a disorder that will be irreversible. The latter situation is the most difficult for the physician and the affected parties. With our present state of knowledge, it is the usual one, nevertheless.

Because there is a danger that labels are proliferating without clear and consistent agreement on their meanings and applications, it seems worthwhile for organizations to push for some realistic guidelines that are clearly defined and communicable to the layperson. This will not only permit more distinct and refined diagnoses but will also allow more precise and understandable communication to the persons most affected by the outcome: the patient and caregiver. It will also bring better focused educational efforts for the general public, thereby expanding awareness and creating a willingness to become involved in substantive efforts (particularly financial) to find ways of preventing the occurrence of dementia in future generations.

CHAPTER FOUR

Technology and Diagnosis

Dementia expresses itself by interfering with the normal or usual pattern of behavior demonstrated by the individual in the past. Essentially, there has been some change that is so marked that a disease or disorder must be presumed to be present. The manifestations of this problem may take any one of a variety of forms, and there may have been a series of unusual events that were neither noted nor responded to. Indeed, the history of the individual might reflect a clear pattern of change had it only been noticed and considered. Unfortunately, such a record is available only retrospectively and then only as the patient and/or caregiver select those items from their recollections that are either recognized or admitted to. That there is a history is unmistakable; the cause of that history, regardless of how well recalled or reported, becomes the focus of medical attention when the patient is brought to a physician for a diagnosis.

One must understand that the physician is at a disadvantage in some respects. There is a complaint that is presented as an acute state but with more intense effects because there is an awareness by both patient and caregiver that the problem has been developing over some time. By now, the patient and caregiver are more than just concerned. To some degree, they may be frightened because a previously healthy person has shown increasing examples of irrational or bizarre behavior, without obvious reason or cause. What seemed to have started as simply instances of "forgetfulness," "foolishness," "pig-headedness," or even "age" has now mushroomed. The psychological distress is intense in most cases, with frustration, anxiety, and/or depression often present in the patient. These same emotional reactions may strongly influence the caregiver as well. What is desired, and perhaps expected, is an examination that will "explain" or even "explain away" what has been and is happening. Physicians, after all, are supposed to work miracles, if not personally, then at least with medications, surgery, and technology.

Unfortunately, reality is different and seldom satisfies expectations and hopes. In the first place, the physician who is consulted usually will be the family doctor, a general practitioner or one specializing in internal medicine. His or her knowledge about the behaviors that comprise the overall complaint and its possible causes will vary with experience, recency and accuracy of education, and interest. Though one might think that every medical doctor in this country is not only aware but also well-trained about the dementias, that belief is unfounded. Certainly, more and more physicians are alert to the consequences called *dementia*, but there remains a considerable range in training and competence.

Furthermore, the issue is compounded by the fact that the complaints presented by the patient and caregiver will be selective and fragmentary. The intake process must be thorough in order to investigate a variety of possibilities and to identify additional incidents not easily faced or remembered. There must be a complete physical examination in order to reduce the number of possible causes of the behaviors presented. Increasingly, we are an aging population with wide variance in information about physical and mental problems that may affect us. The individual must first recognize and accept the difficulty being experienced, and seek competent medical help (see Reifler & Larson, 1985, pp. 11–12). Comprehensive evaluation may identify a cause that is treatable and thereby not only relieve the anxieties of family members but also reduce the inclination toward overreaction. In many instances, of course, the worst fears of the person will be realized. Unfortunately, the diagnostic process is not simple, may take weeks, often is indirect, and frequently does not provide with certainty a sole diagnosis.

If conventional medical tests are not successful in identifying a cause for the behavior changes, there may be a decision to try more sophisticated measures interpreted by specialists. There is an increasing availability of devices used in the process, offering more precise measurement and requiring more expert interpretation. It should be no surprise that the equipment and expertise are accompanied by rapidly escalating costs. One must weigh whether sufficient, precise information will be achieved to warrant the various costs as compared with the demand for exact diagnosis.

Fogel and Faust (1987, pp. 39–44) have described the diagnostic process (as employed by the psychiatrist but not limited to that specialty) as one that requires the setting and testing of hypotheses. This involves using a number of measures and observations pertinent to the complaints and characteristics of the patient. There is, then, no set or "pat" procedure that is followed by rote. However, those authors discuss some standard issues that should be considered by the physician in the decision-making process that will lead to eventual diagnosis. Although presented in the general case, several of these "pearls," as they call them, are pertinent to the use of neurologic measures with dementia.

1. There are indicators that have been shown to be related neurologically to certain causes and conditions: These are called "signs." They may be directly observed and measured or may be inferred. Where there is a brain disorder or disease, demonstration may not be possible in a direct and explicit way. The signs vary in their sensitivity and precision, but the physician must use them to hypothesize about a cause. How effective the procedure is will depend upon the knowledge of the physician about the characteristics and causes of the conditions that produce the signs. In the case of a dementia resulting from Alzheimer's disease, for example, it is almost impossible to have tissue from the brain of the person available for microscopic examination.

If other potential causes of behavioral change have been excluded, the diagnosis must be based upon what is known from other such cases. For example, as mentioned earlier, major depression may be mistaken for dementia and must be differentiated. Pick's disease may be confused with Alzheimer's, though there are ways that help to distinguish the two. Toxic effects of drugs may produce symptoms like those of Huntington's disease. Inferentially, then, the decision may be made that the person suffers from Alzheimer's disease and is demonstrating the resulting mental deterioration. Though accuracy is not assured by this process, it assures greater probability given the experiences to date with other, similar cases. Joynt (1990, p. 929) points out that any neurologic examination has to be evaluated in terms of the age, history, and other findings about the patient. In a few instances, the conclusion may be that the complaints result from some variation in the normal process of aging and are not the expressions of Alzheimer's after all. Part of the diagnostic difficulty is in the fact that norms about aging are not well established, making it difficult to identify the characteristics of a control population (Joynt, 1990, p. 928).

2. There are a number of tests used for screening purposes to ascertain the presence of a possible organic condition. For example, one may ask the patient to respond to questions that indicate orientation to time and place. These kinds of measures are used because they are quick and easy to administer, give immediate feedback, and are believed to have adequate validity. There are other tests, less commonly used because of the cost in time and training, which might give a more complete indication

of the quality of the individual's brain. Fogel and Faust (1987, p. 40) point out that there may be greater differences in validity using these two approaches than is commonly accepted, and they cite research that supports this view. This is not to say that both are not worthwhile under the appropriate circumstances. It is more reasonable to consider more than one possibility in order to avoid the risk of overlooking cases that should in fact be diagnosed (called false negatives).

3. Any examination requires comparison of the results with appropriate norms. If you are given an ability test of some kind, you want to be sure that the results are compared to the results of other persons like you in some essential respects: age, educational level, experiences, and the like. Otherwise there may be bias (either for or against you, depending on the norms group) that should not enter any decisions made. In the same way, a neurological exam should yield results that are compared to the appropriate norms. This may be particularly crucial with the elderly (Fogel & Faust, 1987, p. 42) because of the inherent possibility of decline that occurs, to some degree, with advancing age. Joynt, as mentioned earlier (1990, p. 928), agrees with this caution and reviews some of the difficulties involved.

The issue becomes one of the quality or validity of the norms that are used. The standards that are applied should be realistic. Because neurological examinations center on the quality of the brain, there should be adequate knowledge of the "normal" aging brain as well as of its deviations. In fact, however, such information is not available (Joynt, 1990, p. 927). Further, some behaviors associated with structural changes may show great variability in expression from one person to the next. In this regard, Fogel and Faust (1987, p. 42) point out that gait disturbances may be adjustments to aging factors, while at the same time, gait disturbances indicate central nervous system disease if they are severe enough. The psychiatrist should attempt to discriminate one from the other, particularly because treatment may be possible in some cases. *All* disturbances in the way the older person walks are not indicative of brain disorder, although each should be carefully and completely investigated by the physician.

4. Sources of information used by the physician should be wide-ranging in order to assure as accurate a diagnosis as possible. The psychiatrist who depends only on the current medical examination may miss cues that would be helpful. For example, the history of the case may give as much or more meaningful data as the exam. This situation reflects the idea of hypothesis testing, described earlier. In an area where precision is always a matter of concern, the more comprehensive the basis for diagnosis, generally the better it is. Anecdotal and observational

material supplied by the patient and caregiver can supplement the observations of the physician and combine with the empirical facts from tests. The combined results will probably serve the patient more usefully than any one source alone.

Even with this selective survey of issues surrounding diagnosis of brain disorders, it is apparent that there is no sure procedure or totally trustworthy test. In the final analysis, the decision is often an "educated guess." With sufficient care, however, it is probable that the final decision is most likely the correct one. Indeed, there is some evidence available about the accuracy of diagnosis of brain disorders. For example, there have been reports based upon autopsies of patients who had been labeled "Alzheimer's disease." These studies examined tissue for evidence of neurofibrillary tangles and neuritic plaques, in particular, as the presence of such material would substantiate the diagnosis. Generally, the error rate has been consistent and low (say, 10% or less), though in some instances the error rate has been quite high (Cohen, 1988, pp. 141–142). What must qualify any conclusions from these data must be the fact that *most* cases of Alzheimer's are not autopsied; in fact, only a small percentage have been (Butler, 1990, p. 935). This produces selective bias in either direction to an unknown degree. It should not be surprising, then, that some physicians are becoming increasingly cautious in labeling patients. They are requiring more complete and sophisticated testing and are exercising great care in how they describe their conclusions. Because an aging population is expected to show increases in numbers and percentages of cases of dementia from various sources, this problem of communication and understanding will become greater.

Ideally, this country would be investing heavily in research on the dementias and their causes. However, because there are so many demands on the resources of the population, some priorities have had to be established. Research about dementia has been given a low priority. For example, in Fiscal Year 1990, the total federal budget for Alzheimer's was $148 million, which averages out to about $37 per patient for the year. The average cost to care for such a patient for a year was $22,000 (Eastman, 1991). Butler (1990, p. 933) reports that long-term care costs for SDAT alone exceed *$40 billion per year.* Obviously, answers of any kind will be slow in coming when there is such an imbalance between cost and investment. There are, of course, other sources of research funds, such as private foundations, for example, and the Alzheimer's Association. Still, the overall picture is discouraging. Although one may not be able to buy answers, answers come only through scientifically based models and data collection. These researches are expensive and time-consuming; rarely are the answers derived serendipitously.

In short, the physicians must work with what is available and render the best possible judgment and counsel. The tools at their disposal are increasing and offer substantial improvements over the past. Therefore, a survey of the types of technological advances and their utility seems pertinent.

DATA-GATHERING INSTRUMENTS

In most cases, direct observation and immediate diagnosis of dementia is not possible. Virtually all identification is by exclusion, which not only increases the possibility for error but also compels the use of a variety of techniques and instruments to make the exclusion as definitive as possible. Within the past 20 years or so, there have been major breakthroughs in technology that permit greater assurance that a reversible or alternate cause for behavioral change will not be missed. Each addition to the armamentarium of the neurologist or psychiatrist has been more comprehensive and more sophisticated. Yet, it still is not possible to examine the individual nerve cell with even the best of these instruments, and there seems no chance that such a machine is on the horizon. Even if such an event occurs, the cost may be prohibitive, a factor already militating against widespread use of current technology.

What present data-gathering instruments will allow, then, is more precision and accuracy in excluding identifiable conditions. Not only has use increased in recent years, but there is an accumulating corpus of research which helps define the strengths and limits of the tools. Our survey will describe both their distinct characteristics and the documented benefits from their use.

The Electroencephalogram (EEG)

The measurement of brain "waves" representing electrical output is by no means new technology, of course. The process has been available since the 1930s, though it took the application of technology developed during World War II to enable implementation and routine use. Today, the EEG is a useful tool for a number of conditions, all of which involve the cerebral cortex in some way.

The brain is constantly active and thereby produces continuous electrical impulses that may be measured. These are examined for their quality in general as well as for their features during various states and activities of the individual. During sleep, for example, the "pattern" of impulses differs from that found during a period when one is awake. A brain disease, such as epilepsy, will cause the brain to emit different electrical patterns (at least during seizures) than will a brain not suffering such a condition. There are, then, different levels or degrees of intensity in the electrical impulses that produce differences in patterns according to the brain's electrical activity at the moment. The presence, absence, or deviations of these patterns is reflected in a recording made via electrodes attached to the head.

Four types of brain waves have been identified. They occur separately and according to conditions occurring in the cells of the brain. As the activity of the cerebral cortex fluctuates, the characteristics of the waves will change. However, this does not mean that the brain-wave patterns reflect one of the four. In fact, irregularity is the more general pattern of the EEG (Guyton, 1991, p. 662). Yet, the only meaningful correlations that can be obtained between brain activity and behavior are when one of the four waves is measured. This can only occur in the controlled setting where electrodes are attached to the head and varied experimental conditions are implemented. The accumulation of data reflecting such relationships is increasing and helps to describe certain characteristics that discriminate the brain-wave patterns of dementia patients from those not demented.

One of the expressions measured by the EEG is called the *Alpha wave*. It is rhythmic, with frequencies ranging between 8 and 13 cycles per second. In each second of time, there will be some number of discrete, identifiable expressions between these extremes. Alpha waves are found in almost all normal adults when they are awake but are relaxed and quiet, that is, when there is no major activity in the cerebral cortex (Guyton, 1991, p. 662).

When the Alpha pattern is measured, the most intense electrical signals come from the occipital lobe, but there may also be some measurable activity in the parietal and frontal lobes. When we are sleeping, and particularly in the phase called "deep sleep," Alpha waves are not found. We could say, then, that an Alpha wave pattern is typical of a relaxed, serene, but awake state for the normal person. Should the individual become involved in a more dynamic mental activity, then the pattern will change and produce *Beta waves.*

Beta waves are low voltage and asynchronous, with frequencies of more than 14 cycles per second, sometimes reaching more than 25 cycles per second. Usually, the activity is focused in the parietal and frontal lobes. This pattern is found when there is activity in the central nervous system, that is, under conditions where we are attending to stimuli and using the cortex to interpret and formulate responses. However, Beta patterns also occur under conditions that are not well focused; for example, if we are in a state of tension, this pattern will occur.

Theta waves are expressed in cycles of 4 to 7 per second. In adults, the pattern is found during periods of emotional stress, particularly if the person is frustrated or disappointed. What is more important for our purposes is the fact that this pattern is also found in many cases of brain disorder. It may be a basis for some discrimination and diagnosis, then, particularly if combined with and supported by other kinds of predictive information.

Finally, the *Delta wave* is expressed in all EEG patterns where the cycles occur at 3.5 per seconds or less. The Delta wave occurs most commonly in very deep sleep but has been correlated with cases of serious organic brain disease as well. Thus a connection with dementia may be possible here. Because the Delta wave occurs only in the cortex, it may be independent of activity in lower brain centers, and its expression more predictive of syndromes leading to dementia.

There are some reservations and limitations about measurement of these patterns. First, the mechanical means for observing any of these waves is limited to the condition that many neurons are firing at the time of observation; literally, in the thousands at least and perhaps in the millions (Guyton, 1991, p. 662). Only under these conditions will sufficient electrical energy be expended by the brain for the EEG to record the result. Second, the firing of the neurons and fibers must be in synchrony, that is, they must be firing at the same time. Asynchrony may not produce sufficient energy to yield a measurable pattern.

Several studies have been published that relate performance on the EEG with dementia and other disorders. Brenner, Reynolds, and Ulrich (1989) established several diagnostic groups for comparison of patterns. There were 23 dementia patients who also had symptoms of depression. A second group was comprised of 10 who were depressed and acted in a way that mimicked dementia though they were not in fact demented (pseudodementia). These two groups were compared to several others: One was a group of "probable" Alzheimer's without signs of depression; another had major depressive episodes but did not present symptoms or evidence of dementia; and a third consisted of controls without problems of depression or dementia. A comparison of the differences between these various groups revealed that the group suffering only clinical depression and the one with depression masking as dementia produced normal or near-normal patterns on the EEG. Those diagnosed as only dementia and those who were labeled as dementia plus depression consistently reflected abnormal patterns. In fact, about one-third of the total of these two groups showed moderate-to-severe abnormalities in the EEG.

When the dementia plus depression group was compared to the group with depression that masked as dementia, significant differences in waking EEGs were found. This study supports the contention that dementia patients will produce patterns differing from the norms as compared with nondemented persons or those with a functional disorder such as depression. The sizes of the groups and the lack of significance in some comparisons limits generalization about the utility of an EEG for any precise diagnosis. Nonetheless, the data support the presumption that a dementia includes some adverse effects on brain operation.

A related study has been reported by Coben, Danziger, and Storandt (1985). A group of 40 patients who had been diagnosed as Senile Dementia of the Alzheimer's Type (SDAT) was compared on EEG measures with a control group of 41 individuals. The latter group presented no symptoms that would preclude their being classified as "healthy." The age range of the two groups was very close (between 64 and 83 years in both cases).

Resting EEGs were taken at three different times over a $2\frac{1}{2}$-year period. All four patterns were measured each time along with the strength of each. The authors found that normal changes in the patterns for the healthy older persons included increases in the Delta wave and decreases in Beta. Mean frequency in the patterns also decreased for this group. Theta and Alpha remained unchanged for these controls.

For those with SDAT, however, there were changes with time in each possible comparison. Further analysis considered different developmental stages of SDAT to see if patterns differed. For the sample members in an early developmental level of the disease, both Theta and Beta patterns differed significantly from controls. At a more advanced level, the differences were still present, and there was an additional change in the Alpha pattern as compared to controls. Further in the disease process, Delta also differed for the experimentals as compared with the controls. Such findings are in accord with the position that the disease process will have adverse influences on brain function, including the patterns displayed by brain excitation.

As a final example of research in this area, an earlier study by Coben, Danziger, and Berg (1983) will be described. In this study, there were 40 participants in each of two groups. Group 1 consisted of SDAT patients with only a mild degree of dementia whereas Group 2 had individually matched controls without SDAT. Resting EEGs were obtained for each subject. The authors report significant differences in Theta and Beta wave activity, but there were no differences in Alpha and Delta. These findings fit the change in patterns accompanying disease progression reported and suggest that the effects of dementia are partly developmental. Theta waves were increased, whereas Beta were decreased as compared with controls even in early stages of SDAT. This result is inconsistent with normal aging data.

These studies as well as others offer some support to the notion that the effects of dementia may influence the functioning of the brain in a number of ways. The EEG is sensitive to many of the changes that occur. Such data have not been shown to be valid diagnostically but do suggest that variation from changes in brain-wave patterns found in normally aging persons should lead to determining the possibility of dementia through use of other measures.

Computerized Tomography (CT or "CAT" Scan)

The first of the advanced technologies that have proven to be beneficial to medical diagnostics was the procedure that allowed computer generation of images of detailed features of parts of the body. One of the major benefits is that the CT scan avoids invasive procedures that formerly were necessary, such as biopsies. The patient is certainly better served, and the physician is given, in most instances, accurate information.

The procedure employs X-rays that are absorbed by body structures. The CT scanner converts a series of X-rays into computer-generated videoimages of the structures, sometimes using color to highlight subtle differences between normal and abnormal tissues. It is clear that this permits examination and interpretation superior to standard X-ray images. In addition, the procedure is more sensitive to the density of bodies than is standard X-ray technique and the process usually produces 12 to 15 independent images rather than just one (Haber, 1990, p. 216).

Recent advances now permit three-dimensional (3-D) imaging, so improvements are continuing. The scan gives clearer images, allowing distinction between gray and white matter in the cerebral cortex, basal ganglia, and ventricles. Where dementia is suspected, the procedure may be used to decide if the cause is identifiable and diagnosable (say, a tumor that may be either treatable or nontreatable) or nondiagnosable. Haber (1990, p. 217) reports 95% to 99% success in identification of intracranial tumors. Even more impressive is the diagnosis of stroke, important in decisions related to multiinfarct dementia. Atrophy of tissue in the cerebral cortex is disclosed by the CT scan, though there is still disagreement about the particular meaning of the data. This reflects part of the problem associated with lack of knowledge about the norms of aging: In this case, how much shrinkage is normally expected before it becomes detrimental? At this time, the application of the CT technique in diagnosing causes of dementia, such as Alzheimer's disease, is not possible. The scan will disclose certain changes in the brain but is not capable of detailing the status of nerve cells. The results are used, then, to disclose what isn't a cause, not what is.

The research has yielded somewhat mixed results about the success of the procedure as it is currently used. Wilson, Fox, Huckman, Bacon, and Lobrick (1982a), for example, used the results of CT scans on a sample of 42 patients diagnosed as SDAT. A control group of 38 non-dementia persons of similar age also had been administered CT. The authors report that cerebral atrophy was associated with aging in both samples. There was greater atrophy in the dementia patients, but the amount of the change was unrelated to the degree to which the dementia had progressed. At least for this study, then, it would be dangerous to assume some direct relationship between dementia and brain atrophy (nor is such an assumption accepted by physicians, anyway). Density measures were available for only part of the samples (N = 19 patients and N = 33 for controls). There was no evidence, using data for 14 separate brain regions, that the density figures related either to age or to presence of dementia. The latter finding conflicts with results of some other studies, however. Wilson et al. propose that the scan best serves, and indeed might even be limited to, ruling out brain lesions.

Colgan (1985) has a longitudinal study of a group of 48 persons diagnosed as SDAT. All had CT scans, and each was given a mental status examination and additional memory and orientation tasks. This study, then, offers both the technological measure and psychological ones. A follow-up, conducted 6 months after initial data collection, disclosed that 10 of the sample had died. Colgan examined the performances for these 10 and compared them with the survivors. As far as the scan was concerned, the deceased had lower mean densities than the survivors in the parietal, occipital, and left thalamic regions. This result accords with an hypothesis of such a relationship. It is possible that the loss of density is a measure that may forecast a shorter life span in SDAT patients. It is also of interest, though not so pertinent to this topic, that those who had died performed less well on the cognitive tests used. Colgan believes this may mean that some persons may have a more rapidly progressive form of SDAT that is reflected in the loss of mental competencies. Certainly, we know that some intellectual decline is expected in old age, at least with the instruments (such as the WAIS–R) that currently are popular. More rapid decline, and particularly in mental status, is shown frequently just prior to death in the elderly as a group. Perhaps this finding reflects that relationship in a specific subgroup with dementia.

Haber (1990, p. 213) has prepared a table that describes costs of new technologies as we enter the 1990s. The equipment needed to do a CT scan currently costs from $650,000 to $1,200,000, and installation and site preparation will be about $50,000. Obviously, this is not a machine to be found in each physician's office. More commonly, it is available in a hospital that serves a region or district, as this will allow sharing of costs, more consistent utilization of the hardware, and less expense to the patient. Cost for the scan may run from $200 to $400, depending on the nature and extent of the examination, the interpretation of the results, and ongoing overhead. Once all other diagnostic possibilities have been exhausted, the cost does not seem excessive to help determine what might (or might not, to be more exact) be the cause of behavioral changes.

Positron Emission Tomography (PET)

The more recent invention of the PET scan brought medical diagnostics clearly into the nuclear age. The procedure involves the use of a cyclotron[1] so that a tomogram is produced on a cathode-ray tube (CRT). In this case, the PET scan is a cross-sectional image of metabolic activity in the targeted region. What is depicted are physiological and pharmacological data as they are reflected in cerebral metabolic activity. The procedure is useful to study of the brain because it is sensitive to the conscious alertness of the individual, including mental and physical activities. The PET scan is unique in that it can measure metabolic change even before actual structural change occurs. Fogel and Faust (1987, p. 55) describe research indicating such an outcome for Alzheimer's patients and persons with normal pressure hydrocephalus. In some instances, they point out, the scan may become diagnostic (as for Huntington's disease), whereas for others it is only descriptive (as in Parkinsonism). They point out that the PET scan may well become a useful tool in early diagnosis of brain diseases, but it has yet to prove its place in the routine clinical examination (Fogel & Faust, 1987, p. 56). It is interesting that they maintain the overall cost is significantly higher than for either the CT scan or MRI, which reduces its practical applications. This point is well-taken when one considers costs cited by Haber (1990, p. 213). Equipment will cost $800,000, installation and site preparation some $700,000, and the cyclotron $2,500,000. This totals to $4,000,000—a heavy initial investment indeed unless the resource can be used to the benefit of patients in significant numbers and for significant purposes. Cost per procedure is cited as $700 to $800.

Magnetic Resonance Imaging (MRI)

Among the newest and most impressive of medical technological advances is the MRI. Like the CT scan, it is noninvasive and does not pose a radiation threat. It distinguishes between body fluids (like blood) and tissue (like the white and gray matter of the brain). The tomogram has high spatial resolution (as in the CT scan) and provides metabolic information (as does the PET scan) (Haber, 1989, p. 220). There are no biological side effects that have been reported to date, though the procedure is still quite young and is restricted in use by cost factors.

The MRI discriminates tissues with high fat and water content that cannot be imaged with other procedures and provides information about the chemical composition of tissues as well. For example, gray matter in the brain has about 15% more water in it than white matter (Haber, 1990, p. 220), and this difference is large enough to allow distinction. The importance of the capability lies in the fact that cerebral infarcts, tumors, hemorrhages, and vascular abnormalities can be made visual. Haber (1990, p. 220) states that this technique may even hold the potential for diagnosing Alzheimer's disease as expertise in MRI interpretation increases.

There are some disadvantages, however. Both Haber (1990, p. 220) and Fogel and Faust (1987, pp. 45–46) point out that the procedure may be hazardous for patients with metallic objects (such as aneurysm clips) in the body because the magnetic field may dislodge the object and cause a hemorrhage. Where such dangers to the patient are not present, the MRI poses other problems. Haber (1990, p. 220) specifically mentions that the device must be carefully located because there is the chance for mutual interference with other equipment. The cost of the equipment currently runs from $800,000 to $1,200,000. Installation and site preparation are high—$1.5 to 2.2 million. Total costs then may be between $2.5 and $3.5 million. Cost of the procedure to the patient is $700 to $800 (Haber, 1990, p. 213).

The gains that may be achieved outweigh some of the limitations, particularly those associated with cost. Fogel and Faust (1987, p. 46) cite a number of studies demonstrating that MRI is as efficient at detection of pathology and disclosing lesions as the CT scan. At the same time, it is superior to the CT for detecting certain abnormalities as well as the extent of pathology. These authors caution that the very sensitivity that makes the MRI so promising also requires better understanding of what is "normal" change, especially for the elderly.

At present, the promise is greater than the realization for all of these techniques. There certainly are advantages and advances that are substantial when compared with former techniques for gathering diagnostic information. Yet, even with these changes, the specific information that would make it possible to diagnose accurately and directly the cause of a dementia is lacking. To some degree, each of these technologies reduces the dependency on diagnosis by exclusion. Still, none of them permits examination at the cellular level, and we must await that technology with its unknown costs and possible limitations. Technological research and development must continue in the use, understanding, and extension of current devices, as well as in the search for more sophisticated diagnostic instruments.

DIFFERENTIAL DIAGNOSIS

Given the technological advances of the recent past and the certain progress in the future, there is reason to believe that exact diagnosis for the dementias may someday occur. Meantime, what is available helps reduce the error that might occur because of an inability to identify causes (either treatable or untreatable). There are, of course, some syndromes known to lead to irreversible dementia (e.g., multiinfarct dementia). The present state of the art requires using all possible relevant data to delimit the list of conditions that may be causing the patient's dementia, then generate the probability of each as cause, and, finally, specify *which* condition is most likely responsible. This third step does not offer any particular reassurance because intervention for progressive dementia is most often impossible. However, differential diagnosis is a required procedure and has led to statistics that reflect the incidence and prevalence of major causes of dementia in our society.

The use of data as described has led to the widely held belief that Alzheimer's disease is a common cause of mental incompetence, particularly in the aging segment of the population. Unless there is a major breakthrough, we must expect that the belief will be demonstrated: As more people live longer lives dementia will increase, and AD will show the greatest increases. Some professionals believe that the diagnosis of Alzheimer's has reached "epidemic" proportions in the sense that it is named too-often as the diagnosis. Others take issue with this proposition, maintaining that the estimates are accurate and reflect increased sophistication in the use of technology. Whichever may be the truth, there is no quarrel that the disease is a major threat because it leads to impaired memory and consequent behavior deficits.

Differential diagnosis implies the ability to make *accurate* diagnosis. In the case of AD, this potential has not been reached. The Alzheimer's Association (1987) has pointed out that research currently being done involves identifying a cause, developing a cure, enhancing accuracy of diagnosis, and identifying ancillary treatments. At present, none of these has occurred. Rather, there are several postulations about possible causative conditions.

One line of research involves autopsies of the brains of AD patients. Through such efforts, we have learned that the primary changes occurring in the brain are neurofibrillary tangles in the cell body of the neuron and neuritic plaques. The plaques will interfere with or prevent the reception of signals so that the brain cannot receive the information necessary for the person to continue to function effectively. This condition may be the reason that, even early in the progress of the disease, the patient is unable to encode and respond to current stimuli. For example, while still driving, the person may "run" a stop sign, not because it was not seen but because its significance was not apprehended. Which behaviors will be adversely affected depend on the particular cells that have been affected, so that one individual may show loss in one form of behavior, whereas another individual manifests different symptoms. Thus different persons show different effects, although the outcome of AD is the same for all.

The neurofibrillary tangles in the cell body accumulate and gradually fill the cell, interfering with normal functioning. The nature of the tangles is not fully known, though it may be abnormal protein (Cohen, 1988, p. 22). This possibility has led to increasing efforts to identify the character of the protein and its source. Additionally, there is research to analyze and control protein fragments (called amyloids) in the blood vessels and plaques (Alzheimer's Association, 1987). Yankner (in Alzheimer's Association, 1991c), for example, has some evidence that indicates that a substance called "amyloid beta protein" may be involved in causing the disease to progress. Such data continue to add pieces to the puzzle but with more pieces necessary for solution.

Although study of diseased tissue may eventually explain AD, other scientists believe that biochemistry is the more likely candidate. The focus of research in this case is the chemical that helps transmit the electrical signal that is the "message" to be interpreted. The particular chemical involved in AD is the neurotransmitter acetylcholine (ACh). In particular, ACh assists in carrying the electrical impulse across the synapse from the axon of one cell to the dendrite of another. Research has disclosed very low levels of this substance (but also of other transmitters) in cells that are diseased by tangles and plaques (Alzheimer's Association, 1987).

This could mean that ACh alone is the cause of AD or that the ACh deficiency combines with tangles and plaques as the reason. The result of the neurotransmitter deficit will be an inability to activate sufficient neurons to behave effectively. If we have a person who is responsible for washing dishes, for example, there is the possibility that part of the task will be done effectively, whereas part of it is not remembered. Cells still intact will function, whereas those lacking neurotransmitters will not.

The Alzheimer's Association (1987) also points out the biochemical research that is underway to determine which chemicals in the body act as markers or indicators of specific syndromes. This would allow diagnosis in a straightforward and accurate form. To date, the results are only suggestive albeit promising. In another vein, one of the earliest reported abnormalities in nerve cells was the presence of an excessive amount of aluminum that had been stored. For several years, it was believed that this component was the cause of AD. Now, the position most often taken is that aluminum may be either cause or effect, and research efforts are continuing to determine which is correct.

Still other research is investigating the possibility that AD is the consequence of a "slow-acting" virus, as in Creutzfeldt–Jakob disease. Sunderland (1990, pp. 946–947) points out that the pathological effect in Creutzfeldt–Jakob disease is different from that of AD so that a different virus would be involved. In any event, there is little support for a viral explanation at this point (Alzheimer's Association, 1987).

The problem of diagnosis is being investigated from other directions also. One of these is an attempt to find the elements in common among those who develop the condition (Alzheimer's Association, 1987). In some syndromes, such an approach has disclosed both cause and prevention. For example, tuberculosis occurs in conditions where individuals inhale microorganisms from untreated, active cases. Until this fact was realized earlier in this century, tuberculosis was a major "killer." Now it is well-controlled, though it is still a bigger threat to the elderly than to youth. If scientists could isolate the conditions in which risk is greatest for AD, the cause could more easily be determined and a prevention found.

There is the possibility, of course, that the potential causes discussed focus too closely on the status of nerve cells *after* the causative agent has already forced its consequences. Orr-Rainey (1991), for example, has suggested the possibility that AD results from systemic disorders that were not identified (and perhaps could not be) with eventual progression to brain cells. Whether or not found to be true, the proposal should remind us to keep an open mind even where there are already so many candidates.

Finally, there is the possibility that AD is a heritable condition. This would mean that it is genetically transmitted in some predictable and consistent pattern from one generation to another. With the knowledge that persons with Down's syndrome who lived beyond age 35 or so might develop symptoms much like those with Alzheimer's, this possibility took on added appeal. Cohen (1988, pp. 134–137) has reviewed the literature and concludes that the *reasons* for any relationships are not yet clear. Further and what is important is the fact that he has described the conditions that must hold for a genetic case to be made for any condition. These include, first, the fact that the occurrence of some syndromes in certain families much more often than in others does not necessarily indicate a genetic basis. One of the questions frequently asked by caregivers and family members relates to this position. Not uncommonly, they will "remember" that Grandma Bessie seemed to have the same signs, and Aunt Suzie had problems like this, and so on. To conclude that the cases represented Alzheimer's is dangerous and probably also wrong. Second, Cohen points out that even if there is a genetic relationship, that does not make it hereditary. Perhaps, instead, it is congenital and occurred only because some developmental condition allowed it to be expressed. Third, even when an individual has an inherited predisposition toward a given disorder, unless there are appropriate conditions that allow the expression of this potential, there may never be a manifestation of the disease. At present, there does not seem to be a case to be made for genetic transmission. What is interesting, though, is that it has been shown that the gene that manufactures amyloid is located on Chromosome 21, the chromosome that is involved in Down's syndrome.

A study by Sturt (1986) yields findings that illustrate the complex nature of determining heritability. She investigated the age at which dementia (AD, Pick's or senile dementia) began in relatives of cases diagnosed with a dementia of early onset. She found that female relatives had higher risk than males and brothers were less often affected than fathers of the probands (patients). Relatives of those with Pick's had a slightly higher risk of dementia than those with AD, and this risk increased with age (up to age 80). As has been noted before, there are more older females than males with the disparity increasing with age, and the percentage of persons diagnosed with dementia also increases with age. Thus, her results would seem more concordant with age demographics in the general population than with a case for heritability. She states that "the pattern of the age-related hazard of dementia is due to the nature of the dementing process; that this slow degenerative process is widespread; and that individual differences in the rate of the process are under the influence of genes" (p. 583).

Multiinfarct dementia (MID) seems to offer a greater probability of accuracy in diagnosis and, thus, differentiation from other causes of dementia. For example, the use of magnetic resonance imaging (MRI), if available, can assist in disclosing small infarcts (Slaby & Cullen, 1987, p. 155). Other clinical signs (such as high stroke risk or sudden-onset strokes) combine to make the diagnosis more accurate (Caplan, 1990, p. 971). But, even here, there is the possibility that the decision about cause may be questionable and may require additional diagnostic measures to rule out alternative causes before intervention is implemented.

Research on Diagnosis

In the past decade, the literature on dementia, both in the general sense and for specific conditions, has increased. Typical of the approach has been a subset of articles that review what is known and draw conclusions regarding the present-day status. Storandt (1983), for example, has discussed SDAT in terms of prevalence, changes in brain structure, and causes. She relates the effects from the syndrome to a need for supportive treatment for both patient and caregiver, including assistance to the caregiver. Comfort (1984) has described senility in terms of its pathological influences, including not only structural changes but immunological ones as well. He assesses the genetic connection, "selective" (and often confusing) involvement of areas of the brain, the role and status of neurotransmitters, and the intriguing possibilities of a resemblance to conditions caused by a slow-acting virus. He even coins a term, *Alzheimerism*, to reflect a progressive dementia that interferes with associations and memory along with atrophy of the brain due to a loss of neurons.

Some of the articles that are intended to indicate the present state of knowledge not only approach the same issue from somewhat different directions (as above) but also suggest additional variables for consideration. In this regard, Arie (1984) discusses not only SDAT and MID but also depression because there can be a mimicking of dementia in that functional disorder. Further, he suggests that premorbid personality may be a significant variable and suggests ways in which the person may become more resilient in order to help handle, perhaps even prevent, the mental disorders of old age.

Ban (1989) sees evidence of greater similarity between MID and SDAT than is commonly assumed. In particular, he proposes that cerebral blood flow may be adversely influenced in both. He also reviews studies where chemical treatments have been attempted, with varying results.

Specific Effects of Dementia

There have been several studies about structural changes of specific elements. In 1987, de Ruiter and Uylings compared the dendrites of patients with AD (N = 4) and MID (N = 1) postmortem to a group (N = 5) of controls of similar age. They concluded that degeneration of dendrites is a predominant process in dementia.

The role of specific neurotransmitters and disturbances in their actions have been surveyed by Andrade (1983). He notes that deleterious effects (such as plaques and tangles) have been treated using various chemical substitutes. Levodopa (L-dopa, helpful in controlling tremors in Parkinson's disease), dopamine, and even drugs that work on body systems producing gamma-aminobutyric acid (GABA, the major inhibitory transmitter in the brain) and serotonin (also an inhibitory neurotransmitter) have been used but failed to assist cognitive functioning of patients. Both choline and lecithin have produced conflicting results. Lecithin had a period of great expectations in the past when initial experiments showed some improvements in some patients. Research continues on such drugs, singly and in combinations, but effective drug treatment may be years away. Two major studies have been or are currently ongoing, one with tetrahydroaminoacridine (THA) and the other with physostigmine, a drug that influences the metabolism of ACh but is toxic in larger doses (Heston & White, 1991, p. 100). Various dosage levels are being tested to determine their effects on memory functioning. Either or both may be found to assist retrieval of short-term and/or long-term memory.

Goodnick and Gershon (1984) discuss these drugs and others, pointing to the promise but lack of substance at that time. Gottfries (1985), surveying data on chemical changes in the brains of AD patients, notes that "several attempts have been made to activate[2] the neurotransmitter systems, but the progress of these studies has not been encouraging" (p. 245). When study is extended to other conditions (presenile dementia and MID, for example), pathological changes in biochemical patterns may be expressed in different ways (Degrell, Hellsing, Nagy, and Niklasson, 1989).

Differential diagnosis should include comparisons between changes that occur as a part of "normal" aging and those resulting from disease processes. Winblad, Hardy, Backman, and Nilsson (1985) did this in a study in which they focused on memory function, the central loss found in dementia. They describe the biochemical changes for both groups, as gathered from the literature, and report where differences occur. One interesting area where there are no differences reported is in the cortical motor areas. They relate this finding to the relative success in both groups for memory on tasks involving motor action. They speculate that dopamine may remain stable in the hippocampus, allowing continued performance from memory when a physical action is being carried out.

The concern for accurate differential diagnosis is worldwide. Reports of demographics include attempts to demonstrate identifying charac-teristics, frequently. The results acknowledge the universality of dementia and its expressions. The efforts range from Russia (e.g., Shefer, 1985) to Japan (e.g., Shibayama, Kasahara, and Kobayashi, 1986; Mitsuyama, 1984), and Holland (e.g., Hovestadt, van Woerkom & Hekster, 1986), among several countries. The efforts are not coordinated, but they do focus on similar concerns and issues.

Current Status

Recognizing the differences among the several causes of dementia remains difficult despite the many advances made in technology and rec-ognition of symptoms. Alzheimer's disease, as previously noted, cannot be precisely diagnosed except at autopsy (and even then not always clearly). There are structural changes that identify the condition as distinctly Alzheimer's, but only at the cellular level for which nonintrusive measures into brain tissue are not yet available. The behavioral effects that aid in the diagnosis of AD are shared with other dementias. At present, then, AD remains a diagnosis that is given, based upon as complete information as possible but without the possibility of absolute confirmation.

The evidence for Pick's disease is more clearly shown in CT scans and manifests some differences from AD in behavioral symptoms but still may be confused with it (Sunderland, 1990, p. 946). Thus, autopsy is the only means for a definitive diagnosis. The virus involved in Creutzfeldt–Jakob disease is known and has, in fact, been transmitted to animals in laboratory settings. In these patients, there are changes in the EEG plus involuntary muscle movements. However, other symptoms are common to the state of dementia in general: memory loss, perhaps some apathy and a lack of interest in personal appearance, and even psycho-motor retardation. The progress of the disease is rapid, as compared to AD, usually culminating in death within 24 months.

Huntington's has a clearer clinical presentation that can be identified by the developing motor abnormalities and family histories (Sunderland,

1990, p. 946). On the other hand, in Parkinsonism, diagnosis is made more difficult by the lack of distinctive test results. There are two forms of this disorder. Primary Parkinsonism is the more common, usually occurring after age 50 and involving increasing tremor commonly beginning in the hands. The cause is not known (Yahr & Pang, 1990, pp. 974–976). Secondary (symptomatic) Parkinsonism accompanies a variety of other conditions, such as infections, tumors, and metabolic disorders. CT and MRI scans may show some characteristic brain changes. If the cause is drug-related or associated with a treatable disease, intervention is possible. Generally, however, there is no treatment. The symptoms of dementia do not occur in all cases of Parkinsonism, so that this syndrome is a special case as a cause of loss of mental competencies.

Normal pressure hydrocephalus may present on a CT scan as an enlargement of ventricles but without cerebral atrophy. This finding combined with disturbances in gait and increasing incontinence further delimits the clinical picture. If the usual symptoms of dementia (memory loss, confusion, and disorientation) slowly emerge, the diagnosis of this type of hydrocephalus may be made, but, as Sunderland (1990, p. 946) has noted, the pattern is not a clean one, and variability often occurs.

SUMMARY

Because the brain contains cells that do not regenerate, it is necessary to avoid invasive diagnostic techniques that would damage tissue. At the same time, once a medical examination has been completed without finding a cause for behavioral changes in an individual, it is reasonable to consider some organic pathological state associated with the brain. During this century, noninvasive techniques have been sought that would assist in determining causes and potential for treatment of brain disorders and syndromes.

The efforts have been expressed in the development of technology. The first of these was the electroencephalogram (EEG) that measures brain-wave patterns. Evidence has been collected demonstrating divergence from patterns normally expected when patients are suffering a condition leading to dementia. Such differences, when found, may be included as part of the diagnostic procedure.

In recent years, more sophisticated instruments have been developed and made possible by computer technology. Computerized tomography (CT) yields a series of X-rays of the brain. Each is a "slice" so that several successive (usually 10 to 12) pictures can indicate information about the quality of the structure of that part of the brain to the physician. The utility of this technique is limited by the fact that it discloses narrowly focused data (presence of tumors, evidence of atrophy).

Positron emission tomography (PET) allows depiction of metabolic activity in the brain. This provides information of increased refinement to the diagnostician. The cost of the equipment is very high, however, so that the process is more often used for research than in applied settings at this time.

Currently, magnetic resonance imaging (MRI) is the most sophisticated and promising of the techniques. It delivers data at a level and of a quality not found in any of the others. As costs permit, MRI will be used increasingly to help make a decision about cause of behavioral change. MRI reflects brain structures with different water content. It is superior to CT in terms of contrast for projections of the brain and has a capability for depicting metabolism that equals PET.

Unfortunately, there is no technology that will disclose the status of the individual nerve cell. As a result, in most cases the data are used to identify the status of the brain at a structural level. Differential diagnosis among possible diseases is still partially based on the individual clinician's judgment and intuition rather than on exact test results. Current research is attempting to disclose signs that will help in the process. Until precision and pathognomic signs are available, from whatever form of technology, diagnosis remains judgmental and hypothetical.

CHAPTER FIVE

Dementia and Psychological Testing

The evaluation of test results by psychologists is extensive. Included in the process are a variety of measures that may be used in decision making about the type and degree of mental incompetence found in the dementias. Most of these tests were not *designed* for this specific purpose, but they have either been accepted as appropriate to the purpose or have been adapted to the decision-making process.

These tests are of two types. *Neuropsychological* tests combine evidence of overt behavioral effects due to neuropathology with traditional measurement techniques as substitutes for direct measures of mental events. Groth-Marnot (1990, p. 6) says that these neuropsychological measures were "created to answer such questions as the nature of a person's organic deficits, severity of deficits, localization, and differentiating between functional versus organic impairment." As such, the information gained may be useful in the psychological assessment process for those with mental impairments. Traditionally, a number of tests have been created that use an indirect measure in order to estimate the presence and degree of a trait not directly observable. They may be referred to as *psychometric measures*. They became popular because they appeared to be objective, allowing largely accurate and useful prediction (Groth-Marnot, 1990, p. 3). These tests have been popular for purposes other than the original ones. For example, the Wechsler Scales (Wechsler-Bellevue, Wechsler Adult Intelligence Scale and Wechsler Adult Intelligence Scale–Revised) are intended to estimate the global qualities of intelligence for the individual through the ability to think rationally and act with purpose. In and of itself, such an estimate means little except as a psychometric judgment that the individual should be able to cope effectively in the environment. Indeed, Wechsler built the original scale to be used specifically in a psychiatric setting for clinical decision making about the person. It *was* to be an estimate of one's ability to function, but it was to be used as only one factor, albeit an important one, in the determination about the person's future (usually, commitment or noncommitment to a psychiatric facility). Since that time, the scales have been used for a variety of other purposes. Some of these have been based upon empirical research about the validity of such procedures, but other ways in which the test results have been used are not credible, because there is no research support for such uses. Tests, then, may be useful and accurate, but they may be used also in more or less inaccurate and nonuseful ways.

If there are difficulties associated with tests that are indirect measures, then why use them? The question is legitimate and has several legitimate answers. First, it was concluded in the previous chapter that, despite remarkable progress in the development of technology, diagnosis of causes of dementia is still not precise. Under these circumstances, other data, even though indirect, may assist in assuring that the diagnosis is probably appropriate. This is particularly true when the evidence is gathered independently and different traits that may be affected by dementia are measured. Medicine is concerned with the physical expression of disease and has developed measures to reflect the presence and degree of disease; psychology assesses the behavioral and mental competencies of the individual whether or not influenced by the disease process. Together, they provide more concrete evidence than either does alone. Although it is true that physicians may elect not to ask for or use neuropsychological/psychometric test results, the trend has been toward involving the neuropsychologist[1] in the effort.

Second, there is a need to know the nature and degree of complications from a syndrome more definitively. Medically, the physician can refer to physical changes and their consequences related to the disease. Many times, however, the patient and caregiver will have as great a concern for what the mental and behavioral consequences of the syndrome will be. This is particularly true in a dementia, where problems have already been noted by the patient and family for memory function. The psychological tests can offer information more directly related to these problems and establish expectations of behavioral changes in personality. Periodic retesting may be required or useful in identifying and understanding the continuing changes in behavior.

Finally, the results of psychological testing may be the basis for specifying how the patient and caregiver may deal with problems more effectively. Admittedly, this has been the least successful of the applications of psychological assessments in dementia, but interventions are increasingly noted and included for possible use by those affected (see, e.g., Gruetzner, 1988, pp. 70–139). When the patient and, especially, the caregiver consider the future, they must be concerned with what *may* happen. As time goes on and problems become more frequent and severe, anxiety and worry by the caregiver and patient increase. The burdens experienced by caregivers (see Zarit, Orr, & Zarit, 1985) may become overwhelming, with dwindling resources physically and mentally, leading to a desperation that will not permit capable behavior. Such outcomes, more the rule than the exception, reinforce the need for education, intervention, and support. Particular deficits as well as remaining strengths for the patient may be identified through the testing done. This information, in turn, may suggest interventions to be tried by the caregiver so that the patient will continue to behave as capably as possible. Where the caregiver recognizes the ways the patient may still be competent and is provided with the means to sustain such competence, there may be some relief in the severity of burdens experienced by the caregiver.

Wolfe (1987) has made the same points as sufficient reason to warrant the use of neuropsychological evaluation in association with a neurological evaluation. He proposes that the testing may offer information related to current strengths and weaknesses possessed by the patient. These may lead to planning interventions and estimating possibilities for reversibility. Finally, he concludes that the data may help in the evaluation of the types of support needed and how they may be offered.

la Rue (1986) has described the purpose of neuropsychological evaluation to be determining the type and degree of cognitive problems. There may be included an assessment of emotional disturbance. The procedure should be used only for cases where the deficits will not interfere with reliable and valid measurement. In the most severe cases, testing may even be pointless. Because the measures are to complement neurological examination, they should be reserved to cases where there are still unanswered questions. There are the psychometric issues as well—appropriate age norms for the cases to be tested, time available for testing, and indication of global impairment. Often, a battery of examinations will be used that will include personality variables as well.

Obviously, there are serious difficulties if all the issues which la Rue mentions are to be met. Because an all-purpose, brief, and interesting test has not been developed, there must be compromise. Psychological instruments generally attempt to measure whatever they measure as comprehensively as possible in the least amount of time necessary. However, if a device intended to assess focal brain damage plus a measure of general intelligence plus some scale of personality plus an interview makes up the battery, the total will take several hours. Each test may be appropriate for a particular goal, and each may take only an hour or so to administer. However, the quantity of testing means either dividing the procedure over 2 or more days or taking a chance that the results on later measures may be biased by fatigue and emotional factors. The trade-off may be decided by factors not pertinent to the purpose for which the assessment was intended. In more cases than not, what happens is a selection of a limited number of tests (even only one measure) that appears to be the most pertinent and necessary. Conclusions are limited when this happens, and there may be a danger of inaccuracy due to some relevant data not being collected.

In some instances, of course, a patient may be institutionalized for a sufficient period of time to assure that the most appropriate battery is administered under controlled conditions. For example, a probate court judge may order a 96-hour (4-day) hospitalization, if state law permits. In such a case, medical and psychological evaluations will assist the judge in deciding what is in the best interest for an individual. However, most cases do not reach such legal levels. Decision making (about such matters as institutional placement or support services) becomes the responsibility of the caregiver, based, in part, upon the information provided by the physician and psychologist. Experience shows that many caregivers are not prepared for the intricacies involved insofar as present assessment/diagnostic procedures are concerned.

COMMONLY USED MEASURES

There are two types of tests that are available and more commonly used in the diagnostic setting. *Neuropsychological measures* were devised to evaluate and identify causes for behavior using inferences from test performance. These "causes" will be located in regions or areas of the brain, particularly in the cerebral cortex. The most popular of these examinations are the Halstead–Reitan Neuropsychological Battery and the Luria–Nebraska Neuropsychological Battery. Both have been in use for at least 20 years, and both are believed by psychologists to be suitable for inferring the presence and locus of brain damage. *Psychometric measures* also attempt to demonstrate changes (losses) through indirect measurement but not in terms of a particular location in the brain. Several are screenings for mental incompetence and are brief, easy to administer and interpret. Examples of these are the Mental Status Questionnaire (MSQ) (Kahn, Goldfarb, Pollack, & Peck, 1960) and the Mini-Mental State Examination (MMSE) (Folstein, Folstein, &

McHugh, 1975) that are the most commonly used and the most widely accepted. The Wechsler Adult Intelligence Scale–Revised (WAIS–R) and its immediate predecessor (the WAIS) have been popular for 35 years as an indicator of general intellectual level, but also have been used for identifying specific abilities that may reflect particular diagnostic categories. Wechsler also developed a memory scale (the Wechsler Memory Scale) that was popular and has now been revised (Wechsler Memory Scale–Revised). This test offers, in its current form, information about several types of memory functions. The Bender Gestalt Visual Motor Integration Test (simply called the Bender or Bender Gestalt) has been available for almost 50 years. It has been used as a screening device for a number of disorders, including dementia. Though others could be cited, one can see that the variety may be confusing even to professionals who must make a choice—which one for which purpose. The basis for the selection of tests should be objective, research-based, and appropriate to the specific questions that must be addressed for any given client. However, clinicians often have "favorites" that in some cases may be difficult to defend.

The success rate (in terms of correct diagnosis) depends on several factors beyond the test measures themselves. The psychologist must use caution not to overinterpret or overgeneralize. For example, Edgar Miller (1983), a major contributor to our knowledge about dementia, has criticized a specific logic used by some investigators. In interpreting neuropsychological tests, it may be tempting to assume that if damage to a particular brain structure has already been shown to be related to a particular behavior on the test itself, one may assume that the patient definitely has a lesion in that locus if that test behavior is demonstrated. Although the connection may be correct, there are other possible explanations that must be investigated and disproven first, or there must be some physical evidence that the lesion does in fact exist.

Postmortem confirmation of psychometric prediction has been reported by Hagberg and Gustafson (1985) for 58 persons diagnosed as AD, Pick's, other dementias with degeneration in frontal and temporal lobes, and multiinfarct dementia. At death, the subjects were 62 to 79 years old. The authors had quantitative evidence for vocabulary, ability to attend, block design performance, verbal and spatial memory, and aphasia. They also analyzed behavior and personality to determine their adequacy. The autopsies identified the cases with correct diagnoses, and comparisons were made on both quantitative and qualitative results. They report differences in cognitive profiles, behavior qualities, and psychiatric ratings that were consistent with a diagnosis of AD, MID, or frontal-temporal lobe brain degeneration.

This survey of research indicates some positive evidence for using psychological testing as part of the diagnostic process. The assumptions that the test results are relatively accurate indications of brain damage have some support from findings. However, there need to be more studies to assure reliability of the findings and to distinguish the relationships between test performance and behaviors resulting from the dementing process more clearly.

PSYCHOLOGICAL TESTS AND DEMENTIA

The utility of test data is dependent on the quality of the measure used and the competence of the test administrator. There are two components that must be considered when selecting a measure to suit the task. First, the score(s) obtained for the individual must show *consistency* (called "reliability" in the measurement field). If a person takes a test at one time, a retest at a later time should yield the same score, *unless there has been a change in the person.* For the kinds of measures used with dementia patients, the only expected change will be further deterioration. But most reliability estimates are made with relatively brief periods of time between measures, so that much change would not be anticipated. Unless there is consistency, the test score is meaningful only for that moment in time when it is taken. Normally, we are not much interested in time-limited test scores.

Franzen (1989, p. 13) has pointed out that interpretation with neuropsychological batteries frequently is based on performance by items, not total score. As a result, the use of these tests would be more warranted if item-response reliability were reported. The position seems reasonable as well with psychometric devices. Unfortunately, item-reliability data are not available for the psychologist to use in making a decision about the individual. Reliability for the total test may be computed in several ways, though the principal ones used are called the split-half method and test–retest method. Franzen (1989, pp. 25–27) discusses the effect of the particular type of reliability estimate as an issue to consider in evaluating results as well. In estimating reliability by the split-half method, a test is divided into two parts (say, odd-numbered and even-numbered items), and each person's performance on each half is computed with a correlation coefficient. Because the test has been halved, there are formulas to correct for attenuation, that is, to estimate what the coefficient would be for the 50-item test. The latter type (test–retest) is more rigorous and is more often computed and reported for tests used with dementia patients. In this case, the test is administered to the same persons at two different times. The correlation coefficient is then computed to reflect the stability of performance. In every instance, the sample used to estimate the reliability must be representative of the target population on whom the test will be used. For example, the WAIS–R Manual reports reliability estimates for age groups. The adults used for the purpose were chosen to be representative of all adults in the United States. However, there were no dementia patients included in this procedure. The reliability coefficients, then, may or may not be accurate when the test results are interpreted for a person with dementia. There may be *less* consistency in the scores of demented persons than in other adults. The conclusions drawn from the test performance may be less valid as a result. (It is true, of course, that the results are used to compare the performance of the patient with that of the normal adult population in order to draw conclusions about the current competency level of the person. For this reason, there is less concern about the reliability of the test for dementia patients.)

If there is evidence of consistency, then one must be concerned about the second component. *Validity* is essential to the appropriate use of any scores obtained on the individual. Validity addresses whether the test measures whatever it is assumed to measure. Unless this quality is present, the test scores cannot be used to make relevant or accurate decisions and prediction about the person. In neuropsychological assessment, validity would be demonstrated either by the evidence that the test score differentiates between those with brain impairment and those without or by independent data from autopsy or medical procedures (such as a brain scan) that definitively demonstrate the lesion predicted by battery performance (Franzen, 1989, pp. 29–30). Given the ways that test results are used, the validity of the *inferences* made from scores is more pertinent than the validity of the test itself (Franzen, 1989, p. 35).

Unless there is reliability, it is not possible to have validity. Obtaining adequate evidence of reliability does not assure that the scores will be valid. Interdependent, yes, but the two components are not equivalent. Psychologists select tests for which data are available on both dimensions. Not only will such evidence be gathered as a part of norming and standardizing the test, but ongoing research that confirms or refutes the presence of one or both is (or should be) continuously published. Though this text will not include data on reliability and validity of the measures described, sources that do so will be cited.

TABLE 5.1.

Subtests of the Halstead–Reitan Neuropsychological Battery

Original subtests (1947):

1. Category Test
2. Tactual Performance Test (modified from the Seguin–
   Goddard Form Board)
3. Rhythm Test (originally in Seashore Measures of Musical
   Talent)
4. Speech Sounds Perception Test
5. Finger Oscillation Test (Finger Tapping Test)
6. Critical Flicker Fusion Test
7. Time Sense Test

Research had yielded data that indicate that Subtests 6 and 7
have low reliability for differentiating neurologically impaired
from unimpaired persons. Today, Subtests 1 through 5 comprise
the battery, yielding seven scores. The Tactual Performance Test
is scored for Total Time, Memory, and Location. These scores
are used to calculate an Impairment Index.

Usually, the battery is supported by results on other tests,
particularly the WAIS-R, Minnesota Multiphasic Personality
Inventory, the Trail Making Test, and a measure of aphasia and
sensory-perceptual acuity.

Source. Franzen & Robbins, 1989, p. 91.

The Halstead–Reitan Neuropsychological Battery

Acceptance of the Halstead–Reitan is widespread because it is used
to assess brain dysfunction. Originally there were seven subtests (see
Table 5.1) that were selected because they appeared to discriminate between patients who had lesions in the frontal lobe from those who had
lesions in other areas of the brain. They also seemed appropriate to
distinguish patients who had no brain lesion. From the combination of
scores, an Impairment Index was derived. This index was used to make
clinical judgments, but Franzen and Robbins (1989, p. 92) note that diagnosis about the presence or absence of brain lesions is more accurate
when additional data are included with the Impairment Index.

Currently, there are two "abbreviated" forms (see Table 5.2) that
seem useful and require less testing time (Berg, Franzen, & Wedding,
1987, p. 170). The content differs considerably from the original measure,
with substitution of several subtests. One gain is that the time needed
for administration is about 1 hour. Version II is shorter and requires less
than an hour for administration. So long as reliability and validity are

TABLE 5.2.
Abbreviated Forms of the Halstead–Reitan
Neuropsychological Battery

Abbreviated Halstead–Reitan Screening Battery, Version 1
The tests included are
1. Trail Making Test
2. Aphasia Screening Test
3. Seashore Rhythm Test
4. Speech Sounds Perception Test
5. Stroop Color and Word Test
6. Wechsler Adult Intelligence Test–Revised
a. Block Design
b. Digit Symbol
c. Similarities
d. Object Assembly
Abbreviated Halstead–Reitan Screening Battery, Version 2
The tests included are
1. Trail Making Test
2. Aphasia Screening Test
3. Wechsler Adult Intelligence Test–Revised
a. Block Design
b. Digit Symbol

Source. Berg, Franzen, & Wedding, 1987, pp. 171 and 174.

not significantly reduced, the shorter forms are preferable because they require less involvement by the patient. Whichever form is used, the test must be judged on its capability to demonstrate mental impairment due to cerebral dysfunction. Despite the popularity of the Halstead–Reitan Battery, Franzen and Robbins (1989, p. 107) point out that much research still is needed because reliability and validity evidence is sparse. Cost (the Adult Battery costs $1675.95 currently) and the lack of trained neuropsychologists limit the availability and utility of the test.

The Luria-Nebraska Battery

This test is based partially on a model of the way the brain operates. Intended to furnish a comprehensive neuropsychological assessment, the theory of Alexandr Luria, a Russian neurologist, has been adapted to a psychometric approach (Franzen, 1989, p. 109) by the test authors (Golden, Hammeke, & Purisch, 1985). Luria believed that, although specific areas of the brain control certain behaviors, complex mental activity involves several areas of brain tissue working in harmony. If part of the system fails, the entire system will fail. For example, the ability of the person to recall the verbal label for a common object is not an isolated function in this view. There must be visual recognition of the object, a search for the appropriate label from memory storage, perhaps an awareness of function and use for the object, and the ability to express the label itself verbally, at a minimum. In this chain of mental events, there may be a loss in the search mechanism due to cellular degeneration from a disease like Alzheimer's. The result would be that the individual will be unable to supply the correct label, though other components still function. (The current study of semantic memory focuses on this issue from a somewhat different point of view, as we will see later in the chapter).

The evaluation procedure is intended to find which complex functions have been affected (Fogel & Faust, 1987, p. 70). The Luria–Nebraska is an attempt to utilize this model with a series of 11 scales (see Table 5.3), including motor functions, visual processes, speech competence, educational achievement areas, and intellectual abilities (Franzen, 1989, p.109). Interpretation is complex and may involve several levels (see Table 5.4). The necessary skills and experience needed for the complex task are not often found, even in the limited number of neuropsychologists in this country today (Berg, Franzen & Wedding, 1987, pp. 162–163). In addition, training is not as accessible as is needed. (This criticism they apply to the Halstead–Reitan as well.) Initial costs of the Luria–Nebraska

TABLE 5.3.
Scales in the Luria–Nebraska
Neuropsychological Battery

Form 1 Subscales
1. Motor
2. Tactile
3. Rhythm
4. Visual Processes
5. Receptive Speech
6. Expressive Speech
7. Reading
8. Writing
9. Arithmetic
10. Memory
11. Intellectual Processes

Form II Subscales
The above 11 plus 12. Intermediate Memory
Scale

Source. Franzen, 1989, p. 109.

TABLE 5.4.
Levels of Interpretation of the Luria–Nebraska Neuropsychological Battery

Level	Procedure
1	Using a calculated "critical level" (the score that is the cutoff for impaired performance), find those scales exceeding it.
2	Examine the scatter among scale scores.
3	Compare the "critical level" score to scales for which empirically determined items discriminate persons who have localized deficits.
	Compare the "critical level" score to factors derived by factor-analytic techniques for each scale.
4	Analyze performance on items across scales to locate "patterns" that are consistent with neuropsychological theory about relationships between brain damage and consequent behavior.
5	Examine the quality of the performance by the individual.

Adapted from Franzen, 1989, pp. 111–112.

are about one-third that of the Halstead–Reitan (currently, the test materials and scoring forms cost $365.00).

The decision about utility requires experimental evidence gathered in systematic research. Both of these neuropsychological batteries have been studied under such conditions. Gray, Rattan, and Dean (1986) assessed the ability of the Halstead–Reitan to discriminate between diagnosed groups with dementia, clinical depression, and general neurological impairments. Although this approach satisfies one of the criteria for validity previously cited, the study suffers by lack of a control group. The results for the sample used (N = 80 elderly) clearly distinguished the depressives from the other two groups in terms of score levels, with the depressed sample showing superior performance on most subtests. However, the dementia and neurologically impaired subgroups did not differ on any of the subtests of the Halstead–Reitan. Using neuropsychological variables only, Gray et al. performed a stepwise discriminant analysis for the combined neurologically impaired subgroups and found more significant differentiation from depression. To differentiate psychiatric disorders from organic ones is essential. Reliable discrimination between types of organicity, when related to specific areas of the brain, would be a more supportive finding.

Other studies have combined results on additional tests with the Halstead–Reitan. Alekoumbides, Charter, Adkins, and Seacat (1987), for example, used part of the neuropsychological battery with the WAIS and the Wechsler Memory Scale. One part of the sample consisted of 118 persons (age range 19 to 82) without cerebral lesions. The other

(N = 117) had diffuse or focal lesions, with or without dementia or Korsakoff's. The authors were able to construct tables that helped specify the effects of the kinds of lesions (diffuse or focal) on scores of the tests, including a composite of the subtests taken from the Halstead–Reitan.

In 1988, Charter and Alekoumbides published a follow-up. They had developed an abbreviated version of the scales used in the 1987 study, thereby reducing time for administration but yielding even greater ability to discriminate for diffuse cerebral lesions. The large number of subjects used in the two studies, over 300 persons, makes the results more impressive and suggest that further research in application of the tables is warranted and may indicate the utility of the procedure.

The Halstead–Reitan also is the basis for a retraining program where brain dysfunction has occurred. If the brain is plastic enough (that is, if healthy cells are able to assume functions normally associated with damaged ones) and if damage is not too diffuse, it should be possible for certain areas of the brain to assume functions lost by destruction in other areas, at least partially. The program (called REHABIT) accepts the premise that the Halstead–Reitan measures relationships between the brain and behavior and that retraining is achievable. Brodsky, Brodsky, Lee, and Sever (1986) evaluated this "Brain Impairment Training" with two studies.

The program has five separate but overlapping tracks. Verbal skills and concepts are represented on several tracks, whereas visual–spatial abilities appear on others. Of 26 subjects in the two studies, 23 showed improvement that the authors categorize as mild to "startling." The time taken in the program ranged from 2.5 months to 13 months. The age range of participants for the two studies was from 5 to 56, but the number of "older" persons was limited. As is to be expected, the younger the individual the greater the improvement, an outcome consistent with brain plasticity. The nature of the brain damage of subjects in the study did not conform with syndromes that lead to dementia, however, so the results must be viewed as very limited in terms of the scope of this book.

There have been studies published to test the discriminative value of the Luria–Nebraska also. McCue, Goldstein, and Shelly (1989) used 79 persons between the ages of 60 and 85 years. Of these, some 34 had been designated as "probable" Alzheimer's disease with the other 45 diagnosed as suffering a major depression. The authors report that the Luria–Nebraska distinguished the two clinical groups accurately. As mentioned with the Halstead–Reitan, discriminating between a psychiatric disorder and an organic one is merely a minimum level of achievement for a neuropsychological battery.

The model of Alexandr Luria, as mentioned earlier, underlies the development of the Luria–Nebraska, but the battery is not restricted to that model. A study done in Finland used the Luria Neuropsychological Test Battery (not the Luria–Nebraska) to attempt to discriminate between presenile dementia and senile dementia of the Alzheimer's type. There were 36 patients classified as presenile and 35 who were SDAT. The authors (Sulkava & Amberla, 1982) report that deterioration in memory, intellectual functions, higher visual and motor functions, and orientation was present in both groups. As the disease progressed, the resulting deterioration proceeded gradually. There seemed, then, to be a continuum preserved that indicates that the process is the same regardless of time of life when diagnosis occurs. It is surprising that these authors report that progression was more rapid in *senile* patients, a finding that runs counter to most reports in this country. Perhaps, then, the original Luria battery measures effects in a somewhat different way than the test developed and standardized in this country.

The evidence of reliability and validity of both the Halstead–Reitan and the Luria–Nebraska is more limited in quantity than one would like. Franzen (1989) reviews the literature for both tests extant before the time of publication of his book. Although both tests have proved popular with neuropsychologists, there is little evidence that the popularity is deserved. Until such time as some concerted effort is made to evaluate more rigorously, there will continue to be a certain amount of "faith" that has not been proven to be warranted. Franzen (1989) believes the available literature is supportive for clinical use of the instruments, but he does point out the need for further research efforts (p. 107, pp. 117–118, and p. 120).

The psychometric instruments that have been most popular have a considerable literature about their reliability and some studies reporting on their validity. At the same time, however, the focus of the investigations has been selective so that questions remain about the validity of the tests for purposes of discriminating dementia. The Wechsler–Bellevue, WAIS, and WAIS–R have had widespread use in a variety of diagnostic settings. Indeed, Franzen (1989, p. 59) cites the WAIS/WAIS–R as "a nearly ubiquitous instrument in clinical evaluation settings." But he reports that the utility of the test for neuropsychological evaluation is still debated (p. 60).

The Wechsler Scales

The popularity of the scales devised by David Wechsler is deserved in most respects. As a measure of intellectual ability, it has a history that is impressive. First, the content was chosen to the definition that Wechsler proposed as early as 1932 (Edwards, 1974, p. 12).

> Wechsler proposed a definition which considers the global capacity of the individual as the primary element and the effects of intellectual abilities to act purposefully, to think rationally, and to deal effectively with the environment as outgrowth of this global capacity. Given such a definition, one may hypothesize the interaction of a variety of abilities, only a portion of which may be cognitive in nature. Certainly cognitive abilities such as abstract reasoning, ability to learn, ability to adapt, and ability to solve problems are an important component, but the conative and affective traits of the individual also influence behavior.

Using this defense as a basis, Wechsler proposed a measurement technique that has persisted in his subsequent scales.

> The structure of the Bellevue scale, and the subtests which compose it, reflects the essential elements of this definition. The number of subtests included is somewhat less important than the status that each subtest assumes within the structure. . . . *The content of the test is to act as a medium or language by which the individual can express himself. Some individuals do this better verbally, others by responding to commands, others through manipulation of concrete materials, others by assembling things.* Opportunities to demonstrate competence in any or all of these things are available in a test with the structure of the Bellevue and the following Wechsler scales. It is both most feasible and reasonable to maintain such a structure since *global intelligence,* according to Wechsler, *is multilingual just as is the brain.*
>
> The question becomes: Can the psychologist interpret the score in terms of ability to cope with the environment more validly? (Edwards, 1974, pp. 12–13, italics added.)

This question gets to the heart of using the instrument for diagnosis. If, as Franzen has said, the scale is "nearly ubiquitous," is that application justified? Franzen has also touched on that issue (1989, p. 60) when he says that "the utility of the WAIS–R in neuropsychological evaluation is also a matter of debate. The simplest solution would be to use the WAIS–R as an index of academically related intellectual skills without invoking diagnostic interpretation strategies." Wechsler felt that the test yielded information useful for more than computing an intelligence quotient, as important an indicator of ability as such a score might be. But he also believed that going beyond the basic datum must be inferential, until proven, and that care in generating these inferences must be exercised (Edwards, 1974, pp. 13–16). The scales have stood as the criterion against which other measures of adult intelligence are judged. The care given to norming and standardization justify that reputation but should not mean that whatever is done with the test is automatically correct. Research should indicate the validity of diagnosis beyond that intended by the test author. There are a considerable number of studies, some of which are pertinent to the issue as it applies to dementia.

At the heart of the matter is the meaning of scores obtained on patients who have presented symptoms of dementia. What were they like *before* the condition began to express itself? Have scores been lowered by the disease process and, if so, how much? In virtually every case, there will be no test data available prior to the complaint. One may depend on the patient and/or caregiver to supply information upon which to base an estimate, but the error implicit in such a procedure may be very large. Alternatively, one may assume that the patient was of "normal" or even "above normal" ability, but this could mean exaggerating the amount of change due to the dementia. What may be more reliable is to test "abilities" that are not adversely influenced by dementia and compare those with "abilities" that are. Wechsler advocated such a procedure with certain subtests on his scales. He felt there would be little decline on certain subtests (called "hold" tests), greater decline on others (called "don't hold" tests), depending on the content and the mental activity involved. By comparing the two, some estimate of intellectual loss could be made (Levi, Oppenheim, & Wechsler, 1945).

Yet the central idea is still accepted, that is, some abilities are more influenced by the dementia itself than others. Comparison of the two might allow a better estimate of intellectual decline than less controlled approaches. Crawford (1989) has proposed that "premorbid intelligence" is most accurately estimated when an oral reading test is used. The words should be suitable for adults, reflect previous familiarity with them, yet make only minimal demands on current cognitive capacity. Such a test is available (called the *National Adult Reading Test*, developed by Nelson; see Nelson and O'Connell, 1978). Crawford describes the use of the test in terms of its relation to the WAIS IQ in order to estimate premorbid intellectual level. Continued research efforts should help justify the claim or disclose its shortcomings.

Without attempting to determine the intellectual level of the individual prior to the morbid state, other researchers have looked at the language skills most severely deteriorated as a result of a dementia. This topic will be considered in greater detail later in this chapter.

Still other research has continued to add to our understanding of the use of the Wechsler Scales in differentiating sources of dementia. Loring and Largen (1985) present the position that Alzheimer's disease and senile dementia of the Alzheimer's type differ in more than just the age level[2] at which they occur. They argue that behavior differs clinically between the groups, even though the neuronal changes are the same. To test their position, they compared two groups, one called presenile dementia (N = 13) and one, senile dementia (N = 24). They also included age-matched controls (N = 40). The presenile sample had a mean age of 60, whereas the seniles averaged 72.5 years. All were noninstitutionalized and of mild or moderate degree of dementia.

In addition to the WAIS, several other test measures were included. Unfortunately, for 21 of the patients and 19 of the controls, a short form of the WAIS was used to estimate intelligence (the Satz–Mogel Short Form; see Satz and Mogel, 1962). The results for the WAIS disclosed significant differences between groups on three subtests (Digit Span, Digit Symbol, and Picture Arrangement). On the Digit Span subtest, only Digits Backward discriminated AD and SDAT groups. For these three tests, the *presenile* subjects performed less well. For the other measures included, there were also some statistically significant differences. They state that "patients who develop a degenerative dementia with earlier onset tend to perform significantly more poorly on tests of intelligence, eye-hand coordination and speed, concentration, and embedded figural perception when controlled for normal age differences" (p. 355). The differences could not be explained on the basis of educational level. Their findings need further support, the authors state, but they do advocate continuation of the bifurcation of dementia into presenile and senile variants.

Comparison of WAIS results for different types of dementia was studied by Loring, Meador, Mahurin, and Largen (1986). They used 12 SDAT patients and compared them to 12 multiinfarct patients and 12 controls. Again, age and educational level were matched. Although significant differences were found for Full Scale and Verbal IQ, and for the Picture Completion subtest of the Performance Scale, other differences were not disclosed. They conclude that neuropsychological testing using the WAIS does not discriminate between similar types of dementias. Instead, measures like the WAIS should be used to make inferences about the person's ability to function in an independent way in the environment. These two studies indicate the limited nature of a test designed to serve one purpose when employed to serve another.

The use of "hold" and "don't hold" subtests advocated by Wechsler (Levi et al., 1945) has been reassessed by Larrabee, Largen, and Levin (1985). They found that the two categories did discriminate between normals (N = 25) and dementia of the Alzheimer's type (DAT) patients (N = 25) who were matched on age, education, and sex. Data from performance on Wechsler Memory Scale subtests suggested that they may be used to help make an initial diagnosis, whereas severity of dementia was disclosed better by Information and Digit Symbol subtest results.

The use of the WAIS to distinguish Alzheimer's from MID has been studied by Satz, Van Gorp, Soper, and Mitrushina (1987) as well. Their sample consisted of 149 volunteers in an ongoing study of aging, all between 60 and 94 years of age. In 18 of their cases, they found a subtest pattern that had been reported as more typical of DAT than MID. Given the fact that no members of the sample had shown signs of dementia, the possibility exists that the pattern may have utility as a "marker"—a potential predictor of future development of behaviors resulting from Alzheimer's. They make a case for some restricted situations where, in fact, the pattern may have application. Again, within strict limits, the WAIS may have its place in differential diagnosis.

A study comparing SDAT at a mild level with major depression and a normal group using the WAIS Digit Symbol subtest (Hart, Kwentus, Wade, & Hamer, 1987) did not find differences in psychomotor speed (a trait involved in performance on Digit Symbol) between the clinical groups. However, both groups differed significantly from the controls on raw score (digits correctly matched by symbols within a 90-second time period) and in total time to complete the task. Immediately after completing the total test, each subject was given a copy of the numbers with empty spaces in which they were to insert the appropriate symbol (called an "incidental memory" task). Depressed patients differed from controls on pairs correctly matched but not on ability to recall the symbols whether or not matched correctly. DAT patients differed significantly from depressed and controls on both measures of incidental memory. Hart et al. concluded that incidental memory may differentiate major depression from DAT. "Our findings suggest that the standard administration of the Digit Symbol test has limited potential for distinguishing patients with early DAT from those with depressive pseudodementia. The addition of a brief measure of incidental memory may be clinically useful as part of a comprehensive evaluation." (p. 238).

Schwarb, Koberle, and Spiegel (1988) compared results on an Alzheimer's disease assessment scale designed to differentiate normal elderly from demented ones. Of their 94 subjects, 7 were classified as "clearly or possibly demented" by the procedure, whereas the remaining 87 were considered normal. The correlation coefficient between the assessment scale and WAIS scores obtained earlier was significant. The scale also correlated significantly with the Mini-Mental State Examination. Insofar as both the WAIS and Mini-Mental State are effective identifiers of dementia, the scale might be considered as relatively valid.

In 1984, Fuld published a study that has had a major impact on the use of the WAIS as a diagnostic instrument for dementia. Her premise was that the cholinergic neurotransmitter deficit that is a part of DAT would produce a unique subtest pattern on the WAIS. Further, she hypothesized that this pattern would not be found in dementias resulting from causes other than Alzheimer's disease. She conducted three studies involving young normal subjects (N = 19, age range 19–25) and older persons (N = 77, age range 36–83) who had been referred for neurologic examination. The WAIS was included as a routine part of the neurologic procedure.

One hour prior to testing the normal subjects with the WAIS, she administered scopolamine, a drug that acts as an *anti*cholinergic, thereby reducing the amount of neurotransmitter available for synaptic transmission. Of the 19 normals, 10 of them showed the predicted profile on WAIS performance as compared with 4 of the 22 controls. For those with the "predicted profile," the pattern only needed to be present without regard to magnitude. For the controls, in fact, there were very small differences among pair scores that make up the pattern. Fuld accepted the position that the test profile is associated with cholinergic neurotransmitter dysfunction (Fisher Exact Probability = .0014). She reported also that Performance Scale IQs which are 15 or more points lower than the Verbal Scale IQs are associated with cholinergic dysfunction, based upon similar comparisons to those applied to the subtest scores.

Next, Fuld used the psychometric test procedure with a sample of 61 persons (age range 38–81). From these, she obtained 30 usable WAIS protocols. Of these, 12 had a diagnosis of DAT, 3 of probable DAT, 7 of MID, and 8 with "other" dementias (such as Parkinson's or Korsakoff's). She compared the 15 patients with DAT or probable DAT to the 15 non-DAT for the proposed WAIS pattern, finding 9 in the DAT group who met the criteria to some degree. Only 1 of the 15 non-DAT group did so, yielding a Fisher Exact Probability Test value at the .001 level. Using only those who met DAT criteria (N = 12), 8 had the expected profile. She concluded that the WAIS profile more often is associated with DAT than with other dementias. Direct comparison of this group with the MID group yielded an 8:1 proportion for the profile.

A final study was done for "cross-validation" purposes. She obtained 47 usable protocols, broken down as 21 DAT, 8 probable DAT, 6 mixed cases (DAT *and* MID), 5 MID, and 7 "other" dementias. As before, there were more patients in the DAT and mixed groups (13 of 35) who showed the test profile than in the "other" category (0 of 12). However, the Performance IQ minus Verbal IQ difference of at least 15 points was not found in this study. Fuld proposed that the test profile is the more sensitive and specific discriminant.

She reports that the results indicate that test performance is "relatively preserved" on Vocabulary, Similarities, and Digit Span and "relatively impaired" on Block Design and Digit Symbol—but only for DAT patients. Further, she concluded that there was evidence that cholinergic deficiency found in Alzheimer's patients *may be* the agent responsible for the intellectual changes resulting from the syndrome. Caution must be exercised because the "numbers" reported are far from maximum in either group. There must also be some care taken in presuming the relationship between neurotransmitter deficit and the intellectual decline. Indeed, as cited, one does not know how much "decline" there has been as premorbid intelligence is not known. Despite these concerns, the results are a breakthrough with considerable promise. As a result, several studies have been conducted since Fuld's publication to evaluate the outcomes she reported.

To test the validity of the subtest pattern in distinguishing different causes of dementia, Brinkman and Braun (1984) used a sample of 62 persons, ages 37 through 86 years. Each had received a diagnosis of DAT or MID based upon medical criteria. Of the 23 subjects classified as AD, 13 (57%) were identified correctly by the test pattern on the WAIS. What is more impressive is that 37 of the 39 MID patients (95%) were classified as non-AD in pattern. The Wechsler deterioration quotient (hold–don't hold comparisons), which these authors point out is similar to the Fuld formula, showed a number of false positives (i.e., classified MID patients as AD instead). Further, there was no bias introduced by differences in age, sex, or degree of deterioration. With such positive results, Brinkman and Braun encourage continuation of research efforts.

Heinrichs and Celinski (1987) assessed the power of the subtest pattern with patients who had suffered head trauma. There were 50 males in the sample, with a mean age of 41 years. Only 5 were classified as AD, indicating the proper exclusion occurred in 90% of the cases. The authors point out that this compares favorably with the classification of MID patients when Fuld applied the pattern in her study and supports Fuld's conclusion about a unique test pattern in DAT.

Even normally aging adults have been compared to see if the profile discriminates accurately. Tuokko and Crockett (1987) tested 74 healthy older persons (age range 50 to 90 years) and applied the pattern. Again, the results confirmed the position of Fuld.

To date, then, there have been some encouraging results from research on the power of the Fuld formula. By no means can a strong position be taken with these results, however. There are differences in findings at the same time that the pattern misses a significant number of those *medically* identified as DAT. There is not yet definitive research to indicate the validity of the basic premise of Fuld—the lack of acetylcholine as the principal cause of a loss of mental competence as reflected in WAIS performance. This would not be a problem because research will continue and help delimit the questions remaining, if the test pattern is accepted as a possibility that needs further exploration. Unfortunately, practitioners feel a strong need for tools to assist in decision making, and it does appear that the formula is being used as a basis for psychological decisions. Caution needs to be exercised in these directions.

The research surveyed here is only a fraction of that available on the WAIS and WAIS–R and their appropriate place in testing the demented patient. Yet the sample is sufficient to indicate that results can be useful, particularly if applied judiciously and in concert with other data, both psychological and medical. Given the reputation of the instrument, one may expect continued dependence on WAIS/WAIS–R performance as an integral part of the decision-making process.

The Bender Motor Gestalt Test

The first reference to the Bender Gestalt was in 1938 when the author, Lauretta Bender, published a description of the instrument and its clinical use. In 1946, the test was made available. By that time, it had been used in clinical settings that included World War II so that a considerable body of research was extant. Bender (1946, p. 3) felt the evidence already confirmed its clinical utility to diagnose mental deficiency, aphasias, organic brain disorders, major psychoses, malingering (particularly as it would be observed in armed forces personnel under war conditions), and the psychoneuroses. Indeed, the test promised much—the question became, "What does it deliver?"

Bender (1946) defined "gestalt function" as "that function of the integrated organism whereby it responds to a given constellation of stimuli as a whole, the response itself being a constellation or pattern or gestalt" (p. 3). The procedure is to present a series of cards, each with a pattern that the subject must draw on a piece of blank $8\frac{1}{2}$ in. by 11 in. paper. The drawing is evaluated for accuracy as well as the degree or level of integration. Since its introduction, it has been widely used and highly researched. As Groth-Marnat (1990, p. 158) has pointed out, it is one of the five most frequently used tests by psychologists despite poor reviews and ambiguous research findings. In more recent years, it has been employed (usually with other measures) in diagnosing dementia.

Proponents of the Bender Gestalt would point to the position that it is "organicity" that reveals itself in performance on the test. The term usually means some set of behaviors that is allowed if the brain has integrity. Franzen (1989, pp. 241–242) has described the problems involved with demonstrating the validity of this instrument for such a purpose. However, the tacit acceptance of this integrity hypothesis remains active in the use of the instrument. Indeed, there are various scoring methods and modifications intended to improve the capabilities of the test to perform its functions. Delaney (1982) evaluated one such procedure and found it lacking in some respects. In this study, he employed an adaptation proposed by Canter that called for standard administration of the Bender followed by readministration with the drawings to be made on paper that had curved and intersecting lines as background interference. Canter and others who have used this technique believe that the testing adaptation is helpful in screening for organicity. Delaney used the procedure with epileptics, certainly a group for whom interference in organic integrity exists. The results were insignificant when the comparison was made with control subjects. Delaney proposes that, as promising as the Canter modification appears to be, it is useful only with significant cerebral disorders such as stroke, or acute and chronic brain disorders. Persons with seizures would be missed (false negatives) in the screening and thus judged to have brain integrity. Advocating caution from such results, Delaney proposes that various assessment procedures be employed "based upon the background, referral, and best clinical judgment in each case" (p. 846). Again, there is evidence that psychological evaluation and prediction is not yet precise enough to depend upon a limited set of measures.

It is not easy to explain the great popularity of the Bender Gestalt. Certainly, as Groth-Marnat (1990, p. 155) has pointed out, "it is brief, economical, flexible, nonthreatening, nonverbal, and extensively researched." Considering the seriousness of decisions affecting the person being tested, the last of these should be the major criterion. Unfortunately, the results of studies have not been kind to the employment of the test. Practitioners should be required to justify their choice of the Bender on more legitimate grounds than are commonly cited.

The Mini-Mental State Examination (MMSE)

This screening device (the work of Folstein, Folstein, and McHugh, 1975) has been very popular with psychologists because it offers evidence about orientation in time and space, short-term memory, mental skills like calculation, and language function. Yet only 30 items are used to reflect these five abilities that are so frequently affected in a dementia. Orientation questions about time and place, for example, might include asking the person to name the street on which the psychologist's building is located. (This is not one of the questions actually used.) The ability to recall such items is a reflection of the awareness of the individual about relationships with the environment.

A second area requires the patient to retain the labels of three concrete objects common to the environment but not related to each other. This task measures short-term memory, the ability to hold in storage a few items for almost immediate use. In the absence of such ability, the person will not be able to function capably with environmental demands. A third area of questioning requires the individual to count backwards, say from 50 by 3s (50, 47, 44, etc.). This is a somewhat more demanding task both of memory and of arithmetical skills, and concentration is required. It is not unusual that this will prove too difficult for the dementia patient who has progressed beyond the mild state. Since some persons will find this task a threat that is too stressful, an alternate may be used: spelling a word backwards. This alternate samples the same skills.

Storage of information is next checked by asking the patient to repeat the three labels recited a few moments before. Because the individual was not instructed to remember them, this task points to the level of incidental learning that may be possible for the person. Finally, there are several language tasks, requiring recall of the names of objects, repeating a sentence, following a three-stage command, obeying a written command, writing a sentence, and copying a design. This array of verbal tasks can help pinpoint particular language functions already affected by the disease, so that inferences may be drawn about the competencies remaining to the individual that may be used as a part of staying mentally alert.

Overall, the MMSE is not so much "diagnostic" of a syndrome as it is a screening device that helps locate strengths and limitations of the patient. This issue is more practical than one of specifying the cause of a person's mental problems if the intent is to decide what interventions are appropriate to assist the patient to behave as competently as possible. The popularity, then, is deserved so long as the test permits discrete and accurate identification of competencies. Further, it may assume a more essential role if it permits the charting of activities and involvement that allow the patient to remain as mentally involved with life as the progress of the disease permits. There are no norms for the MMSE in the psychometric sense, nor are they needed, because an ability is judged present or absent by the nature of the response elicited from the person.

Reliability has been less often reported than evidences of validity, as some representative studies show.

Teng, Chui, Schneider, and Metzger (1987) looked at performance on the MMSE by diagnosed Alzheimer's patients in three ways. First, they analyzed performance on the individual items. Second, they examined performance decline in relation to duration of the illness (i.e., since the diagnosis was made, not since the disease process might have started). Third, they compared performance by patients according to the age at the time the diagnosis was made. Their sample consisted of 141 subjects (48 male and 93 female) with DAT. There were no significant differences between the sexes on age, education, age of symptom onset, duration of illness, or test performance itself. Thus the results could be considered for the total sample without regard to sex. The mean age of the group was 73, with a range from 53 to 96 years. The standard procedure for administration was used (see Folstein, Folstein, & McHugh, 1975) except for a few substitutions that Teng et al. felt were equivalent. For the short term memory task for three words, they added cued recall for missed items; if still missed, they allowed recognition by showing alternatives that the patient could point to. This procedure was done not only to assure a measure but to see if aids might be helpful in eliciting labels that could not be recalled under normal conditions. They elected not to use the serial subtraction task and so used only the spelling of a word backwards.

Their results were based on correlations of scores on items with the several dependent variables. They found a significant effect with duration of illness (the longer since diagnosis, the poorer the performance). Duration of illness also correlated significantly with age of onset (the longer the duration, the younger the age at which it was diagnosed). The authors subdivided the sample into those diagnosed prior to age 65 ($N = 51$) and those over age 65 ($N = 90$). There was a fairly regular decline in performance on some items (for example, naming three objects), whereas other items showed a stepwise decline (for example, orientation to time). If such differences are consistently found, the meaning of performance on the MMSE may take on somewhat different implications than for nondemented persons. Nevertheless, performance on all items did show negative correlations with duration of illness (thus the longer since diagnosis the less competent the performance of the patient). Though not true for all items, on most the earlier the onset of the dementia, the poorer the performance. This accords with other findings on "presenile" and "senile" dementia. The authors state that "the finding that only 3% of 141 Alzheimer's patients passed both the 'recall' [delayed recall of three items] and the 'copy a design' items suggests that the combined use of these two items could be useful in screening for Alzheimer's disease" (p. 99). In addition, the "findings suggest that patients with younger age of onset have more severe dysfunction of both cerebral hemispheres" (p. 99). This study offers some evidence on how scores relate to significant variables that are independent of the process, as well as what significance the performance of the individual may have for functioning in life. Such data support the use of the MMSE for these practical questions.

Validity has been assessed by correlations with other measures as well. Rai, Scott, and Beston (1989) administered the MMSE and two automated psychometrics requiring classification and digit recall to a sample of older persons with dementia. One subgroup had been labeled DAT (N = 27); the other, MID (N = 20). The MMSE correlated significantly with both automated tests for both subgroups. The authors observe that the MMSE is an objective measure of the mental capabilities of dementia patients. Nelson, Fogel, and Faust (1986) reviewed the effectiveness of five screening devices, labeling them "bedside tests" because they may be administered in almost any situation. Among these was the MMSE. Interrater and test–retest reliability were found to be satisfactory, and scores corresponded to medical diagnosis of condition (including dementia). The authors do report high false-negative rates (that is, patients would not be judged to have a disorder by one of these tests), particularly for persons with focal lesion in the right hemisphere. In addition, such tests miss some types of deficit that can be influential for differential diagnosis and case management. Given a brief, "bedside" instrument, high false negatives seem more likely. Once again, here is evidence that there is no single, all-purpose test, and decisions should be made upon multiple sources.

The Mental Status Questionnaire

Another screening device that focuses exclusively on orientation in time and space is the Mental Status Questionnaire (MSQ) (Kahn, Goldfarb, Pollack, & Peck, 1960). There are 10 questions, designed to determine if the individual is aware of the place where she or he is, items relating to current time (day of the week, for example), one's own history in time (one's age, for example), and common facts of significance to appreciating time–space relationships (for example, "who is our president?"). This device has been extremely popular also, and Zarit (1980, pp. 141–143) has pointed out that responses may indicate language changes that are relevant to assessment.

> A patient who is asked these mental status questions can give three possible responses. He can answer correctly, suggesting intact brain

functioning. He may respond that he does not know or give a wrong answer, which is often indicative of dementia. Or the person may respond to connative, rather than denotative, aspects of the question. (Zarit, 1980, p. 142)

Although there are only 10 questions and although these questions seem simplistic to a nondemented adult, there is information elicited that far exceeds what might seem possible with the MSQ. The person with an intact brain will have little, if any, difficulty with such questions. As there is loss of competence, the picture changes. Even though language use is still present and may sound appropriate, it is often shallow and re-stricted. One patient, who was unable to answer any of the MSQ ques-tions, made the observation, "You know, it's just like sticking a pin in me. I know these things, and I know I should be able to tell you about them, but I just can't get it out."

The literature most often reports utility and limitations to that utility for the MSQ. Robertson, Rockwood, and Stolee (1982) administered the test to a sample of 49 elderly persons (age range 67–97 years). They report that performance identified moderate and severe impairment in the sample but was not adequate for mild loss as compared with normals. False positives and false negatives were not excessive. They felt that the scoring method used was too restrictive to identify the more subtle signs. In fact, cutoff points suggested by Kahn et al. (1960) are necessarily loose. With only 10 items, no more than a suggestion of degree of severity is possible. Of course, if all items are missed, the loss would seem major, a fact that may be confirmed or denied by the caregiver. Where moderate loss shades into severe and, what is more important, where mild shades into moderate is debatable, not only for the MSQ but for any other diagnostic system. How much loss of competence is only "mild" or "moderate" anyway? Robertson et al. (1982) have offered this as an appropriate criticism, but it is not one that is apt to be corrected.

There are additional questions that the psychologist may use to help in the assessment process with the MSQ. These added items are not part of the scored procedure, however. They sample the awareness of the patient for the immediate relationship between her or him and the examiner. To assure that such information has been provided, the patient must have been informed fully about whom she or he will be seeing and why.

With older persons, there is always the chance that other factors may be the cause of an inability to answer correctly. Kahn et al. (1960) suggest that, if the person makes three or more errors, the psychologist must be sure that there is no hearing loss. Weinstein and Amsel (1986) tested 30 institutionalized dementia patients (age range 58 to 92 years) with the MSQ and also did a complete audiological evaluation. All subjects had been diagnosed as AD. They found that over half their sample had moderate to severe hearing loss. A sample of 30 age-matched controls showed 40% with hearing loss. The MSQ scores correlated with severity of hearing loss and, in some cases, providing amplification improved performance on the MSQ.

There are other factors that may adversely influence performance on the MSQ unless identified and controlled. Among those specifically cited by Kahn et al. are medications (frequently a source of difficulty in functioning of the elderly even when appropriate and needed), the progress of the condition (acute or chronic), educational level, primary language (English or some other), and personality factors (anxiety level, for example). These are not frequent so often that they invalidate the use of the instrument, but the psychologist needs to be sure that what is observed is in fact a valid measure. Of course, such factors must be considered for their effects on performance for other tests as well.

The Wechsler Memory Scale

Memory is a trait of such dominance in our daily activities that we are apt to underestimate its importance. The store of experience we possess allows us to interact with the environment in an increasingly competent manner. The system itself permits augmenting the store as new environmental encounters occur. Redundancy in behavior may even bring responses in the absence of a repetition of a stimulus. Though human intellect is memory plus other things, the ability to assess memory in its unique qualities can be a first significant step to understanding human behavior.

Wechsler (1961) had concluded that memory assumes different emphases at different age periods. Even though there is evidence of the impairment in certain forms of memory with age, he maintained that the elderly person is *more* dependent on it than the younger one (Wechsler, 1961, p. 157). Indeed, mental traits must change with age, he thought (1955), at the same time that the significance of each trait will be altered at different ages. This means that common test materials yielding common responses from different age groups do not necessarily reflect the same psychological parameters. In this view, the meaning of "memory" is as dependent on the criteria used to evaluate the trait as it is on the storage and retrieval system in the brain itself.

The Wechsler Memory Scale (Wechsler & Stone, 1973) was designed to fit the structure of the WAIS. This means that there were several subtests, each allowing the person to demonstrate a type of memory. Though each of these might have meaning for clinical judgments, it was the total score that measured the functional status of the individual. Indeed, this total score was a "Memory Quotient" that had been age-corrected to allow comparisons by rankings. The process of assuming consistency between different measures by summing them, though understandable, may have veiled the potential inherent in subtests of different types of "memory." At the same time, the scale has been popular, at least partly because it conforms to an already-accepted format. Research has not been kind to the instrument insofar as evidence of validity is concerned (Franzen, 1989, p. 179). Its popularity, however, has led to several attempts to improve it.

In 1987, a revision of the scale (Wechsler, 1987) was published. Now there are several scores intended to reflect performance on different types of memory tasks, again in the quotient format equivalent to the WAIS–R. Only as research is conducted and published will it be possible to evaluate the quality of the scale as a measure of memory function and change or in terms of its ability to discriminate memory dysfunction caused by specific syndromes.

There are other, somewhat less popular, psychological tests that are used as part of the diagnostic procedure. The ones surveyed here are certainly the more accepted ones. It is somewhat surprising that there is so little compelling evidence of the validity of these instruments for the decision-making process. The role of clinical intuition and experience becomes important in the consequent judgment. Part of the problem of validity lies in the fact that all such measures are indirect. In the hands of an experienced, competent, and conservative psychologist, the dependence on intuition may be justified. It will assume more acceptance as the decision is made on the basis of additional data from other sources. It is critical, however, that the estimate of mental competence not be confused for a reality. Test scores are subject to error, as shown statistically in reliability and validity estimates. However, even high reliability and validity coefficients are not sufficient. There must be the monitoring from the test setting to the life setting that provides evidence that the judgments made are accurate.

VERBAL MEMORY AND DEMENTIA

There is another approach to the study of outcomes of dementias as they may be related to empirical relationships. Though more experimental, this approach is no less psychological than the clinical one. As an alternative viewpoint, with some potential application to understanding the behavioral effects of dementia, a brief survey seems warranted.

In verbal learning, there has been a considerable study of long-term memory. It is currently believed that there are two kinds of such memories. One is called *semantic* memory, and it is associated with the role of language. With verbal experience, we acquire knowledge about words: what they mean, how they are related to one another, and how they may be used to communicate. This type of memory is felt to be stable so that little forgetting will occur over the course of our lifetimes. The other kind of long-term memory is labeled *episodic*, and it focuses on specific events in our lives, including dates, places, and people. Supposedly, forgetting of these kinds of episodes is more likely, under appropriate circumstances, so that the episodes that make up the texture of our retention will vary with circumstances and importance. The two are not independent, but they are clearly distinguishable in most cases.

Applying these concepts to the memories of dementia patients seems a reasonable and potentially rewarding enterprise. We might hypothesize that a loss in semantic memory will indicate not only the presence of an alteration in the memory system but also something about its severity and meaning for everyday behavior. An inability to recall the meanings of words, particularly common ones, is a sign of some severe loss. If labels for common objects are no longer remembered, the person will be at a more severe disadvantage. Being unable to repeat the name of one's children or spouse will indicate rather extensive functional deterioration.

At the same time, there may be alterations in episodic memory due to the disease process. This would mean a loss of historic events that would normally be available to the person. Particularly as major incidents in life are lost, a case may be made that the disease process has selectively influenced the ability of the patient to use experience. This type of memory loss may be harder to demonstrate because it requires a knowledge of events and some evidence of their importance to the individual. Perhaps some such episodes as marriage, the birth of a child, the death of a parent, and the like will fit the criteria for episodic memory.

Memory impairment is considered a definitive feature of dementia in the *Diagnostic and Statistical Manual*–III, Revised (DSM-III-R). Schultz, Schmitt, Logue, and Rubin (1986, p. 77) point out that the result has been an emphasis on loss in episodic memory when a clinical diagnosis is being made. In studies comparing patients diagnosed with AD with nondemented elderly, Nebes (1989, p. 377) states that most results indicate that semantic memory is severely disrupted by the disease, whereas it remains virtually intact in normal aging. The two positions are not antithetical, but they indicate that there are possible differences in the type of memory that is most severely altered in dementia, depending on factors that need explanation.

The experimentalist may be concerned by possible confounding factors in a way that the clinician may not. Schultz et al. (1986) explicitly mention the neglected role of ability to attend in making estimates of memory capabilities. When a severe memory disturbance is found by testing, there is the possibility that the score is some combination of inability to attend or concentrate plus memory loss. If only the latter is considered, the patient may be diagnosed as more limited than in fact she or he is. When one adds in the effects of motivation and emotion, only loosely controlled usually, the meaning of the score is less clear. Thus the experimentalist prefers to deal with data that reflect the processing in the memory system, as reflected in rehearsal techniques or use of the semantic structure (Schultz et al., 1986, p. 78). This is not to say that there are not problems involved in such investigations, but the results are apt to correspond to more meaningful changes that occur in memory from various syndromes. Indeed, as the authors state, the systematic approach might assist diagnostic accuracy as well.

With this background, Schultz et al. (1986) propose that recall tasks that use prose material may be analyzed in terms of both syntactic and semantic structures. The result may yield better understanding of different kinds of memory failures that have been observed in older persons with clinical problems. In effect, "although there appear to be marked decrements and perhaps wide differences between clinical populations in the nature of memory performance, *episodic and semantic memory systems may be differentially disrupted by different clinical entities*" (Schultz et al., 1986, p. 79, italics added). The contrast between the syntactic/semantic structure and the clinical views is marked. Instead of the use of particular measures of memory (like digit span, or counting backwards by 5s, or other tasks accepted and used over the years as memory tests), the focus is on the structure of memory based upon a model that defines memory systems and how they express themselves. The two approaches (clinical and experimental) may in fact converge and support each other. Only research can determine that possibility.

The literature from the verbal learning group is growing and includes a body dealing specifically with dementia. Schultz et al. (1986) used the Wechsler Memory Scale and an adaptation of it by Russell (1975) to compare the quality of what is remembered with the quantitative (how much is remembered). Such an approach would help control for variables like attention without affecting inferences about memory processing. Their sample contained six groups. The first consisted of 69 AD patients; the second, of 13 MID; the third, 14 cases of persons with closed head injuries; the fourth, 15 individuals with metabolic disorders; the fifth, 14 persons with an affective disorder; and the sixth, 37 normal controls. It should be possible to compare both differing conditions and similar ones. Though not tested statistically, there were apparently differences between groups on age (a mean of 40 years for head injury patients and 66.5 for the controls). There were lesser differences in education with the MID cases having a mean of about 11 years, whereas the affective group had an average of 13.5 years. There were 77 males and 85 females with some differences by sex in the diagnosis assigned.

Memory was tested with a subtest from the WMS in the form adapted by Russell (RWMS) and scored in such a way as to allow partial credits where verbatim recall was not exact. Clinical patients were also given the WAIS and portions of the Halstead–Reitan during a delay period of 30 minutes before delayed recall was assessed. The control group had the interval filled with a variety of different activities.

Among the results, there were differences between the groups in amount recalled. Controls and those with affective disorders recalled the most, whereas MID and AD recalled the least. This accords with the usual findings, as does the fact that clinical groups were differentiated from controls by their performances. As might be expected, the poorer the recall scores of a group initially, the greater the loss over the 30-minute retention interval. But the greater interest in the results of this study lies in the analysis of the particular elements or units that were recalled. Schultz et al. (1986, p. 83) report that the different groups tended to recall or fail the *same* units, at either retention trial. This means there were differences in amount, as has been demonstrated in a number of clinical studies, but not differences in the *kinds* of things remembered or forgotten. As the authors state:

> The simple conclusion derived from the data is that the clinical groups cannot be differentiated from one another or from the normal control group on the basis of which particular units are recalled. *The A.D. patient recalls much less than the normal older individual but recalls essentially the same major ideas.* (Schultz et al., 1986, p. 85, italics added)

The reason for this outcome is not clear, but the result is intriguing. If such an outcome is verified by other studies, we must consider the possibility that different kinds of memory losses will be found in the dementias depending not on the locus and extent of damage so much as the kinds of memories themselves. In that sense, the differences between nondemented and demented would be quantitative only, not qualitative.

The issue is far from settled, and other research may help codify both the strengths and limitations involved. Nebes (1989) has surveyed studies done on semantic memory of Alzheimer's patients in an attempt to identify themes and consistencies. As he points out, there is evidence to indicate that semantic memory is severely disrupted in AD patients, but it remains virtually intact in the normally aging individual. For example, those who are not demented do not show decline in performance on such subtests as Vocabulary, Information, and Comprehension of the WAIS–R. However, much less competent performance is found in those with Alzheimer's and other dementing diseases. Nebes reviewed over 50 studies done in recent years that used semantic tasks with demented patients.

Nebes categorized the results of the studies in four general areas. Briefly summarizing each in turn:

1. Word finding (i.e., retrieving the correct label for an object). The research done in this area (17 studies were reviewed) shows that AD patients are less competent than controls. There seems to be no question that AD victims have difficulties finding the correct word on demand. In the tasks used, the labels required (and the stimulus qualities presented) are very common and usual. The results are highly predictable, but *why* the patients have such difficulties is unknown. Nebes says that the hypothesis that patients cannot use information about semantic attributes of a stimulus to determine the identity of the stimulus is an attractive one. Even if true, we would still not know whether the information is "lost" and irretrievable or if the information is unavailable to a search directed by the experiment and required of the subject. In this area, the agreement between findings of clinicians and experimentalists is consistent: Retrieval of labels with high semantic level is deteriorated in the dementia patient. What needs testing now are hypotheses that might identify the *why*.

2. Knowledge of concept meaning (10 studies surveyed). Though labeling skills may be affected, it appears that knowledge about the category to which an object belongs and its more prominent defining qualities (such as physical features and functions) remains, even in AD. Whether or not this truly benefits the patient may be questioned, Nebes points out, because such knowledge is less accessible than in normals. Indeed, the evidence indicates that patients have difficulty answering direct questions about the features of an item, that is, retrieving a specific piece of information about a concept when it is demanded by the experimenter.

3. Effect of semantic context (19 studies reviewed). The studies indicate that there is an effect in this area, but it seems limited to situations where it is unnecessary to remember the specific word. Processing of

presented stimuli is appropriate in this instance. If the word must be found and used, we're back to the first area above.

4. Impact of semantic memory on episodic memory performance (6 studies). Results here indicate that demented persons may be as successful at using semantic structure to improve episodic memory as are nondemented. When it comes to using the same semantic structure in the form of a categorized word list or object attributes, patients are less successful. Nebes suggests that reading text is such an overlearned skill in most of us that the information in connected text retains its benefits. Thus the dementia patient may be able to encode semantic information only to the extent that the encoding is induced and directed by the stimulus material itself. When it is necessary for the person to encode as an intentional act, the patient cannot implement the necessary skills.

Nebes concludes that AD patients are severely impaired on a number of semantic memory tasks that do not cause problems as a normal part of aging. The magnitude and nature of the deficit is strongly influenced by stimulus and task variables, however. From the data he proposes several possibilities requiring solution. First, an explanation is needed for the obvious semantic impairments that evolve from the AD. Perhaps they are due to some loss of semantic material so that there is no longer anything to retrieve. On the other hand, the semantic problems may be symptomatic, reflecting the presence of other cognitive deficits that limit the person's ability to access and appropriately use semantic information that is in place and available. If the former, the disease process includes a direct effect on the language function. If the latter, there must be identified which "deficits" are responsible and a decision made about possible intervention. At present, there is no answer and, seemingly, none forthcoming. Second, perhaps there is no loss of semantic information from AD but a disruption in the way the material is now organized. There are no studies bearing on this issue at present. Projects need to be designed that demonstrate whether or not some components of semantic memory remain intact even as the disease process continues. Third, there is the appealing possibility that the problem is one of retrieval. In this case, at least some aspects of semantic memory must be intact, but the patient is unable to "get it out." The case study mentioned earlier of the patient's awareness that he had answers to orientation questions but that he was unable to retrieve them is relevant here. Nebes reports that some evidence supports the retrieval loss idea, but he feels that it will not be a likely candidate to explain all semantic problems. He is left with the position that "at present, there is no one simple explanation for why Alzheimer's patients are severely impaired on some semantic memory tasks but perform quite normally on others" (Nebes, 1989, p. 392).

Language Function in Dementia

A parallel line of research has investigated the use of language by those diagnosed as demented. Several of these have looked at the labeling problem that patients demonstrate when required to retrieve names even for very common objects. Barker and Lawson (1968) noted that patients who could not retrieve a label without difficulty were able to demonstrate how the object might be used. This demonstration of use then facilitated the naming of the object. Further, they observed that if the object label functioned both as a verb and a noun (e.g., a "comb" and "to comb") there was a greater likelihood of a correct response. To test the validity of the role of such variables, they designed a study using 100 patients diagnosed as "organic dementia" (70 females, 30 males). Their mean age was 74.5 years. A control group of 40 adults (12 males, 28 females) with a mean age of 71 years was compared on performance. They created a list of 24 names of objects, controlled for familiarity in six separate lists of four objects each. Half of the objects had their use demonstrated during the presentation; the other half did not. Half were both verbs and nouns; the other half were nouns only. The variables of concern were thus present in equal proportions throughout the list.

Their results confirmed the greater failure rate of the dementia victims. The familiarity variable was significant also, with an interaction that was explained on the basis of the uncommon occurrence of some words in the list. Where a demonstration occurred, there were significantly fewer errors but only for the patients. The demonstration seemed equally effective for both common and uncommon words. If the word served as both verb and noun, the patient group was more successful than if the word was a noun only. Their conclusions pointed to the difficulty in word finding that is so common in dementia (but not so well illustrated at the time of this study). They also felt that demonstration may help patients to label more easily. In addition, they believe there is the possibility that this technique might be useful as a diagnostic procedure. As to the cause of the failure to name, it "may be attributed on the one hand to the perceptual deficit of failure to identify the object or alternatively to the cognitive deficit of impaired word finding" (Barker & Lawson, 1968, p. 1355). It is of more than passing interest that, over 20 years later, Nebes has to speculate in a similar fashion.

More recently, Skelton-Robinson and Jones (1984) used a similar procedure. They stated as their purpose the attempt to discover if there is a direct relationship between *degree* of senile dementia and the severity of naming difficulties. Further, they wanted to determine, if possible, whether naming problems may be explained on the basis of brain damage itself. Their sample consisted of 20 persons diagnosed as "dementia." Their age range was 69 to 88, with a mean of 79 years. Several psychometric measures were used, but one consisted of a large number of items that were presented as objects (nouns) or actions (verbs) to be named by the subject. Some of these items served as both verbs and nouns. If the patient could not supply the name after 30 seconds, the experimenter described the use of the item or, if a verb, an occasion when the action occurs. If, after another 30 seconds, there was no correct response, the subject was presented with a choice between the correct answer and one in the same semantic category. Neither of these latter two techniques benefitted the patients. The group was subdivided into "less demented" and "more demented" (10 in each group), and the former subgroup performed better than the latter. The frequency of occurrence of a word in the language had a significant effect on the ability to name. They concluded that verbal agnosia (loss of ability to recognize familiar objects, principally due to brain damage) is relatively much less important than the language defects of demented persons in causing naming errors.

Bayles (1982) compared normal controls with senile dementia patients on five language tasks. There were 28 controls and 35 demented persons, all age 60 or over. The dementia group was subdivided on the basis of severity: mild, moderate, or severe. The last had to be dropped from the study because the subjects could not perform well enough to achieve a comparative score. Among the language tests, there was a naming task (15 color photos of common objects); story retelling; sentence correction (made by the subject); verbal expression (creative use of language); and sentence disambiguation (does sentence have more than one meaning?).

There was some overlap between the controls and patients. These consisted of "normal subjects whose overall performance was below the mean for normals but above the mean for the demented group, and senile dementia patients whose overall performance was above the mean of the demented group but below the mean of the normals" (p. 672). Such persons would be misclassified (either as false positives or false negatives). Bayles speculates that there may be a performance level where reliable diagnosis may not be in doubt. On every comparison, the normals and dementia patients differed significantly. "The semantic system emerged as most vulnerable to the ravages of senile dementia" (p. 273). Greatest impairment was noted for those with moderate degrees of dementia, particularly on story retelling, verbal expression, and nonsense-syllable learning. Of course, the severely demented probably would have performed even less well if their performance had permitted quantification.

Bayles notes that "age did not adversely affect the language–speech skills necessary for normal communication, whereas age-related senile dementia significantly altered language function though generally sparing speech production" (p. 278). Those who must live with a patient who is deteriorating (and those who work with them) will attest to this inexplicable outcome.

Finally, Wilson, Kaszniak, Bacon, Fox, and Kelly (1982) investigated nonverbal functioning to see if similar effects and outcomes were obtained. They used unfamiliar faces as stimulus material. They first looked at 48 pictures for 5 seconds each. Retention was tested with a combination of these 48 plus 48 distractor photos, with the subjects asked to identify whether each picture was a "new" or "old" one. For comparison purposes, a verbal naming task was employed also, using the same technique. For each choice on the retention test, the subject gave a confidence rating of her or his assignment.

A control group of 41 persons was compared to an experimental group of 29 dementia patients. Age and educational levels were equivalent. Differences were significant between the groups. Wilson et al. (1982) report that "amnesia of SDAT is not limited to verbal material" (p.334) and that

> verbal and facial memory deficits in SDAT are dissociable. First, performance in the two areas is relatively unrelated. Second, the nature of verbal and facial memory deficits appears to differ. . . . [V]erbal memory impairment in SDAT is a complex deficit involving linguistic and encoding abilities in addition to memory proper. The facial memory deficit . . . appears relatively uncomplicated by perceptual factors, response bias, or linguistic ability. (p. 334)

Among the conclusions drawn by Wilson et al., one relates to the dissociation found between verbal and facial memory performance. The outcome indicates to them that the pattern of cognitive decline in SDAT may not be uniform for all patients. Perhaps that is due to differences in strengths and weaknesses in cognitive abilities present before the disease process began. There is the alternative, though, that there is an uneven distribution of degenerative changes in the brains of AD patients. Only more sophisticated research projects (and models) will bring an answer.

SUMMARY

Although the history of psychological testing is relatively short, the influence and effects have been profound. Knowledge of causes of human actions is not often directly available so that inferences become necessary. Tests supply scores that may be used for such inferences.

As with other aspects of human behavior, consequences of disease process are often obvious in dementia, but appreciating the reasons for such consequences is difficult. Psychological tests that might help in that understanding have been available for years. In some instances, tests have been developed specifically to identify difficulties and/or diagnose causes.

The tests used are normally classified as neuropsychological, which are devised to identify brain dysfunctions of specific types and locations, or psychometric, which are intended to measure traits indirectly that are not directly accessible. In either case, inference is the rule most often, and the differences between the two are less marked than the distinction would imply.

A number of psychological tests are surveyed in this chapter with a sampling of the research done on their applications and utility. The popularity of the instruments is not always warranted by empirical results, but the need is so great that their use will continue until something better is available.

An alternative to the clinical use of tests is through experimentation in verbal learning. Because memory is so adversely affected in the dementias, part of this research has focused on the structure of memory and its alterations by the disease. Research on semantic memory, particularly, but with reference to implications for episodic memory is included and discussed. To date, more questions than answers have resulted, but increasing sophistication in investigation may permit a resolution in future.

At some point, clinicians and experimentalists need to begin conversing with one another for the benefit of dementia patients!

CHAPTER SIX

Dementia and Psychiatric Disorders

The consequences of dementia resulting from some structural changes in the brain would seem to be sufficient penalty for both patient and caregiver. There exists, however, the possibility that psychological disorders that may already be present will become aggravated. An example of this would be an exaggeration of anxiety states in a person already subject to worry. Further, dysfunctional conditions new to the individual may develop, in part as a reaction to negative events accumulating in the life of the person and in part as an attempt to adapt to difficult events. In this case, we might see a patient and caregiver become increasingly depressed as the patient's status worsens and introduces new problems that seem impossible to remedy. There is the additional possibility that structural and/or chemical changes in the brain may alter the personality. Thus the psychological dimensions should not be underestimated or ignored because there is suffering that may be unnecessary if diagnosed and treated.

These conditions are often designated as "functional disorders" because they have no known organic or physical cause (Zarit, 1980, p. 214).[1] They are disorders when they interfere with the abilities of the person to interact successfully with life. Under stress, the individual may have difficulty identifying the nature of problems accurately, thinking rationally about their solutions, and/or pursuing a course that will lead to appropriate and effective resolution. An individual's responses to stressors may confound and complicate what is already a dysfunctional situation. The brain syndrome may be untreatable and irreversible and a resulting dementia may be progressive. Therefore, the psychological correlates of brain deterioration should be identified and distinguished from any reactive (functional) psychological expressions. This distinction often is difficult;

sometimes, impossible. However, immediate, effective treatment of the functional disorders may give substantial relief both to the patient and caregiver. For this reason alone, they deserve special attention.

The functional disorders[2] are of several types and subtypes. In considering dementia, the three that are most pertinent are anxiety, depression, and delusional behavior. Of these, depression is the most often recognized and discussed, but the others deserve attention. In addition, the symptoms of depression may include suicidal thinking and signals, so it will be worthwhile to include the topic of suicide (for both patient and caregiver). The point to remember is that all three disorders are subject to treatment with psychotherapy, medications, or both. Any or all of these may develop or be exacerbated in the patient and/or caregiver given the exigencies of life that are concomitant with a dementia. Awareness and understanding of the manifestations of these physical disorders should assist in their identification and treatment.

ANXIETY

Anxiety is a common experience. At various times and under certain circumstances, probably all of us suffer some anxious moments. However, for dementia patients and caregivers, the disorder assumes more intense ramifications and expressions than merely temporary discomfort. The DSM-III-R (American Psychiatric Association, 1987, p. 235) describes the characteristic features of the Anxiety Disorders as symptoms of anxiety and avoidance behavior. Panic Disorder is expressed through recurrent panic attacks, accompanied by autonomic nervous system activity (such as shortness of breath, accelerated heart rate, sweating, dizziness, and trembling) as well as psychological expressions (such as fear of dying or going crazy and depersonalization) (DSM-III-R, 1987, p. 237). A Generalized Anxiety Disorder reflects unrealistic or excessive anxiety and worry about at least two circumstances in one's life. These expressions must have been present for 6 months or longer, with the person showing concern more days than not. There will be evidence of motor tension, autonomic hyperactivity, and vigilance features (DSM-III-R, 1987, p. 244). The psychological and physical manifestations are powerful influencers of behavior that may be appropriate or inappropriate to the circumstance. When they interfere with the individual's effective functioning in relationships, society, or work, they are labeled *disorders*.

Blazer (1990, p. 1008) points out that the panic disorder is more often found during youth and young adulthood with symptoms declining as the individual ages. The Generalized Anxiety Disorder, however, is more frequent in late life, perhaps reaching an incidence of 5% of that population. One can appreciate that aging persons, as they encounter increasing difficulties and losses in various aspects of life, might worry about potential problems and additional losses more than younger persons. They thus might develop an "anticipatory" or "presumptive" pattern of defense that is manifested as symptoms and signs of Generalized Anxiety Disorder. In the case of dementia, Blazer (1990, p. 1008) states that primary degenerative dementia may well be the most common cause of functional anxiety in older persons.

> Early recognition of cognitive dysfunction and memory loss in individuals with continued social demands frequently leads to generalized anxiety, with periodic episodes of panic. This, in turn, contributes to social withdrawal and isolation. The severe and traumatic behavioral changes that result from this anxiety syndrome frequently mask the underlying dementia. (Blazer, 1990, p. 1008)

The opposite state of affairs is possible also, that is, the dementia may mask the anxiety felt by the person. With attention paid only to the dementia, a treatable condition (anxiety) may be ignored. The possibility of anxiety must be investigated by the clinician because older persons have reason to worry about many life circumstances. Living on a fixed income, physical decline, death of spouse, friends, and family, and so on often assume a larger role in the lives of the elderly than the lives of younger adults.

Treatment of Anxiety Disorder may consist of medication, psychotherapy, or a combination of both. Where drugs are used, there is always the possibility of overmedication and even side effects with the elderly. Blazer (p. 1010) says that the issue is a real one with treatment of anxiety, although the response to the anxiolytic drugs usually will be satisfactory. If the person is demented, then particular care and monitoring are essential if these medications are used. Psychotherapy has limitations as well, but Blazer (p. 1010) says that short-term, insight-oriented therapy (reflecting the current circumstances in the patient's life) is more useful. Biofeedback may help the person control symptoms, and a paced exercise program can assist those who feel loss of control over parts of their lives (Blazer, 1990, p. 1011). Overall, the returns for any of these approaches is limited, and perhaps especially so for patients. Somewhat better results may occur in caregivers because they will have more capabilities to bring to the task.

The literature on anxiety and dementia is more limited than one might expect or hope. However, there has been recognition of the potential concurrence of anxiety and depression with its importance to the well-being of the individual. Schmidt (1986), for example, points to a need for sensitivity to what is "normal" functioning in an elderly population as it relates to the complex interrelationships between medical and psychological conditions. The vulnerability of the aged requires awareness by professionals and specialized mental health services of the behaviors commonly found in the elderly.

Lader (1982) not only reiterates the association between physical states and anxiety but also posits that anxiety often accompanies the early development of dementia. This association may be implicit in the argument that, as the patient becomes aware of memory loss and confusion, there may be the fear that further incidents will occur. Lader believes that, although the anxiety experienced by the patient will have an individual content, so long as it is sustained it becomes more and more debilitating. The "individual content" alluded to by Lader is demonstrated in an observation by Hess (1987). He describes what he refers to as a "King Lear syndrome" in the anxiety of old age. This phenomenon is shown in the dread of being abandoned and becoming totally helpless. The incidence of this syndrome is particularly related to catastrophic events like dementia. When it occurs, the defense used by the patient is usually some form of tyrannical control to assure meeting of needs that are fundamentally narcissistic, according to Hess. The plausibility of the King Lear syndrome fits with the complaints of some caregivers who find more and more demands from the patient with less and less empathy and concern for the caregiver. Unless the caregiver is unusually psychologically strong, the burden can become overwhelming. The concern for the well-being of the caregiver must be a consideration for the psychologist. Unless there can be some balance between demand from the patient and personal well-being of the caregiver, mental health will suffer. As for the patient, there may be less effectiveness in intervention attempted by the caregiver. What must be resolved and accepted by both the patient and caregiver is that reasonable demands will be met, whereas tyrannical, self-centered ones will not. This clearly is easier to state than it is to achieve because the caregiver often will experience guilt, if she or he is not able to meet the needs and demands of the patient, and shame, at wanting to impose limitations. At the same time, the caregiver must take care of her/himself, especially in the face of the patient's losses. With support and education, many caregivers experiencing the role of Cordelia (the "good" daughter who was so tyrannized and rejected by Lear) will be able to understand and adjust to the situation.

The "masking" phenomenon whereby complaints may lead to a mistaken diagnosis is illustrated in a case study (Barclay, Blass, & Lee, 1984). The authors describe a 75-year-old attorney, still actively practicing, who complained to his physician about forgetfulness, a condition representing a major threat to his livelihood. The complaint might represent a cerebral illness but, if there is no deterioration in cognitive function, there may be mimicking of anxiety. Barclay et al. report that eventually cerebral lesions were discovered so that, in fact, masking had been present but was undetected.

Programs to assist persons to find relief from their anxieties have been reported both for patients and caregivers. Schwab, Rader, and Doan (1985) report an effort to enhance the self-esteem of patients who experience fear and anxiety as a result of confusion and disorientation. They developed a program incorporating exercise and relaxation. Their goal was to assist the residents in achieving more order in a disoriented world. As might be expected, the results were mixed. Some residents showed large improvements, others were more modest in outcome, and some were failures in the sense of no improvement. One outcome of considerable importance was the spinoff of more positive attitudes by staff members toward the residents and their problems. This alone can have benefits for the well-being of the demented group members.

Overall, anxiety, particularly of the generalized type, may be part of the adjustment patterns of patients (see Blazer, 1990, p. 1008) as well as for caregivers. This is due in part to the fact that Generalized Anxiety Disorder is relatively common in old age (Blazer, 1990, p. 1008) but also in part to the specific nature of stressors present with dementia. For the patient, anxiety probably occurs earlier in the process and will be greatly reduced as the deterioration in competence increases. Eventually, there may be no anxiety found, simply because the patient is no longer capable of anticipating and understanding the conditions that lead to anxiety. For the caregiver, the occurrence of anxiety may start fairly early, as disturbing behavior changes are noted in the patient, and become more pronounced and more interfering as the dementia progresses. Interventions medically with anxiolytic drugs leave some symptoms of generalized anxiety unchanged though some relief is experienced (Blazer, 1990, p. 1010). Side effects from such drugs are often reported. The development of socially based, problem-centered programs will be helpful to some patients and caregivers but may not relieve the anxiety level to any significant degree.

DEPRESSION

Like anxiety, depression is a condition widely prevalent across all ages. Its manifestations may differ somewhat between age groups, however. In its milder forms, one may feel sad and dejected but continue to function reasonably well. As the number and/or severity of the depressive symptoms increases, however, it becomes increasingly debilitating. In its most severe form, called Major Depression, it can be disabling, with marked deterioration in the individual's personal, social, and occupational functioning.

The DSM-III-R (1987, pp. 218–221) states that a loss of interest or pleasure (called anhedonia) in all or almost all activities is a primary symptom of Major Depression. Sleep disturbance is cited as a frequent expression, along with loss of appetite, changes in weight, loss of energy, feelings of guilt or worthlessness, and difficulty in concentrating. There also may be suicidal thoughts, delusions, hallucinations, or paranoid thinking. Blazer (1982, p. 273) points out that "the current diagnostic system is not suited to an elderly population, in whom depression may express itself differently, is hidden or expressed through 'equivalents,' is often denied, and possesses a special 'relationship' with physical illness and loss." He would put greater emphasis on depressive symptoms in the elderly and certainly differentiate these symptoms from Major Depression (Blazer, 1982, p. 273).

One reason for care in using criteria of the DSM-III-R with older persons is the complaint that the individual presents. Most often, this complaint is couched in terms of a physical illness, or problems in relationships, or difficulties financially (Blazer, 1982, p. 20). The clinician must consider these grievances in their own right but also question the older person in order to disclose symptoms that, in fact, are related to depression (Blazer, 1982, p. 20). Blazer (1982, pp. 19–30) has described and discussed symptoms and signs in the elderly as they may be presented and as they should be interpreted vis-à-vis depression.

The condition, then, may mean the same *consequences* across age groups but is not necessarily *diagnosed* or *treated* as it is with younger adults. Blazer (1990, p. 1014) maintains that depressive disorders are one of the most frequent psychiatric problems found in the elderly. The incidence in that subgroup alone may run as high as 15%, at the same time that prevalence is less in old age than in other age groups. These facts may represent a cohort effect (Blazer, 1990, p. 1015) because today's older generations have experienced less depressions than generations before them. Still, as current young adults age, there may be a higher prevalence than currently because of the history of the generation (Blazer, 1990, p. 1015).

Treatment may consist of antidepressant drugs (the so-called tricyclics and newer drugs such as Nortriptyline, Desipramine, and Doxepin), or psychotherapy, or both. Side effects represent a real danger for the elderly, and so the drug of choice should be the one with the *least* adverse effects (Blazer, 1990, p. 1017). Therapy is usually more successful if it focuses on behaviors and thoughts in the current life of the person, so that behavioral and cognitive therapies are more often successful. The more traditional psychotherapies like psychoanalytic theory are not necessarily appropriate. Major depression and dementia may coexist in a patient but, with progression of the dementia, depressive symptoms will remit (Blazer, 1990, p. 1017).

The possibility that dementia and depression may occur simultaneously reinforces the need for diagnostic caution so that each may be recognized and dealt with properly. This opens the possibility that one condition may appear to be the other, with a consequent misdiagnosis. The term *pseudodementia* has been coined to describe the mistaking of symptoms of depression for those of dementia (Zarit, 1980, p. 158). Because confusion of the two states may occur, the diagnostician must look at such events as more sudden onset (typical of Major Depression), history of episodes, and mental status test performance (depressives do not make errors typical of a dementia patient).

Henderson (1989) points out that improved methods in epidemiological research will make comparative studies of depression more meaningful. In addition to cross-cultural research on the prevalence of dementias, an outcome may well be clearer distinctions between dementia and pseudodementia. Gershon and Herman (1982) maintain that, though AD and MID are usually untreatable, pseudodementia must be differentiated as it can be reversed.

The similarities between the behaviors representing each condition permit some confusion (Whall, 1986). However, the depressive should have more accurate short-term memory (as reflected on the MMSE, for example) that will help in making the distinction. This possibility is demonstrated in a study by Wands, Mersky, Hachinski, Fishman, Fox, and Boniferro (1990) that used a sample of 50 patients diagnosed as demented and measured their anxiety and depression levels with a scale devised to discriminate the two conditions. A comparison was made with 134 age-matched controls. There were marked differences between the groups in anxiety and depression, with the patients showing the higher levels. In fact, the patients showed rates for the two functional disorders higher than those found in the general population.

The rates found depend on samples and measures, and therefore all demographic studies do not agree. Wands et al. found that 28% of their sample presented symptoms of depression. Griffiths, Good, Watson, O'Donnell, Fell, and Shakespeare (1987) report an 18% rate of depression in a sample of 200 older persons in a rural community. The studies agree on the possibility of relationship between anxiety and depression. Griffiths et al. found that a mental test score was related to both syndromes for persons age 60 and over, whereas the score was not related to depression alone in older persons. The ability to distinguish conditions on a mental status test is underscored by this finding.

The problems associated with distinguishing dementia and depression are not limited to the United States, of course. Surveys have been done to compare presence and rates of various conditions between cultures over the world. Gurland, Copeland, Kuriansky, Kelleher, Sharpe, and Dean (1983) compared the incidence and diagnosis of depression and organic mental disorders in New York and London in *The Mind and Mood of Aging*. More recently, Henderson (1990) has examined the role of social factors in how mental disorders are perceived and diagnosed among the elderly. The increase in incidence of AD with age seems to be common to different cultures, but with great differences in prevalence rates between cultures. Henderson speculates that there may be a true difference in prevalence among regions of the world. There is the possibility, of course, that such diagnostic differences as occur may reflect personal experience and training. Gurland et al. presented evidence that might be interpreted in this way.

Henderson (1990) reports that his survey of research done in various countries indicates a case for lower rates of depression with age. Perhaps this reflects the criteria used for diagnosis. The DSM-III-R cites eight symptoms, four of which must be present to qualify for the psychiatric label. In addition, duration of the symptoms is considered, though frequency and severity are not. To make matters worse, geropsychologists and geriatric psychiatrists do not agree that depression expresses itself in old age as it does in youth and young adulthood (see, for example, Blazer, 1990, p. 1016; Alexopoulos, 1989). Criteria must be described and maintained, but it may become necessary, in the future, to determine data on variables such as the age cohort to which the individual belongs as well as by symptoms. Henderson concludes that those individuals who have many social relationships are apt to live longer and healthier lives, both mentally and physically. Such a conclusion, extended worldwide, accords with gerontological experience and theory in most instances. Such conditions may affect the incidence of depressive symptoms in the future.

The experience of dementia being masked by depression (and vice versa), as well as the fact that they may coexist has led to some attempts to classify in a more orderly fashion. Reifler (1986) has proposed two types of cognitive–affective disorders in old age. Type 1 would be used with those who have depression, of whatever type and degree, as the sole diagnosis. In these cases, when the depression is treated, whatever cognitive deficits appeared to be present are resolved. Type 2 would include those who have both conditions present to some degree, that is, they are demented *and* depressed. Here, when the depression is identified and treated properly, there will be amelioration of the symptoms of the mood disorder, but the cognitive deficits that reflect the dementia will remain (and, in all probability, worsen with time). This Type 1 versus Type 2 distinction seems reasonable and already is used by clinicians to achieve differentiation and improve intervention. What is most interesting about Reifler's model is that he proposes that the number of Type 1 cases has been *over*estimated, whereas the number of Type 2 cases has been *under*estimated. If he is correct, there should indeed be less depression in the elderly as a group but with a secondary depression where dementia is found. Dementia increases with age, with Reifler's assertion suggesting that accompanying depression should be anticipated, identified, and treated as and when it is present. Kim and Hershey (1988) inject a note of caution, however. They have described problems in the diagnosis of depression in older persons, including depressive symptoms that accompany SDAT. So long as such diagnostic difficulties exist, and insofar as they are confounding, models may be less realistic than we would like.

Other authors have taken a more positive approach. Ancill (1989) believes that depression in especially common in old age, although its features are presented differently than at younger ages. More to the point, he asserts that depression is often associated with dementia and supports the idea of a "cognitive–affective disorder." In the case of the depression, Ancill cautions that mood disorders may be highly treatable, but the drugs available often prove toxic to many older persons. If severe enough, electroconvulsive therapy (shock treatments) may be a viable approach, he believes, because ECT appears to be successful and reasonably well-tolerated. For dementia, even if one finds improvement in cognitive abilities, they tend to be short-lived and unpredictable. Again, we have the suggestion that treatment, at least for depression, is plausible and successful. The optimistic attitude is tempered by the effects, and side effects, of such treatments in older persons. This dilemma remains a crucial one in decisions about intervention.

This survey of publications about copresentation of depression and dementia, the diagnosis of each, and possible treatments could continue. Perhaps the issues involved are best reflected in Stoudemire, Hill, Gulley, and Morris (1989). They point out that there is no single technique that is sufficient to assure differentiating the contribution of depression and dementia to the cognitive dysfunction found in a patient's behavior. What must be decided by the diagnostician is whether the cognitive symptoms reflect depression alone or reflect a true dementia, or both. This position reinforces the idea that currently medicine and psychology are still at a level that is more art than science. That fact must be realized by practitioners and the public.

There is no consensus about the depression/dementia relationship. Knesevich, Martin, Berg, and Danziger (1983) used two measures of depression with a group of 30 mildly demented and 30 nondemented individuals, testing each twice over a 1-year interval. They found no differences in depression between the two groups; in fact, they both had mean scores in the nondepressed range. Although the dementia patients were more likely to show depression on one of the scales, a single item (dealing with "work and activities" on the Hamilton Rating Scale for Depression) accounted for some of them being rated as "mildly depressed." As a result, Knesevich et al. conclude that depressive states may be independent of DAT and might be considered rarely associated with it. They suggest that any depressive syndrome noted in a dementia patient should receive "aggressive" treatment even at the risk of anticholinergic effects of the usual drugs used.

What is the process of intervention once differential diagnosis has occurred? Because the lives of the patient and caregiver become involved so totally in the problem behaviors, it would seem plausible to expect that program planning will include elements related directly and indirectly to the consequences of the problem. Representative of this perspective is a study by Lindsey and Murphy (1989). With a sample of 99 persons aged 65 and older diagnosed as demented, they investigated the relationship between depression, supports offered in the home, and admission to institutional care. None of the sample was institutionalized at the time of the study. Within their sample, 44 received routine care, and 55 were given extra home support. The symptoms of depression—apathy, agitation, irritability, and early waking—interfered with the home support techniques. The behavioral symptoms of depression make the demands and burdens of caring for a dementia patient with concurrent depression in the home all the more difficult and may well lead to earlier institutional placement than the caregiver would like.

Treatment outcomes may range from effective to limited for depression, depending in part on the intervention used (drugs or psychotherapy or both), the condition of the patient (in general health as well as demented state), and the intensity or degree of the depressive state. As depicted in Figure 6.1, the treatment outcome has the greatest likelihood of "success" when the problem is one of depression only. Admittedly, drug side effects may lead to lack of improvement even in this case. Depression with pseudodementia permits reversal of the symptoms of

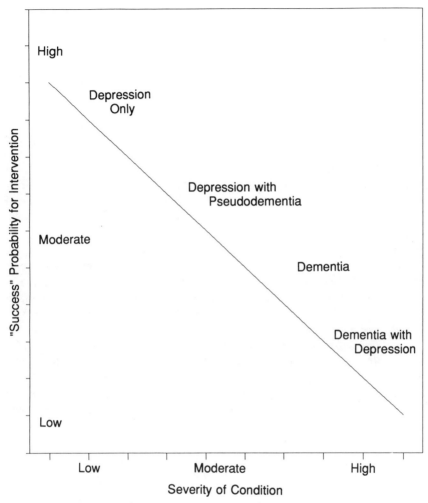

FIGURE 6.1. Treatment success as related to condition.

dementia when proper treatment is employed. Unfortunately, adverse side effects of drugs may be more prominent when some degree of dementia is present because there is already nerve cell degeneration. Any drug that contributes to confusion and disorientation under the ideal circumstance must be even more suspect in such a case.

If the problem is one of dementia without depression, certainly the conventional interventions must be eschewed. They will not only be inappropriate but may lead to greater confusion and emotional distress on the part of the patient. Most difficult is the case when both the dementia and the depression are present. Though treatment must be attempted, the probability of success is weighted in the direction of limited and even ineffective outcomes. This is a discouraging picture, surely, but a realistic one that must be accepted given current intervention possibilities.

One area of interest is the effect of depression that presents as dementia (often called "depression of dementia" or DOD) as compared to dementia alone. O'Boyle and Amadeo (1989) approached the comparison by examining performance on the MMSE at admission and just before discharge from a medical unit. Those who received a diagnosis of dementia ($N = 20$, mean age = 76 years) scored significantly lower on the screening device than those with depression that presented with signs of dementia ($N = 11$, mean age = 68.5 years).

The authors took the additional step of examining performance for the number of answers of "I don't know" by the patients. There was no difference between the groups, even though the demented subjects made more errors on orientation questions. This would reflect the effort of patients to supply an answer to questions even when that answer is inappropriate or incorrect. Experience reinforces this view that the person does try to answer questions often. There is the issue of why such a result? Perhaps the effects of the syndrome do not leave the individual with an awareness of the insufficiency in answering. Almost childlike, then, the patient attempts to deal with some reality presented but not necessarily interpreted accurately. Conversely, the patient may feel that the answer she or he supplies is correct, that is, reality is altered to accommodate the abilities of the person. From still a different viewpoint, perhaps the individual has no comprehension of what is asked or answered. Verbal behavior patterns have been so well rehearsed over so many years that a response is generated that is literate if not accurate. This would conform to the redundancy theory whereby responding may occur in the absence of a stimulus. Because we have so little knowledge of the way in which dementia operates, any of these (and perhaps others unstated) may represent the reason for the observed behavior in the patient. Unfortunately, words used in some correct context by an adult who has been mentally competent may be accepted with face validity (something that *appears* valid even if it isn't) rather than as some reflection of a reality that is different from what we think is the stimulus.[3]

Whatever the explanation, the symptoms of dementia, actual or imposed, are often demonstrated. Speedie, Rabins, Pearlson, and Moberg

(1990) compared three groups: elderly persons (N = 61) hospitalized with major depression, reversible DOD, or irreversible dementia. A control group consisted of 17 spouses of the subjects. Several memory tasks were used, and the controls were superior in performance to all patient groups. Among the patients, those with DOD scored less well than depressives on free recall, delayed recall, and verbal delayed memory tasks. The differences between DOD and dementia groups were less apparent, with both groups showing great difficulties in both speed of response and accuracy on a confrontation naming task. Somewhat different results are reported by O'Connor, Pollitt, Roth, Brook, and Reiss (1990). Their control group consisted of 213 "normal" persons who were compared to 36 depressed and 135 mildly to moderately demented older persons on memory tasks from a standardized test. In only two of seven instances significant differences were found between depressed and normal persons, and the former group showed performance above the mean for the total sample. The demented subjects were well below the other groups in performance. The authors report that depressed patients in their study reported being indecisive and unable to concentrate (typical symptoms of depression) as well as mental slowdown and difficulty in efforts. The demented group did not report such problems. This finding shows a greater disparity between normal and depressed groups as compared with the dementia patients than the Speedie et al study. Why? One possibility lies in the characteristics of the sample. Control groups are obviously very different, and not only in size. Using spouses as Speedie et al. did might produce some bias in results because wives and husbands are sharing a problem that must produce adverse effects; the difference between a spouse with possible depressive symptoms and his or her spouse diagnosed as depressed with dementia may not be so great as the difference between normal controls and depressed subjects as selected by O'Connor et al. There are also differences in the test materials used that must influence the results obtained to some degree.

Finally, there may be differences in the degree to which the dementia has progressed in the subjects in the two studies. Differences in results more often reflect sample selection criteria, measurement devices used, and diagnostic criteria than they do "true" effects. This does not necessarily invalidate results, nor does it signify that researchers don't know what they are doing. Rather, interpreting the meaning of outcomes requires consideration of all the factors that might have influenced the results. Admittedly, it would be helpful if there were some standardized procedures applied to studies investigating the same phenomenon, but that is not likely to occur.

Comparisons with Technology

In a few instances, studies have included data from scans as part of the procedure to evaluate the relative dimensions of Major Depression and dementia. Ames, Dolan, and Mann (1990) used 34 older persons (ages 69 to 97) who showed depressive symptoms or had been given a diagnosis either of dementia or depression. Computerized tomography (CT scan) was administered to each subject. The results were not encouraging to the procedure because the scan did not disclose differences between the groups. Perhaps the technology used is not sufficiently sophisticated to disclose such differences, a position that accords with other data about the utility of CT scans. What is more surprising is that there were no differences between groups on psychometric measures either. Follow-ups after 1 and 2 years indicated that only five persons had improved in their depressive symptoms. Ames et al. conclude that their data indicate that there may be neither validity nor clinical usefulness in a distinction between depression and dementia in very old age. These outcomes are in disagreement with other studies.

At variance with the study above is one by Pearlson, Rabins, Kim, Speedie, Moberg, Burns, and Bascom (1989). A sample of 26 persons over age 60 who had been diagnosed as having Major Depression were compared on CT scans with 13 patients diagnosed as probable AD and 31 controls. Of the depressed persons, 15 were labeled as DOD from use of the MMSE. Results indicated that depressives had CT values between those of the Alzheimer and normal subjects, with the DOD subgroup being closer to the AD patients. They also had cognitive losses more like the dementia sample. This might suggest that DOD patients may be in progression to a true dementia, but Pearlson et al. did not find evidence of that outcome, at least over the short term.

The issue becomes one of the relationship, if any, between measurable changes in structural and chemical integrity of the brain and the presence of conditions mimicking dementia. If there is, then an intermediate step between a functional disorder and developing structural change may have been identified. Research to test the plausibility of this hypothesis is sparse, but Zubenko and Moossy (1988) have offered some evidence using postmortem data. The brains of 37 persons who had had diagnoses of primary degenerative dementia were compared with the brains of seven elderly controls. Degenerative changes in portions of the brain (the locus ceruleus and substantia nigra) were associated with depression reported in the clinical picture of the dementia patients. The authors believe their study offers some evidence about the interaction of neurotransmitter mechanisms in the development of primary degenerative dementia. In this case, noradrenaline and dopamine are the brain chemicals involved. Though only a limited beginning, the study is intriguing in its potential. One deterrent lies in the fact that the association of depressive symptoms and brain locus did not permit prediction of depression from significant degeneration in either area alone. This represents an example of correlative data, where relationship is present with no evidence of cause and effect.

The "chemical connection" has been demonstrated in a study by Zubenko, Moossy, and Kopp (1990). The brains of 37 patients with primary degenerative dementia (apparently the same sample as above) were studied for neurochemical changes and compared to 10 brains of elderly controls. They found a "profile" of neurochemical changes in dementia plus depression that was qualitatively different from that in dementia alone. Depression seems to involve noradrenergic, serotonergic, and cholinergic systems. Amine and acetylcholine neurotransmitters influence the cortex and subcortical areas in distinct ways when major depression is present. As further research is conducted, our understanding of brain–behavior relationships will be expanded even more.

A picture of the structural processes involved is hinted at in a discussion by McHugh (1989). He considered three conditions—dyskinesia, dementia, and depression—as they occur in individuals with disorders in the basal ganglia region of the brain. In Huntington's disease, all three are found, and McHugh believes pathology in the basal ganglia is the explanation. What may happen is that in nondiseased brain "neural loops" (patterns between nerve cells) from the motor and sensory cortex, the association areas, and the limbic system form pathways that are parallel in the basal ganglia. These parallel loops influence each other (he speaks of "communicating") in the basal ganglia as various functions interact and become integrated. If this complex but essential relationship is disturbed by pathological changes in nerve cells involved in the processes, the result may be the dyskinesia, dementia, and depression that typify cases of Huntington's. Yet to be proven, the logic of his argument is appealing.

Treatment for Patients

Given a patient with DOD or with dementia plus depression, intervention should be attempted to improve the condition as much as possible. Such an attempt was tried by Pearson, Teri, Reifler, and Raskind (1989). They had a sample of 50 dementia patients, all of whom still lived in the community. Twenty of them were also diagnosed with Major

Depression; the remaining 30 were not. Pearson et al. evaluated cognitive status with the MMSE and functional status with a report by a family member on the ability of the patient to carry out activities of daily living (dressing, cooking, cleaning, etc.). Those with depression were found to be less impaired, as reflected by the MMSE, on cognitive functioning. Using a statistical technique to control for cognitive status, Pearson et al. report that there was an effect on the degree of functional impairment. They conclude that the treatment and alleviation of the symptoms of depression might have positive effects on the quality of activities of daily living.

The positive effects of treatment have been noted by others. Kral and Emery (1989), for example, identified a sample of 44 older persons who were experiencing DOD. They were treated intensively for their depression. As the symptoms ameliorated, cognitive competencies returned to their level before the episodes began. The sample was seen again at 6-month intervals over a time period that lasted from 4 to 18 years, with an average of 8 years. For some individuals, there was recurrence of depression at some point, but treatment again was successful. What makes this study applicable to the discussion here is that, eventually, 39 (89%) of the sample were diagnosed as dementia of the Alzheimer type. Perhaps there is a case to be made for the probability that DOD, if followed carefully, may be a marker or precursor of a true dementia.

A study by Goldwasser, Auerbach, and Harkins (1987) used behavioral interventions to test their effects with depression. Their sample of 27 nursing home residents diagnosed as demented was divided into three subgroups: Nine of them received reminiscence group therapy, another nine were given supportive group therapy, whereas the other nine had no treatment. The first of these interventions is based on the use of life review, where the participant expresses feelings about her or his life as death is approaching (see Chapter Ten for a more complete description). In some instances, the review is reflected in nostalgia and some regrets, whereas at some times it may be stressful, with anxiety, guilt, and depression being major elements. Though its qualities therapeutically have not been well investigated (Blazer, 1982, p. 203), it is popular in some institutional settings as a means of reinforcing feelings of self-worth. Supportive group therapy, in turn, is based on the support provided by group members for the need of the person to express feelings and to be received in a nonthreatening and nonjudgmental way. Although solutions frequently are not possible, it is presumed that the speaker does feel the psychological relief that accompanies confronting and admitting difficulties.

All subjects were administered the MMSE, a depression scale, and an index of activities of daily living. Self-reports on depression were positive for the reminiscence group as compared with the support group approach or no treatment, but no effects on cognitive or behavioral functioning were found. Essentially, the gains made must be judged on feelings and mood rather than on physical or intellectual changes.

In determining the presence or absence of depression with dementia, one technique is to identify a sample diagnosed as demented and then determine the existence, if any, of depressive symptoms. Lazarus, Newton, Cohler, Lesser, and Schweon (1987) followed this procedure with 44 persons presumed to have primary degenerative dementia. A control group of 42 individuals of about the same age was compared with them on a depression rating scale (the Hamilton Rating Scale for Depression) and a clinical assessment–geriatric scale. They found that the patient group had significantly higher scores than the control group on items of the scales that reflect depressed mood, anxiety, and feelings of helplessness, hopelessness, and worthlessness. Differences in vegetative symptoms of depression were not significant. They suggest that professionals should be alert to depressive symptoms in patients with primary degenerative dementia.

Depression in Caregivers

The demands and burdens of caregiving must inevitably take a toll on the caregiver. In most instances of dementia in the elderly, this will usually mean a spouse or a middle-aged child. As the patient shows greater and greater deterioration and dependence, the "wear and tear" on the family is tremendous. There may be reports of physical exhaustion because of lack of sleep, accompanied by feelings of loss of control, lack of resources, and need for respite. Psychological exhaustion is just as likely as irritability occurs, followed by guilt and some mixture of love and hate. Such conditions include symptoms of depression, and a Major Depressive Episode would not be unexpected. The dementia has thus had its effects on at least one other party and has begun a ripple effect that probably will not end during the lifetime of the patient. The need for respite and support cannot be overstated if the caregiver is to cope effectively. The study of depression in caregiving therefore normally includes some attention to coping methods, education, and support systems.

All caregivers do not necessarily develop emotional problems, including depression. Men, perhaps because they are more apt to find respite through a job or by hiring assistance, less frequently participate in support groups and other aids to mental health. However, the prevalence of dementia, the intensity of the problems, and the changing structure of families will eventually require many caregivers of either sex to make alternate arrangements, probably nursing home care, for the patient.

The incidence of depression in caregivers has not received the attention it may deserve, but some information is available. Lichtenberg and Barth (1989) interviewed 70 older spouse caregivers and followed-up with a second interview of 40 of them. They found that, using the Geriatric Depression Scale (Brink, Yesavage, Lum, Heersema, Adey, & Rose, 1982; Yesavage, Brink, Rose, Lum, Huang, Adey, & Leirer, 1983) and the Hypochondriasis scale from the Minnesota Multiphasic Personality Inventory, about half the original sample showed evidence of mental health problems. The follow-up indicated an increase to 66% during the earlier periods after caregiving ended. Apparently, some caregivers adapt because the percentage of mental health problems disclosed by the measures dropped to 33% after longer postcaregiving experience.

Dura, Haywood-Niler, and Kiecolt-Glaser (1990) surveyed "distress" in caregivers of SDAT patients, where they hypothesized that distress would be a primary component, and in caregivers of Parkinson's disease, where they thought distress would be a secondary component. There were 23 spousal caregivers in each group compared to a control group ($N = 23$). They used two measures of depression, to quantify distress, and found that both caregiver groups showed evidence of greater depression than the control group. The two were comparable in the amount of distress expressed, which might be interpreted to mean that whether depression is primary or secondary is of little significance to its effects.

Whether interventions will assist the caregiver is an issue that has been seldom tested. The study by Mohide et al. (1990) described earlier in this chapter was just such an attempt. Unfortunately, the assists provided to caregivers did not affect levels of depression or anxiety. The authors did gather some evidence that supports the idea that caregivers felt better about their lives and were able to tolerate demands a bit better (shown through the longer period of care before institutionalization). They perceived their roles in caring for the patient as less difficult. Such results are tenuous but are typical of outcomes with such interventions as these.

A large sample of caregiving spouses ($N = 318$) was sampled by Moritz, Kasl, and Berkman (1989) with somewhat surprising results. All patients were living at home, and the sample consisted only of persons over age 65. Their results indicated that where wives had the dementia, there was a significant relationship with symptoms of depression in the husband. By contrast, where the husband was the demented member, there was only a small correlation with depressive symptomatology in the wives. This would suggest that women may be better able to tolerate the effects of dementia even if unable to escape some of the burdens. Moritz et al. note also that whether the spouse, male or female, participated in social events depended largely on the cognitive abilities remaining to the patient. It seems that the relationship between wives' loss of competencies and the husbands' depressive symptoms was most affected by the availability of financial resources from relatives and friends as perceived by the husband.

The ability of the caregiver to cope effectively is enhanced by access to resources available or provided to that individual. Haley, Levine, Brown, and Bartolucci (1987) report that caregiver appraisal of problems, coping responses, social support, and activity were significant predictors of whether the caregiver developed depressive symptoms, and their attitudes held toward life and health. There was no one pattern that would be successful for all caregivers; in fact, their analysis indicated great diversity in individual patterns of appraisal and coping. There was also wide difference in what constituted both the amount of social support and activity and the types utilized. Overall, however, Haley et al. advocate developing some model of stress and coping in caregiving in order to assist the caregiver in dealing with stress.

Support groups for caregivers have been and are popular in this country. The effectiveness of such groups is not certain because they vary widely in purpose, size, frequency of meetings, content of meetings, and competency of the facilitator or therapist. Haley, Brown, and Levine (1987a) found that such groups seemed to have little effect on depression, life satisfaction, social support, or coping behaviors. Yet, caregivers did report positive attitudes toward the group meetings and rated the groups as "quite helpful." Such a result signifies that attitude is the major variable affected. The therapeutic efficacy would seem to be quite limited also. Perhaps the caregiver feels some relief by the mere act of attending a session designed to "help" in some abstract way. Perhaps there is a certain amount of appreciation that someone cares enough to conduct such meetings. Perhaps there is some effect from the realization that others also have great stress.

Ancillary Effects and Dementia

Both dementia and depression may show expressions from brain function in ways that will permit discrete measurement and prediction.

For example, Reynolds, Kupfer, Houck, Hoch, Stark, Berman, and Zimmer (1988) measured sleep patterns in 67 depressed persons without dementia, 49 with probable DAT, 42 with depression and dementia, and 77 controls. Ages ranged from 49 to 89. They report that depressed patients could be discriminated from demented ones on four measures: REM (rapid eye movement) sleep percentage that was higher in depressives; NREM (non-rapid eye movement) sleep percentage that was higher in dementia; REM sleep latency that was lower in depressives; and sleep maintenance or early morning awakening that was higher in depressives. For those clearly depressed only or demented only, the pattern correctly identified about 80%. Classification functions derived for nondemented depressives and nondepressed demented subjects were applied to a group with mixed symptoms (N = 42). Overall, 27 of these patients (64%) with either pseudo-dementia or dementia with depression were classified correctly using the same four predictor variables. Hoch, Reynolds, Kupfer, Houck, Berman, and Stack (1986) had already obtained data that indicated a higher percentage of nonrapid eye movement for AD patients where apnea (difficulty or irregularity in breathing while asleep) was present. What is more important is that they report a greater presence of sleep-disordered breathing in Alzheimer's patients but not in elderly depressed persons or those with mixed depression and cognitive impairment. Among the AD patients, those who were apnea-positive spent less time in sleep than those who were apnea-negative. There was a significant positive relationship between the apnea index and the severity of the dementia. Those with AD who were apnea-positive had a higher NREM sleep percentage also.

There have been other variables that might influence or might reflect the dementia/depression complex. Emery and Breslau (1989), for example, have reported a study where language processing was investigated in SDAT patients, nondemented persons with depression, and a control group. The samples were fairly small (Ns of 23, 20, and 20); the mean ages were all in their 70s. The authors used measures of aphasia and syntax to investigate language processing. The depressed patients performed on most tasks at a significantly better level than the dementia patients. They also displayed better language-processing skills on certain tasks. However, they performed at a significantly lower level than the controls on 3 of the 11 measures that were used. The important element for these latter differences seemed to be complexity of task. Emery and Breslau suggest that their findings may mean that, where language deficits occur in Major Depression, there may be some organic reason just as there is in dementia. The possibilities are intriguing when we consider the relationships with neurotransmitters discussed earlier and some results from a few studies yet to be described.

In this regard, Gilles, Ryckaert, de Mol, de Maertelaere, and Mendle-wicz (1989) analyzed the actions of the chemical clonidine on growth-hormone-using elderly depressives (N = 6, ages 64–81) and persons with SDAT (N = 8, ages 70–81). Gilles et al. report no differences in the effects of the chemical on the two groups. They conclude that, in combination with results from studies by others on secretion of growth hormone in SDAT, there is an accentuation of the effects of aging on reaction to growth hormone for patients with the dementia.

Consolidating findings from different fields, even when investigating the same major variable, is both difficult and dangerous. However, there should be some awareness of the *variety* of research that is being conducted relative to dementia, its effects, and some of its associations. With increases in knowledge through controlled data collection, the current picture of dementia will be more complete and more useful. At present, those involved most directly with the effects of the condition, including the patients, their caregivers, and the professionals, are forced to contend with a plethora of problems with only limited knowledge. It is encouraging to think that the situation may be changing for the better, although the research efforts are still too restricted.

SUICIDE

Major depression may have a fearful consequence beyond its inherent misery—ending one's life. In fact, suicide is 20 times more likely in depressed individuals than in the population at large (Kermis, 1986, p. 200). The highest rate for suicide is found in white males over age 65, and the incidence is greatest in persons over age 60 regardless of sex or race. Blazer (1982, p. 34) reports that 23% of all suicides occurred in those over age 60, though this group was only 18.5% of the total population using 1975 figures. More recently, the data for 1986 indicate that there are 21.6 suicides per 100,000 for those over age 65, whereas the overall rate is 12.8. Such figures in all probability are underestimates because they represent cases classified under a specific definition. Blazer (1982, p. 34) quotes Stengel in this regard: A suicidal act is any deliberate act of self damage which the person committing the act could not be sure to survive. In most instances, this is interpreted to mean sudden and volatile acts, but there are many ways to cause one's death, and the elderly may practice more of them than even the statistics reflect (Zarit, 1980, p. 227).

Whatever the definition and classification scheme, the depression that so often accompanies the early development of a dementia would seem to imply a need to investigate the incidence of suicide among demented persons. At the same time, the diagnostic criteria used by physicians should be expanded to include detection of suicidal potential (Shamoian, 1985). Where there is concurrent depression, the treatment used must be considered for its relationship to suicide. Gerner (1987), for example, has described the advantages of the use of the antidepressant Trazodone, including its extremely low relationship to incidence of suicide.

In the literature on aging, there is more service to the potential for danger than there is to an investigation and discussion of incidence. Charatan (1985) includes reference to "problems involving suicide" among a variety of other topics. Gurland and Cross (1982) make a case for the association of mental disorders in the elderly with such outcomes as suicide. Alerting professionals to such possible relationships is essential, but there needs to be data that document the problem and its extent. There is a particular paucity of studies of suicide among those with dementia.

Pierce (1987) has published a survey of 145 cases involving what he calls "deliberate self-harm." These occurred over a 12-year period and were collected from a district general hospital in Wales. Among the elderly, he found no differences in "self-harm" between the sexes in the local population. However, the male to female ratio of hospitalized cases of self-harm was 1:1.5. Over 90% of the hospitalized had symptoms of depression, and 3% had been diagnosed with some form of dementia. In only about 10% had there been earlier attempts at self-harm. The relationship between self-destructive behavior and depression (90%) is consistent with estimates. Because only cases seen in a hospital setting were included, we may be seeing only the tip of the iceberg, at that.

The available literature on dementia and/or caregiving and suicide attempts/successes is disappointing. Indeed, our knowledge about suicide in the general population needs to be increased. The problem is a major one, not only for individuals but for society at large. The need for research is manifest.

DELUSIONAL IDEATION AND BEHAVIOR

The DSM-III-R describes Delusional Disorder (called Paranoid Disorder in earlier DSMs) as being demonstrated in a persistent but nonbizarre delusion (DSM-III-R, 1987, p. 199). The delusion is a false belief that persists despite evidence to the contrary. The individual with this disorder then interprets reality in ways that are consonant with the delusion. The delusion is usually restricted to only a narrow portion of one's life, so that in most aspects the person does not differ from others. The individual may feel persecuted or demonstrate morbid jealousy or grandiosity, for example. Although such a condition might not seem pertinent to the evolution of dementia, it is clear that some patients will react to the changes they are encountering with misinterpretations that may be labeled *delusional*, and often the theme is paranoid (persecutory).

Even if the relationship between a developing dementia and delusional behavior is slight, there is the possibility for misunderstanding by caregiver and family members. Part of the education provided (in whatever form and by whomever) should include the awareness that some delusional thinking may occur. The symptoms and types should be explained, so that caregivers may be able to identify such behavior and report it to appropriate professionals for treatment. Where other family members are available and involved in contact with the patient, they must be prepared for understanding patient behavior (see Schmidt, 1989, for a discussion of the approach in its general contexts).

Proulx and Campbell (1986) have described a case study where a 78-year-old male with MID suffered apparent paranoia. A behavioral program was established with the caregiver, and appropriate interventions were instituted. The authors report that there were significant changes in both confused and paranoid behaviors.

However, even in the limited literature available, there is not agreement that paranoia may accompany dementia. Brink, Carter, Janson, Love, Menn, and Peratis (1985) compared paranoid and nonparanoid elderly on a test for dementia. The task involved recognition to assess short-term memory. Paranoids had slightly lower scores, but the differences were not significant, even statistically. As a result, the authors argue that there is no case to be made for a correlation between dementia and paranoia, at least with their data. Perhaps, they say, paranoia may represent a defense mechanism against the losses of old age and, as such, occur as a part of many mental disorders. This argument does not preclude the possibility that a dementia patient may develop paranoid adjustments to the radical changes occurring in life.

SUMMARY

Dementia is reflected in the loss of mental competencies of a patient. At the same time, there can be psychological effects that are debilitating in their own right, though they may be treatable, even reversible. These effects may occur both for patient and caregiver, and include anxiety, depression and suicide, and paranoid behaviors.

The survey of literature on these topics is not evenly distributed. There are many books and articles on depression as it may accompany the dementing process and as it affects patient behavior. Similarly, the burdens of caregivers may be antecedents of depressive episodes so that a considerable literature is available here as well. What is surprising is that little attention has been paid to suicide in patients and caregivers. Until more data are available, the topic remains open.

Anxiety is such a common occurrence that it should be expected in conditions where dementia exists. In this case, the less common, generalized state is more often reported for both patients and caregivers. Such states occur earlier in the process for patients and seem to be an inverted U-shaped function for caregivers. More precise attention to anxiety as such would seem warranted.

There is a chance that delusional behavior, particularly in patients at some period of the decline in competence, should be relatively common. If so, investigation of incidence, effects, and interventions is needed. Unfortunately, very little study has been done and, where done, there is some debate about its prevalence and meaning.

CHAPTER SEVEN

Dementia and the Patient—I

The conditions that produce demented behavior in older persons were described briefly in Chapter One. A more detailed and precise examination is necessary to appreciate the distinctions and similarities that are known at this time as well as the relationships that may be assumed between diagnostic label and both current and future behavioral outcomes. For this purpose, we will return to each of the several syndromes (Alzheimer's disease, Multiinfarct Dementia, Pick's disease, Creutzfeldt–Jakob disease, Huntington's Chorea, Parkinson's disease, and normal pressure hydrocephalus). For each, the extant literature will be surveyed for cause, course, and outcomes. Finally, the research on drug intervention in progress (almost totally being conducted for Alzheimer's disease) will be examined and evaluated. Much of the material in this chapter will reflect our knowledge (and lack of it) about Alzheimer's, primarily because this is where the research efforts have been focused but also because medical diagnosis most often uses the label. In this sense, then, Alzheimer's disease (AD) stands as the prototype or model for the various causes of dementia. This role accords with the fact that AD is considered most prevalent and, to a lesser extent, to the demonstration of accuracy of diagnosis at autopsy.

The former—prevalence—must receive reserved judgment if Katzman (1985, p. 13) may be generalized. He reports that, when stringent diagnostic criteria are employed (such as the DSM-III-R), the likelihood of a correct diagnosis, confirmed by histological data, will be about 90%. The problem is that many patients will not meet such criteria. For 100 consecutive cases referred for evaluation for dementia, he found that 55 seemed to be probable cases of Alzheimer's, but only 32 actually met the criteria. The remaining 23 persons were described as presenting "unusual clinical features" ($N = 11$) or a coexistent disease that could produce dementia that was treatable ($N = 12$). In the latter case, treatment should resolve the dementia, but that outcome did not occur for these cases.

The second reason for using Alzheimer's as the prototype—accuracy of diagnosis at autopsy—involves two dimensions. In the first, the issue is one of assuring that the diagnosis is confirmed. In most instances, as much as 90% accuracy has been claimed (Katzman, 1985, p. 18). Some studies have not agreed with such a high probability, with error rates at autopsy reported between 10% and 30%. For the second dimension, one must be concerned about the percentage of cases diagnosed as "dementia" that are, in the specific case, Alzheimer's. Swash, Smith, and Hart (1985, p. 1) report that about 70% of the cases examined postmortem (sample size not stated) where dementia had been diagnosed have been shown to be Alzheimer's alone or in combination with vascular disease. Though one might wish even greater accuracy, the results are still impressive. They would seem to support a position that the syndrome does stand as a prototype, both in terms of diagnostic frequency and in terms of accuracy.

Dementia remains, however, as a more comprehensive concept that includes but is not restricted solely to Alzheimer's disease. This position is in accord with that of Pearce and Flowers (1985, pp. 19–23). They point out that definitions used for a term like *dementia* tend to reflect the disciplinary preference of the individual. This allows some differences in meaning that may confuse laypersons and even professionals. Further, they note that several of the terms employed in describing (or defining) the concept are debatable in their application. For example, these authors cite the "irreversibility" often included in a definition of dementia and point out that there are sufficient exceptions such that the term *irreversible* should not be included. As yet another example, they propose that the equation of Alzheimer's disease with dementia rules out other disorders and is not helpful. With similar rationales, they discuss the problems involved with other popular descriptors: "progressive," "decline in intelligence," and "global." The solution, they believe, is in precision and detail, and so they separate primary and secondary factors in dementia (Pearce & Flowers, 1985, p. 23). The primary factors are structural, cognitive, and behavioral, whereas the secondary ones are medical and social (see Figure 7.1 for an adaptation of their schema). Even so, they advocate that still other variables should be included in order to permit more rigorous research to be conducted. Such additions would include premorbid personality traits as well as environmental and personal conditions affecting the status and well-being of the patient, both from past history and the present.

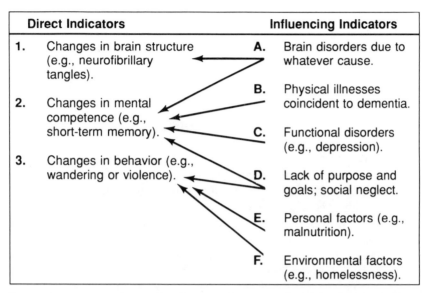

Direct Indicators	Influencing Indicators
1. Changes in brain structure (e.g., neurofibrillary tangles).	A. Brain disorders due to whatever cause.
2. Changes in mental competence (e.g., short-term memory).	B. Physical illnesses coincident to dementia.
	C. Functional disorders (e.g., depression).
3. Changes in behavior (e.g., wandering or violence).	D. Lack of purpose and goals; social neglect.
	E. Personal factors (e.g., malnutrition).
	F. Environmental factors (e.g., homelessness).

FIGURE 7.1. Primary and secondary factors in dementia. Adapted from Pearce & Flowers (1985). Reprinted by permission of Karger, Basel, Switzerland.

Caird (1985) has advocated that even the term dementia itself presents problems already recognized in concepts like "senile" or "arteriosclerotic." Because such terms may become stereotypic, he proposes, instead, the label *brain failure* as an alternative to this terminology. Further, this alternative will fit with other physical conditions (such as respiratory failure) that have been coined to represent processes rather than static conditions, with the possibility that progression may or may not occur. One benefit is that acute and chronic brain failure may present with different symptomatology. The greatest gain, he feels, is that the notion of irreversibility would no longer be a necessary component. He does admit to problems with the term, a major one being that physicians are comfortable with current diagnostic labels and are not apt to change easily. Further, the concept must be expanded to include behaviors, a function not consistently found with medical conditions like respiratory failure. His proposal may eventually be employed; at present, it serves primarily to restrain our too-ready acceptance of medical, psychiatric, and psychological labels that lack evidence of credence at times and at others are overly inclusive.

Resolution of such issues is not at hand, and so this text will continue with the use of "dementia" to represent the outcomes of the several medical syndromes that produce the systematic and deleterious changes noted in patients. As mentioned previously, cause and prognosis, course, and outcomes will be described, as well as is known at present, for each of the causative syndromes.

ALZHEIMER'S DISEASE

The history of the condition labeled "Alzheimer's disease" (AD) is restricted to the twentieth century. Although there can be no doubt that a dementia due to this causative agent must have had a prior—and probably long—history, the recognition of a specific syndrome occurred only with the observation of Alois Alzheimer, a German neuropathologist. Fields (1985, pp. 12–17) has described the history of vascular disease and dementia beginning with the seminal compendium on psychiatric disorders published by Kraepelin in 1883. Alzheimer enters the picture in 1899, with a citation in which he proposed that there was the possibility of a "noninfarct dementia" that also was due to vascular disease but involving arterioles rather than arteries. His proposal generated no interest or acceptance at the time.

In 1906, Alzheimer presented a paper that made a more definitive case for a presenile dementia that was due to a disease process of the neurons. He demonstrated his position with data from microscopic study of brain tissue of two women patients of his who had developed severe dementia in their 50s and who had died at a relatively early age. Alzheimer maintained that there was a distinctive disease process responsible for such senility at such a time period in life. Kraepelin accepted and noted the position in 1912, and the label "Alzheimer's disease" was accepted for those cases where neuronal deterioration was involved (Fields, 1985, p. 13). The principal evidence cited by Alzheimer was the accumulation of neurofibrillary tangles in cell bodies. He believed these were unique to the condition he described but, since then, such alterations have been found to be present in other syndromes. Indeed, a complicating factor is that tangles are found in brain cells of older persons who have led seemingly normal and dementia-free lives. Nevertheless, the point had been made that, at least in presenile dementia, there were certain instances that illustrated that healthy neurons may be altered in a systematic way that affects the behavioral competencies of the person and produces mental changes expected only in the very old. These "changes" principally include memory inadequacy but also confusion and disorientation.[1] However, his proposal did not lead to any emphasis about this possibility within the medical community even though a few cases were reported over the next four decades. In fact, the syndrome reached prominence only as there was the notable increase in the number of aging persons in our society and increasing complaints about problems they were experiencing. Among those problems were cases like those reported by Alzheimer, but in *those who were in their 70s and 80s and beyond.* This led not only to increasing recognition of cases where mental competencies seemed to decrease with age but also to differential labeling. There was the distinction, first, between presenile and senile dementia; then there was the separation of Alzheimer's disease and senile dementia of the Alzheimer's type (SDAT). Such distinctions may not have great importance, ultimately, when we consider the devastation in the lives of patients and caregivers that results from the consequences, regardless of how labeled. Fisk (1981, p. 45) has noted that there may be only a single disease, showing itself in a few cases during middle age and in many more patients in old age. The former may be called presenile dementia (or Alzheimer's disease) and the latter senile dementia (or senile dementia, Alzheimer's type), but he seems to opt for the general label of Alzheimer's disease for both, apparently based upon the position that they are the same disease. The argument is appealing, though increasing suggestions that AD may be more than one syndrome after all compel some degree of caution.

Whatever the ultimate designation, the effects on the structure of the brain are seemingly clear. Pfeiffer (1978, p. 171) describes the brain as the "organ of adaptation." There is cell destruction throughout life, but this occurrence should not put the person at risk, of course, given the large number of neurons. However, as Pfeiffer says, the remaining cells are at greater risk to adverse influences, particularly in old age. Perhaps this is the reason that the probabilities of AD increase with advancing years: The disease process finds a brain that has less integrity and is thereby more susceptible to adverse influences than was true at younger ages.[2] The problem results, not from age as such, but from an aging body that puts more stress on all its components. As Pfieffer has said so succinctly: "The healthy older brain is like a man walking along the edge of a cliff: he remains quite safe and intact in the absence of any disturbing influence" (1978, p. 171).

Those persons autopsied with a diagnosis of SDAT show general atrophy and loss of nerve cells. As many as half of the cells may be affected in certain parts of the brain, with the possibility of a 70% loss in the most severe cases (Fisk, 1981, p. 46). Generally, the brain is atrophied (i.e., there has been shrinkage of tissue mass as compared with normal expectations), particularly in the frontal and temporal lobes.

This leads to greater spacing between the brain folds and increased ventricular fluid. The meaning of the atrophy is not clear, especially because the brains of persons who have not had SDAT show similar atrophy.

Microscopic examination of brain cells has revealed two characteristic findings in SDAT patients. First, there are bundles of proteinlike material, called neurofibrillary tangles, in the cell bodies (see Iqbal, Grunde-Iqbal, & Wisniewski, 1985, pp. 98–105, for the biochemical properties). Second, there will be neuritic plaques in the cytoplasm of the cell. The plaque is composed of amyloid, a starchlike substance (see Kidd, Allsop, & Landon, 1985, pp. 114–126, for a histopathological description). Both conditions are found with other syndromes leading to dementia, as well as in cells of "normal" aging persons but to a lesser degree (Fisk, 1981, p. 48). In the hippocampus, there may be found a further evidence of degeneration in the cells. Given the fact that such cellular changes occur in several syndromes producing dementia and even in normally aging people, Fisk (1981, p. 48) has noted that "Although much has been done to elucidate the ultrastructure of the brains of patients with senile dementia, and there are findings that indicate that this is probably a distinct disease entity, the exact meaning of these neurofibrillary tangles and senile plaques is unknown."

Cause and Prognosis

The cause of AD is not understood at the present time, which dictates that research efforts must take several directions, including any that offer a promise of describing, ultimately, a specific cause. Wisniewski, Merz, and Carp (1985, p. 45) propose three distinct possibilities. The first is aluminum, based upon the finding of accumulation of large amounts of the metal in sufficient quantities to be toxic. There is evidence to support the conclusion that high amounts of aluminum can interfere with mental competence, but these authors believe the evidence does not support the position that aluminum *causes* SDAT. The second is a genetic explanation. There are limited data to support such a predisposition, but Wisniewski et al. also state that the evidence is insufficient to accept it as the cause of SDAT.

Finally, they point to an infectious agent, similar to the kind involved in Creutzfeldt–Jakob disease. This explanation seems most viable to them, and they present a defense, based on scientific data currently available, for their choice.

Others involved in research do not accept the conclusions of Wisniewski et al. so completely. Whalley, Wright, and St. Clair (1985, pp. 18–31) have surveyed the literature on the connection with Down's syndrome and find some similarities, particularly for cases of presenile dementia. Down's syndrome (at one time called "mongolism" from some of the physical attributes of the condition) is known to be associated with a genetic error; specifically, a trisomy on Chromosome 21. With improved conditions for longevity, Down's patients who at one time rarely lived beyond age 30 are, in increasing numbers, living to be older. This event has led to descriptions of a relatively large percentage of cases of dementia in the aging Down's person. The fact that aging persons without Down's also show increases in the percentage with SDAT has led to speculation and research on a genetic factor as a cause of AD. Whalley et al. caution that there is only "a superficial similarity to the degenerative changes found in Alzheimer's disease" (p. 25) in terms of the shared disposition toward loss of dendrites. As a result, they propose that a different mechanism is involved in the two conditions. Though far from certain, there is the possibility that DNA damage provides a stronger clue to the relationship. Butler (1990, pp. 933–934) states that AD seems to have a genetic cause in about 50% of the cases, the other 50% being due to "sporadic" etiology. Miller (1977, p. 9) agrees that relatives of those who develop senile dementia are at higher risk of showing the same effects, but the mechanisms involved are not yet known. Overall, the evidence for a genetic cause of SDAT is far from compelling at the same time that there are sufficient data to require continuing investigation.

Yet another "connection" that may lead to evidence of causation is the relationship to neurotransmitters. The millions of neurons throughout the body are independent of each other in the sense that they do not touch. A small gap—the synapse—occurs from the axonal ending of one cell to the dendritic section of another. The electrical signal that represents a "message" of sensation to be interpreted in the brain (or spinal cord) must make its way through the appropriate cells to the site where it can be translated and a reaction dictated. This system, which is complex and only partially understood, depends upon appropriate relationships: healthy cells, adequate dendrites and axons, and a chemical to assist the passage of the signal across the synapse. This chemical, the neurotransmitter, is secreted at the axonal part of the cell. It attaches to the receiving portion of the synapse and acts either to assist transmission across the synapse (excitatory) or to prevent it (inhibitory). There are a number of neurotransmitters, but in the discussion of AD, the important one seems to be acetylcholine (ACh). ACh assists the nerve impulse in transmission to another cell in a sequence. Under normal circumstances, the chemical is present as needed at the axonal ending. However, there must be a counterbalance because almost constant firing would be detrimental to the cell. An enzyme called cholinesterase that destroys acetylcholine is present. The balance is delicate, and for most of us, there is never a problem of imbalance, and so we can act with assurance and efficiency. If there is a reduction in ACh, the relative roles are changed: Cholinesterase becomes more dominant. Current drug research is focused on both chemicals. On the one hand, a drug is sought that will increase ACh to a level that restores the balance with cholinesterase. On the other, a chemical may be developed that suppresses cholinesterase so that the ACh that is present, despite its diminished quantity, will have a better chance to express itself.

With AD, an insufficiency of acetylcholine at the synapses has been found. *Why* this insufficiency occurs is not known, and it has become the basis of research efforts in the belief that discovery of the cause may help define AD itself. For example, if there is insufficient acetylcholine, it may be due to the role of cholinesterase. There have even been attempts to bolster the amount of acetylcholine available to diseased brain cells by means of a pump placed in the chest cavity. To date, such efforts have not been successful because the brain will not take up an artificial substitute for acetylcholine as it will for certain other neurotransmitters. The present status of the relationship of neurotransmitters to AD is still essentially exploratory. (For more detailed discussion and description, see, e.g., Reinikainen, Soininen, Kosma, Halonen, Jolkkonen, & Riekkinen 1985, pp. 184–197; Rosser, Mountjoy, Roth, and Reynolds, 1985, pp. 198–212; Bowen, Davison, Francis, Palmer, & Pearce, 1985, pp. 156–174).

As is apparent, the attempts to discover the cause of AD are diverse and basic. Although there may be a major breakthrough in the near future, the chances are greater that we are still years away from success. It is important to continue the search because only as the cause is known can prevention be assured. Eventually, society should like to insure that no person need fear the destruction of AD, just as society wishes to prevent cancer, heart disease, or any other condition threatening the well-being of citizens. Without prevention, the search must be for cure or, more realistically, for stabilization and control of the effects of the syndrome. These are also matters under investigation that we will consider at the end of the next chapter. Given the lack of knowledge of cause and the inability to prevent, prognosis for the AD patient is poor. Over some period of time, differing from person to person, there will be continued and gradual degeneration in mental competences until the patient is totally dependent on a caregiver. As the brain has less and less integrity, there will be an inability to receive and deal with .stimulation so that the person begins to manifest physical deterioration as well. Death results from more conventional causes in the elderly, such as pneumonia, and is only indirectly due to the disease itself.

Course

As stated, the course of AD is a degenerative one. In terms of neurons, there is increasing invasion and destruction of cells throughout the brain, though the hippocampus is apparently the first focal area involved. Memory loss, specifically for recent events, is frequently reported as the first "sign" of a problem. With time, greater memory loss accrues, and there is a lack of ability to deal with ordinary aspects of life, indicating continuing effect on the hippocampus with spread to cells in the association areas as well.

Such general description must be made because the course of the *effect* of the disease—dementia—is irregular in its presentation and expression from one patient to another. Yet, there have been attempts to specify "stages" in the process, tied to developmental events. Butler (1990, pp. 934–935) has described such a model, but with the strong caution that "*there is great variability and the progression of stages often is not as orderly as the . . . description implies.*" With this caveat, he details some three such degrees. The "early stage" is a pronounced loss for recent memories. This has its effects upon the ability to deal with new events as they occur, much to the distress of the patient and of the caregiver.

As this "early stage" continues, the patient may find greater difficulty in successfully carrying out even routine tasks that have never before posed a real problem. This may induce irritation and hostility, with subsequent lashing out at the environment and family members. As Butler points out, however, the social skills of the patient are much less affected and she or he may interact with friends and neighbors, even strangers, in a way that seems normal. This can confuse and frustrate the caregiver who now may feel that she or he is living with a Jekyll and Hyde personality.

The "intermediate stage" reflects continued and increased losses in mental competence. Now the patient is unable to deal effectively with any new demands or tasks. The amount of confusion and orientation becomes pronounced, and the person may not even be able to remember specifics of well-rehearsed behaviors. For example, even if the patient remembers the location of the bathroom, she or he may not be able to remember where one urinates while in the bathroom. Is it the lavatory, the commode, the bathtub, the waste basket? Under the pressure for relief, any of these may be used for the purpose. The effects on the caregiver, who is faced with unpredictable events and consequent demanding chores, can be intense.

Gradually, too, there will be losses for more remote memories. The patient may be able to recall several specific events while other memories are no longer available. As a result, the individual will rehearse those well-remembered ones over and over, apparently without awareness of the repetition or the lack of continuity with other life events. At this point, dependency becomes greater. The caregiver has to provide more and more supervision; sometimes, she or he must even perform the needed action. For example, if the patient is to be bathed, the caregiver must assist as though dealing with a child. Dressing may become a chore because the patient not only may not remember to put on underwear *under* outer clothing (and not vice versa) but may even utilize the clothing of the caregiver if not properly supervised. Caregivers must become alert and anticipate a variety of potential problems under these circumstances. The awareness of reality may be lost, and the patient may wander aimlessly or deny knowledge of family members or resist any attempts at assistance. Orientation in time and place is likely to be very poor, if present at all.

The "severe stage" reduces the patient to the level of an infant in at least some respects. There is no memory for how to walk, or to talk, or to realize the correct actions to be continent. Memory may be so altered that the patient may not even be able to swallow, with an adverse effect on nutrition. It is possible now for the disease that is called "the old person's friend" to occur—pneumonia, leading to death. Almost certainly, there will be malnutrition, and there may be other physical consequences. The patient is totally dependent.

The problem with attempting to specify stages has two aspects. First, there is the confounding of disease with outcome. What part of each stage represents a progression of the syndrome and what part is exemplification of the outcomes associated with dementia is difficult to discriminate. Second, there is the implication that the course of AD and its outcome, dementia, is a regular one with clearly differentiated developments and discrete sets of behaviors. Even when disclaimers are given, as Butler has done, there is a tendency to ignore the warnings and ascribe greater validity to the stages than they deserve. Caregivers often ask about progression; they would like to know what to expect and when to expect it. Honesty requires admitting to ignorance about a pattern and explaining only in generalities. Experience has shown that more often, however, some stage model will be presented and treated as though it were valid. The consequent effect, more often than not, is that caregivers find the model inadequate, and they may question the competencies of the professional who has informed them about it.

There may be, of course, some regular events or changes that can be documented. Research that attempts to chart such changes is available, although there is some marked discordance in procedures and results. To demonstrate the state of knowledge about regularity and patterns, a brief survey of such studies is worthwhile.

As described in Chapter Four, technology is an increasing part of the diagnostic procedure. One of the benefits of this technology is to allow disclosure of systematic changes identified by the technique. Due to the nature of the technology, the changes demonstrated will be structural, not behavioral. Nevertheless, the findings are pertinent to our understanding of the progression in AD. Thus Stigsby (1988) examined electroencephalographic (EEG) readings for patients with AD and found slowly progressing abnormalities in the brain-wave patterns. Generally, these fit with the usual finding of a diffuse atrophy in the cortex of patients. So far as the use of computerized axial tomography (CT or CAT) is concerned, Benson (1984) reports that Alzheimer's does not have a distinct scan pattern. On the other hand, positron emission tomography (PET) has disclosed rather clear patterns for several disorders and, in particular, has shown the decreases that occur in cerebral blood flow and glucose metabolism in demented persons. Benson believes too little has been done with magnetic resonance imaging (MRI) to take a definitive stand but that the procedure has great potential and may yield the most valuable results.

The potential for diagnostic differentiation with such techniques is encouraged by reports such as that of Kamo, McGeer, Harrop, McGeer, Kalne, Martin, and Pate (1987). They did pre- and postmortem examinations of a 75-year-old man with severe dementia. Among their techniques was the use of PET scans. With this patient, it appeared possible to identify a pattern distinctive enough to discriminate Alzheimer's from Pick's disease *premortem.* More extensive use is necessary, of course, but the promise warrants the effort. In neither condition is intervention possible at present, but the ability to make more accurate diagnosis of cause is a progressive step.

Even more encouraging is the study reported by Ihl, Eilles, Frlich, Maurer, Dierks, and Perisic (1989). Using both PET and EEG scans, they examined 15 older persons with probable AD. The results were compared with 15 matched controls. They found distinct differences in patterns, with the possibility of temporoparietal damage in DAT patients as compared with controls. The Alzheimer patients also showed greater activity in the frontal lobe, an outcome that they suggest may indicate that the frontal areas will assume certain functions when other regions experience difficulty. Of course, eventually this action will be overcome as the disease progresses. But it does signify the adaptability of the brain, if substantiated with further study, and underscores the utility of redundancy in the neurons. Ihl et al. also state that certain findings (in this case, increased activity in Beta waves) may be useful as early markers for DAT. This suggestion fits with the research underway to find evidence of measurable physical phenomena that are correlated with later expression of AD. Such signs are called "markers" and could be used to anticipate (and begin intervention and planning) for later disease evidence. Again, the eventual course of the syndrome would not be changed by consistent markers, but many professionals believe that the earlier the condition can be anticipated or identified the more realistic and helpful the various interventions can be—medical, psychological, and social.

The most promising of the new technologies, MRI, has been tested to some degree. Harrell, Callaway, and Sekar (1987), for example, had a sample of seven patients, all between 64 and 78 years of age, who had been found to have primary degenerative dementia (either Alzheimer's or Pick's) based on clinical, laboratory, and CT data. They used MRI with these patients and found additional evidence of infarctions in the white matter of the cerebrum. This intimated to them that MRI may be a useful way to discriminate multiinfarct dementia (MID) from either AD or Pick's, though the procedure will not differentiate the latter two.

As seems evident from this survey of the research, the use of technological advances to assist the diagnostic process and to delineate the structural changes occurring with dementing diseases has only begun. Part of the outcome may well be a systematic charting of the progressive degeneration in specific parts of the brain. As such data accumulate, there will be clearer understanding of the physical properties of the disease that may be correlated with behavioral changes.

Meanwhile, there is continuing research on the structural changes either with or without technology. Such evidence comes from autopsies so that they usually reflect the end stage of the process rather than the developmental one. Nevertheless, such data are helpful.

In the behavioral sphere, studies have been reported that attempt to describe systematically the mental decline that occurs and its relation to dementia. Rinn (1988) makes a case for a generalized, subclinical type of dementia that occurs in all of us as we age. Using data from the WAIS–R, which shows decline with age, and particularly with old age, he speaks of a life-span deterioration that begins during early adulthood. He proposes that such a decline is unrelated to slowing of mental and motor processes or educational disadvantage. Neither is it merely a cohort effect that may or may not be found in future aging generations. Instead, he maintains that there are small pathological changes in the brain due to a variety of conditions (some of which are treatable if detected) that slowly but surely accumulate and produce adverse behavioral effects. If he is correct, all of us must suffer some degree of dementia. The problem becomes one of degree, not of presence or absence. Such a stance also opens the door to a wider view that includes but is not restricted to medical models based on disease processes.

Whether Rinn is correct may be debatable, but there is an empirical relationship implied. The age at which the disease process and consequent dementia begins may be a significant variable in explaining effects and outcomes. In consideration of various diseases, Kontiola, Laaksonen, Sulkava, and Erkinjuntti (1990) found different effects on language impairment for different diagnoses. With a sample of AD patients (N = 33), MID (N = 52) and controls (N = 86), they not only report differences between controls and demented subjects but between types of dementias as well. They suggest that examination of language function may help in differential diagnosis. This study offers some evidence, then, that the type of syndrome has an effect on language capabilities of demented patients.

An important tool for carrying on normal activity is awareness and ability to respond to independent living demands. DeBettignies, Mahurin, and Pirozzolo (1990) examined insight for independent living skills in AD patients (N = 12), MID (N = 12) and normal controls (N = 12). They had both the patient and an informant (say, a caregiver) respond. Comparisons were made between what the patient reported as activity and competence with what the informant reported as the actual occurrence. The Alzheimer's patients showed significantly greater loss of insight than MID patients. There was no relationship with age, education, mental status, or depressive states. However, there was a significant relationship with the degree of burden reported by the caregiver. Thus the less aware the patient becomes, the more burden placed on the caregiver in both the physical and mental sense.

In the residential setting (e.g., a nursing home), behavioral problems are no less likely, usually interfering with independence and adjustment. Taft (1989) has observed the agitation found in the dementia patient. Because it is no longer possible to use the mental competencies of the individual to reduce the agitated behavior, there must be special management techniques, developed on a case by case basis, to help staff. Agitation is a problem not only for control in the nursing home setting but also for the well-being and contentment of the resident. For these reasons, Taft proposes methods that may be legitimately used by personnel.

Just as home caregivers experience increasing burden in dealing with the effects of AD, so staff members develop stress in residential settings. Benjamin and Spector (1990) measured stress in 27 personnel who were involved in the care of 36 demented residents in a hospital setting. Some were in a short-stay ward of a general hospital, others were in a long-term unit of a psychiatric hospital, and still others were in social service bungalows intended for dementia patients. The authors found that stress was related to characteristics of the staff as individuals (personality), the residents (in terms of the degree of dementia), and the environment (characteristics interfering with helping behaviors).

When we speak of the "course" of a syndrome like AD and the consequent dementia effects, it is obvious that there are medical, social, and psychological factors to be considered. There is an interaction among these that complicates understanding and treatment. Further, there is a "ripple effect" such that others than the patient become involved and are both a part of the problem and part of the solution.

Outcomes

As stated about prognosis, the degeneration that increases the dementia in an Alzheimer's patient assures death by some partially related cause such as pneumonia. The process from inception to termination (or, at least, from diagnosis to termination) is a varied and complex one. It involves the patient directly and other persons indirectly. The progression is not a linear one, either. Indeed, factors of involvement and progression are highly idiosyncratic at the same time that they are predictable in some generalized form.

For the patient, the pattern must begin with some awareness as unaccountable behaviors occur. During the period before diagnosis, though not documented, there probably is a series of events involving recent memory that will be noticeable to the patient if not to others. However, the events may be isolated and well separated in time so that it is plausible for the aging individual to "explain them away." After all, the stereotype of a mind losing its sharpness is accepted still, and perhaps particularly when it will help a person avoid confronting reality that implies deterioration. It may be self-explained, then, as just a little forgetfulness that happens to all of us as we age. With time (the exact amount differing from one patient to another), incidents will be more often, closer together, and more noteworthy. It would seem reasonable to expect certain reactions to such events: fear, perhaps terror at times; denial; irritation; oversensitivity to reasonable mistakes; and/or projection of problems onto others, especially those close to the patient. Eventually, there must come some incident that is critical to the recognition of a severe mental problem. Such incidents that force awareness have been described (e.g., Butler, 1990, pp. 934–935; Gruetzner, 1988, pp. 69–73), but there are far more possibilities than could be included in any listing. With diagnosis, the medical involvement begins (and sometimes ends, depending on the physician, patient, and caregiver). Because there is no treatment, intervention in the conventional medical sense is not possible. The burden now shifts to the caregiver for the decisions that must be made. The patient may be placed in a residential setting at this point, but this is not the usual step. Most caregivers prefer to keep the patient at home, primarily because the relationship is long-standing but also because they feel some responsibility beyond the medical reality. A part of this position may be economic because placement will mean expenditures not anticipated in routine planning for retirement. Some recognition that the caregiver does not know the problems that lie ahead also must be included. Or there may be some belief that the diagnosis is wrong, or that this patient will not develop the severe problems others report, or some dogged adherence to duty. Whatever the motives and their interactions, the caregiver becomes a part of the problem—immediately or later—as well as a part of the solution in terms of care. Caregivers may become involved with support groups at some point, though many are not ready at the time of diagnosis. Others persevere without respite until the patient is finally placed in an institution, or dies, or the caregiver collapses or dies. With a decline in mental competence, patients will not experience stress and may become physically stronger than the caregiver. We can see an intersecting relationship, then, between the strengths of the two parties. At the same time, the decline in mental vigor by the patient on the one hand and physical stamina of the caregiver on the other portends only increasing demand and burden (see Figure 7.2a and b). Yet, there are apparently a few caregivers who escape many of the tangles of the relationship, though literature about such individuals is not extant.

The tone of these comments may leave the impression that little or nothing can or should be done for and with the dementia patient. As Miller (1977, p. 142) has cogently pointed out: "It is appropriate that the search of ways to halt the physical progress of the disease should be matched by complementary research into methods to modify and to compensate for psychological deficits." There have been major efforts in this direction in recent years and, though far from complete or even satis-

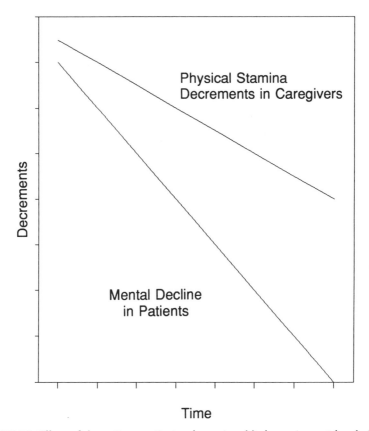

FIGURE 7.2. Effects of dementia on patient and caregiver (a) change in mental and physical states; and (b) stress expression in patients and caregivers.

factory, a variety of techniques and tools are available today. Taught to the caregiver, they may lead to less burdensome problems even though they cannot change the eventual outcome.

MULTIINFARCT DEMENTIA

Considered the second most common cause of dementia (Hughes, 1978, p. 201), multiinfarct dementia (MID) results from vascular disease leading to strokes and subsequent cell destruction. The principal mechanism is arteriosclerosis, a chronic disease that causes thickening and hard-

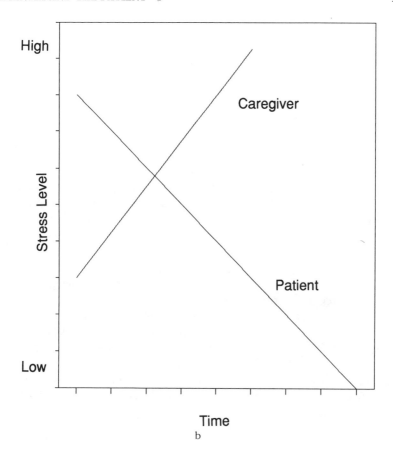

Time

b

ening of the walls of the arteries. There is a consequent loss of elasticity in the artery, and blood flow will be adversely affected. Neurons are highly susceptible to insufficient blood supply because they have higher metabolism and energy requirements than other brain cells (Torack, 1978, p. 105). Inadequate blood flow may mean inadequate nutrition for the cell, and the neuron may be altered or destroyed. The process is a stroke, either major or minor (called "silent") with the complete destruction (called an infarct) of some amount of tissue. Where the damage occurs is crucial to its effects. Torack (1978, p. 102) proposes three forms of cerebral arteriosclerosis that may result in dementia: (a) large infarcts with attendant disability that can be identified medically; (b) small infarcts that are not noticeable in their effects; and (c) destruction of nerve cells in restricted areas but with no evidence of any infarction. Though the first two are both associated with dementia, it is the second (accumulation from silent strokes) that is most often the cause of MID.

Because arteriosclerosis is considered the principal component leading to strokes, the issues of treatment and reversibility are more meaningful in MID than in AD. Caplan (1990, p. 971) notes that those with vascular dementia frequently suffer high-stroke-risk diseases, such as hypertension, diabetes, coronary and peripheral vascular occlusive disease, heart disease, and hyperlipidemia. Their history includes transient ischemic attacks (TIAs) and/or strokes, and there are neurological signs that are measurable (e.g., exaggerated reflexes or visual field defects). Because several of the risk factors are treatable, even preventable, there has been medical emphasis on identifying conditions like hypertension as early as possible in adulthood. Treatment includes a modified diet, with controlled intake of fat and cholesterol and weight reduction as needed. Exercise programs can assist in controlling the hypertension as well as assure physical fitness. If such efforts do not succeed in reducing blood pressure readings to an acceptable level, medications are used as well. When the appropriate recommendations are followed, the risk of stroke is usually reduced and sometimes avoided altogether. The difficulty in this case is that *major* strokes may be avoided. In MID, the more common cause is believed to be small, silent strokes that may be unnoticed by the patient and undiagnosed as a result. In the presence of hypertension, adequate treatment may be instituted and the argument made that the occurrence of silent strokes should be reduced to a minimal level as well. Unfortunately, there are no data to prove the point.[3]

Torack (1978, pp. 102–103) points out that infarcts resulting from arteriosclerosis can occur anywhere in the brain so that the result of stroke may or may not be dementia. Where dementia occurs, it is described as a stepwise deterioration of mental competences. There should be, as a consequence, focal neurological deficits.

Unfortunately, there has not been the recognition of the relationship of strokes to dementing outcomes that might be expected (Torack, 1978, p. 103). Hypertension is closely associated with lacunar infarcts, where the locus of destruction seems to be related to small areas of destruction in an artery (Torack, 1978, p. 104). In a small stroke, there is blockage of one or more arteries, usually only briefly, leading to physical symptoms. The person may feel numb for a period of time or unable to use some part of the body effectively or show speech defects with problems in thought. There may even be dizziness and nausea. What effect is felt depends upon the place where the stroke occurs and the degree of involvement. Because the episode is temporary, perhaps only seconds or minutes, and will not reoccur until another stroke is experienced, the episode may be dismissed as unimportant. The symptoms may be so mild that they won't even be noticed. But any damage done to cell bodies in the brain is permanent, so that over time reoccurrence of strokes in critical areas may bring about demented behavior. Predicting when the next "step" will occur and the depth of that step is not possible. Untreated, the process may move more rapidly, but even with treatment there may still be progression to dementia.

This general picture is widely accepted, but there remains some unease with the validity of the stepwise description. As a result, the literature does include discussion about proving that, indeed, cognitive impairment does result from repetitions of cerebral infarcts (see, e.g., Kase, 1986). As an extension of that issue is the incidence of MID. Jorm, Korten, and Henderson (1987) analyzed data from 47 studies done between 1945 and 1985. They found differences in prevalence rates that were explained on the basis of methodological diversity between the studies. Even so, the correlation of age and incidence of dementia was consistent for the various studies, with the rates *doubling* about every 5 years. Either there was some true increase, or greater awareness on the part of diagnosticians, or an increasing bias to see dementia as the diagnosis of first choice. Of course, the more probable fact is that the changes are a function of all three possibilities. Jorm et al. also found that MID was more commonly diagnosed in men. For incidence, Japanese and Russian studies showed greater prevalence for MID over AD, whereas Finnish and American studies reported no differences between prevalence rates for the two conditions. In western European countries, AD was more commonly diagnosed than MID. The meaning of such figures is difficult to deduce. Perhaps they represent nothing more than an indication of a lack of agreement both on characteristics involved and methods of diagnosis. Certainly we must exercise some caution about statements that indicate scientific validity about conditions so little understood.

Even racial differences have been reported for types of dementia (de la Monte, Hutchins, & Moore, 1989). Based upon 6,000 autopsies performed from 1973 to 1986, these authors identified 144 cases with some form of dementia, 78 of whom were white and 66 were black. MID was more commonly found in blacks. Taken with differences found for other causes of dementia (AD, e.g., was found 2.6 times more often in whites), de la Monte et al. propose that the evidence supports a strong case that there must be a genetic transmission involved in the sporadic incidence of AD. Because the data come from actual examination of brain tissue, the argument must be given greater credence, though the proof of the hereditary link is not present in such facts. Given the results that AD and Parkinson's were more prevalent in whites, whereas

MID and dementia associated with ethanol abuse showed higher frequencies in blacks, they point to a paradox of some importance.

> Although the frequency of MID may have been higher among blacks because of the higher incidence of systemic hypertension in this population, the significantly lower frequency of AD in blacks cannot be explained on this basis. (de la Monte et al., 1989, p. 651)

The picture concerning MID seems clearer than for other diseases, then. Cause is medically identifiable and either preventable or treatable. The number of cases of MID should be reduced and perhaps avoided altogether, as more persons assume responsibility for healthier lives. In recent years, a decline in the incidence of heart disease as a "killer" has been reported for the very reason that diet and exercise regimens are better understood and followed by Americans. There should be a decrease in the number of cases of MID as well, if the assumption of a direct relationship between risk factors and disease is accurate. There are no clear indications of this in the literature, however. Meanwhile, MID continues as the second leading cause of dementia.

Cause and Prognosis

Evidence of the correlation between MID and hypertension has been increasing in recent years. Whether direct cause or not, cardiac disease and hypertension have been found commonly in persons with MID, whereas low rates are reported in AD (Tresch, Folstein, Rabins, & Hazzard, 1985). In addition, some studies have disclosed specific components in both relationships. Rogers, Meyer, Mortel, Mahurin, and Judd (1986) followed 181 neurologically normal older adults over a 7-year period to determine the onset of dementias. Within that time period, six members of their sample developed SDAT; this equates to an incidence of about one-half of 1% per year. By contrast, 10 persons were diagnosed with MID, an incidence of more than three-quarters of 1% per year.[4] The authors explain that the difference probably lies in selection bias. Of 88 individuals who were at risk of stroke, 10 of them (11.4%) developed MID. An interesting sidelight is that cerebral blood flow began to decline about 2 years before symptoms of MID were presented. By contrast, blood-flow levels in SDAT were normal to the time of reported dementia symptoms.

As an antidote to the emphasis on the relationship with hypertension, mention of a study by Sulkava and Erkinjuntti (1987) is worthwhile. They describe six patients with cardiac arrhythmias and *low* blood pressure (hypotension) who were in a group of 133 vascular dementia patients (and thus, about 4.5% of the total. The conditions led to a lack of cerebral blood flow that produces the same effect—MID. Though the reported incidence is small, the outcome of hypotension may be as debilitating when it does occur. Such reports also remind us of the limitations of correlative data.

Several studies have reported postmortem analysis of brain tissue to confirm diagnosis and indicate locus and degree of damage. Predescu, Alexianu, Tudorache, and Tudor (1983) examined tissue from 14 persons who had vascular dementia. Their findings substantiated the clinical data used to make the diagnosis initially. The extent or the number of lesions was not a significant factor in the presence of the dementia. By contrast, Alexianu, Tudorache, and Dumitrescu (1985), examining the brains of 30 patients, found that 9 cases had lesions on vascular walls but no cerebral changes. An additional 4 had a single lesion in the cerebrum where the tissue was destroyed. As a result, Alexianu et al. report that only 17 of the 30 could be accurately classified as MID regardless of the earlier diagnosis. Again, locus and number of lesions was not a significant factor.

Accuracy of diagnosis remains an issue, particularly where autopsies are not performed. Reding, Haycox, Wigforss, Brush, and Blass (1984) have defended the clinic as a reliable source for diagnosis. They followed 85 older persons referred to a rehabilitation service for a 4-year period. Physicians (a neurologist, psychiatrist, and internist) examined each person, and data were collected on neurological tests. Reding et al. report that, of 56 cases predicted as possible dementia victims, 55 progressed to that level during the 4 years. Mortality rate was highest for MID, with the differences in death rates for different diagnoses (AD and "mixed") supporting the clinical expectations. It is interesting that they also conclude that intellectual deterioration may be a poor prognostic sign in the elderly. Where impairment is shown, or even anxiety about impairment, the professional should be more alert to illness in general rather than dementia alone.

The stepwise progression cited as a characteristic of MID has been questioned by Zubenko (1990). He found that SDAT and MID could not be differentiated in 124 patients with diagnoses of dementia using a criterion of stepwise versus insidious increments. In fact, among patients with two or more cerebral infarctions, only 6 of 40 showed the expected decline pattern. As for diagnostic agreement and accuracy, Boller, Lopez, and Moossy (1989) had two neurologists independently predict the diagnosis of 54 demented persons who had been autopsied. Most of the cases had AD (N = 39), but the remaining ones (N = 15) included MID. The physicians reviewed the medical records without knowing the diagnosis or outcomes of autopsy. Boller et al. report that at least one of the two accurately inferred the true diagnosis in about 80% of the cases. Though encouraging, the results still indicate considerable error. In fact, in only 34 cases (63%) were both clinicians correct. In nine (17%), one was correct, and in 11 (20%) neither was correct (thus yielding the "80% accuracy" figure). Boller et al. maintain that these results indicate that, in patients with a clinical diagnosis of dementia, etiology cannot be accurately predicted during life. That statement depends on the two clinicians used being representative of all clinicians.

The problem occurs with psychological measures as well (Hagberg & Gustafson, 1985). Where postmortem data were available to indicate an accurate diagnosis, a comparison with various psychometric and psychiatric data disclosed variability among the anatomically identified conditions. The problem extends even to models developed over years and refined by members of a discipline in the field. Thus la Rue (1986) describes the misclassification of MID that occurs when the DSM-III is used as the basis for diagnosis. He believes that the criteria specified are not sensitive enough to the condition and, in fact, are not sufficiently specific, at least in terms of the procedure followed in classifying clinical conditions. Earlier, Liston and la Rue (1983) had called for a reliable and valid set of criteria to differentiate primary degenerative dementia (as in AD) from MID. Efforts to that time were not supported by research, even though criteria were employed and accepted. They described more explicitly the problems involved when research in the literature was examined (Liston & la Rue, 1983). Methodological problems were cited as common so that the validity of the findings in a given study often were debatable. Comparisons between studies confounded the problems even further. Clinical diagnosis of MID was particularly suspect, they thought, an issue they reiterate in the 1986 article.

Despite these criticisms, there is a predictive efficiency beyond chance when postmortem analysis is conducted. Thus Molsa, Poljarvi, Rinne, Rinne, and Sako (1985) found that both AD and MID had been diagnosed correctly in over 70% of the cases, though mixed cases were diagnostically unreliable. One discriminator was developed by Hachinski (Hachinski, Iliff, Zhilka, Du Boulay, McAllister, Marshall, Russell, and Symon, 1975). Widely quoted and used, it has been found to be useful and reasonably accurate. However, often it is modified by some weighting procedure to improve its discriminative value.

The cause of MID remains, then, a mixed bag because there is rather common agreement about the involvement with vascular disease and, particularly, hypertension. Some research results support such a relationship, whereas others are less supportive. A criterion of a minimum of two infarcts is also widely accepted but has not always been found consistently. Clear differentiation from AD is as often not found as it is substantiated. Postmortem studies have reported accuracy in diagnosis above chance but still with error rates high enough to warrant concern.

Prognosis is poor. Apparently, MID occurs more often in men, occurs earlier in life on average than does AD, and has a more rapid course of decline. Stepwise deterioration is often described but has been questioned by some authors.

As with AD, the current technology has increasingly been used as part of the diagnostic picture. A survey of research using these techniques may help to clarify some of the confusion. EEG patterns were examined by Leuchter, Spar, Walter, and Weiner (1987). They compared 6 patients with MID with 12 DAT and 6 controls. They found electrical activity in the left temporal lobe distinguished dementia victims from controls, except in three cases of mild DAT. When coherence in the EEG pattern was examined, DAT and MID cases were distinguished. With a larger sample in Finland, Soininen, Partanen, Helkala, and Riekkinen (1982) also distinguished demented patients (DAT and MID) from normal controls but not from each other. The MID patients showed greater asymmetry in patterns than did DAT, but Soininen et al. conclude this was not sufficient for high accuracy in differentiation. Striano, Meo, and Bilo are somewhat between the two (1988). They have described differences in brain activity as recorded on the EEG that indicate differential diagnosis is possible. What is concluded may depend on what procedure is followed in reading patterns. Loring, Sheer, and Largen (1985), for example, used patients at rest and during two problem-solving tasks. They found differences between DAT patients and both normals and MID under both conditions. Persons with MID differed from normals in electrical activity during one of the problem-solving tasks. They conclude that EEG activity at the level used by them is of possible utility in early diagnosis of DAT, and the rhythm at that level discriminates similar patterns of dementia.

The combination of EEG with CT scan and clinical features was used by Ettlin, Staehelin, Kischka, Ulrich, Scollo-Lavizzari, Wiggli, and Seiler (1989). Their cases represented SDAT, MID, or a mixture of the two. All were autopsied ($N = 32$). Though there were somewhat positive results for SDAT, they report that MID was more successfully diagnosed using clinical criteria than either the CT scan or EEG. The mixed cases were missed by all three methods.

Computerized tomography (CT) would seem to have an advantage for diagnostic purposes over EEG because it will provide evidence of structural changes that can be visually examined. Indeed, Erkinjuntti,

Ketonen, Sulkava, Vuorialho, and Palo (1987) report the ability to discriminate MID and "probable vascular dementia" from AD on the basis of infarcts and white matter low attenuation disclosed in the scan. Although brain atrophy correlated positively with degree of dementia, regardless of type, it was not useful for discrimination between the types. Comparison of MID patients with controls ($N = 30$ of each) by Jayakumar, Taly, Shanmugam, Nagaraja, and Arya (1989) disclosed a strong relationship between atrophy and the presence of dementia. This finding accords with that of Erkinjuntti et al.

Single photon emission computed tomography (SPECT) has been used to examine cerebral blood flow as a differential element between MID and DAT.[5] Gemmell, Sharp, Smith, Besson, Ebmeier, Davidson, Evans, Roeda, Newton, and Mallard (1989) report highly significant differences between the two but with some overlap in the cerebral bloodflow patterns, thereby suggesting some limitations. Jagust, Budinger, and Reed (1987) compared SPECT and PET on blood flow in the temporoparietal region. They found a similar effect and were able to differentiate MID and control subjects from AD. A caution has been advocated by Deisenhammer, Reisecker, Leblhuber, Markut, Hoell, Trenkler, and Steinheusel (1989). They found that SPECT showed a discrete pattern for AD patients but the same pattern in about one-third of a sample of MID persons. They advocate that SPECT be used to help support clinical classifications of dementia but not serve as a diagnostic procedure.

Magnetic Resonance Imaging (MRI) has its advocates for differential diagnosis as well. Besson, Corrigan, Foreman, Eastwood, Smith, and Ashcroft (1985) believe it may serve not only to distinguish SDAT and MID but also to localize regions of brain damage for more specific effects. In this regard, Christie, Kean, Douglas, Engelman, St. Clair, and Blackburn (1988) have described neuropathological change for AD, MID, and Korsakoff's patients as compared with controls. They point out that, at least for AD, magnetic resonance imaging shows little relationship to neuropsychological deficits. A further study (Besson, Crawford, Parker, and Smith, 1989) disclosed differences in parts of the brain between several dementia groups (AD, MID, alcoholic dementia, and Korsakoff's) when compared with controls. Further, the various dementia groups differed except for Korsakoff's and alcoholic dementia.

As was true with the use of technology in studying AD, there is promise—though major efforts must continue to assess the utility of the techniques both for diagnosis and differentiation. At present, the evidence is mixed and inconclusive.

Course

The course of MID has been described as stepwise deterioration, correlated with the occurrence of small strokes. The risk factors center on hypertension but include various other possibilities as well. Thus heart disease, cigarette smoking, and diabetes mellitus become dangers. Meyer, McClintic, Rogers, Sims, and Mortel (1988) focused on the types of cerebrovascular lesions that occurred when such factors were present. Most often, they report, the result is multiple lacunar infarctions of the brain. Men suffer MID more often than women, they say, and the location of infarcts is correlated with cognitive impairments more than is the amount of infarction over the brain. Similarly, Erkinjuntti (1987a) found that about 89% of a group of persons with MID and 41% of those with "probable vascular disease" showed infarcts on CT scans. The same author (Erkinjuntti, 1987b) has described two possible types of MID. He labels one of these cortical MID, brought on by strokes and producing motosensory hemiparesis, rather severe aphasia, and abrupt onset of cognitive loss. The other type, called subcortical MID, is accompanied by lacunar strokes, some dysarthria, motor hemiparesis, depression, and emotional instability. Even though there are some signs signifying differences, whether the outcomes represent clinical distinctions is not known. He concludes:

> Thus, it is still an open question whether cortical MID and subcortical MID, including the lacunar state and Binswanger's disease, are two distinct entities or merely represent the expression of biological variation while having the same etiopathogenesis. (Erkinjuntti, 1987b, p. 391)

In two studies using CT scans with MID patients, evidence was found that white matter brain tissue shows greater involvement in MID than in AD (e.g., London, deLeon, George, Englund, Ferris, Gentes, and Reisberg, 1986; Kato, Sugawara, Ito, and Kogure, 1990). London et al. note that the effect does not help particularly in making differential diagnoses. Kato et al. believe the white matter disturbance may be related to dementia through its disturbance of axonal conduction.

There have been efforts to determine if cerebrospinal fluid is affected by dementia. Nonspecific enolase in the fluid was lower for MID patients than for AD or controls in a study by Sulkava, Viinikka, Erkinjuntti, and Roine (1988). (Enolase is an enzyme that assists in the metabolism of carbohydrates. What the meaning of such a finding may be for the course of MID is not known.) Degrell and Niklasson (1988) have presented evidence that purine levels in cerebrospinal fluid differ among causes of dementia and may be used for differential diagnosis.

Deutsch and Tweedy (1987) examined cerebral blood flow of AD and MID patients, controlling for age and severity of dementia. They found that under these circumstances AD had significantly lower mean blood flow than MID. Because most studies do not control for severity, they feel their finding helps clarify discrepancies in results previously reported. With such controls, diagnosticians may use either global or left parietal flow to discriminate the two conditions. The results will be 87% accurate, according to their data. Judd, Meyer, Rogers, Gandhi, Tanahashi, Mortel, and Tawaklna (1986) found that loss of cerebral vasomotor responsiveness in MID patients, a biological marker of cerebrovascular disease, gives positive evidence of the vascular etiology of MID and helps differentiate MID from AD.

A considerable body of literature is accumulating that looks at structural changes accompanying the course of MID. The lack of focus and the inability to relate the findings to a significant understanding of MID reduce the practicality of the results. It is still true, however, that amassing data of scientific validity even though application is unknown is part of the process that will eventually lead to a comprehensive picture.

Even without knowing the exact nature of process, there can be intervention and treatment. All such treatments need not be sophisticated, either. For example, Meyer, Rogers, McClintic, Mortel, and Lotfi (1989) divided MID patients into two groups, matched on risk factors for stroke as well as cerebral blood-flow values and cognitive abilities. One group (N = 37) received aspirin, whereas the other did not. Evaluations were conducted on blood flow through the brain cells and on cognition at each of three yearly intervals. On both measures, the aspirin-treated group showed significantly greater improvement than the control group. Apparently the aspirin assists blood flow so that cells are nourished to a higher degree than would be possible without the aspirin. By no means a cure for MID, for certain patients, at least, there may be some slowdown of dementia when this drug is used. More sophisticated drug therapy has yielded positive effects on such outcomes as social behavior, sensory impairment, central noradrenergic output, and memory test performance (see, e.g., Ban, Conti, Morey, Lazzerini, Cornelli, Postiglione, & Grossi, 1987; Passeri & Cucinotta, 1989; Corona, Cucchi, Frattini, Santagostino, Schinelli, Romani, Pola, Zerbi, & Savoldi, 1989; Hagstadius, Gustafson, & Risberg, 1984). Continued experimentation with drug therapy may assist the patient in functioning at higher levels for longer periods of time even though the eventual deterioration is inevitable. What is just as important is that caregivers may benefit in having a patient who is more tractable and malleable.

Outcomes

MID appears to proceed more rapidly than AD with the eventual cause of death being one of the usual forms (such as pneumonia), though an acute cerebrovascular accident will occur with a moderate degree of probability. Thus Molsa, Marttila, and Rinne (1986) reported a 33% incidence of death in MID patients from such accidents. Overall, the survival prognosis is less favorable for MID than for AD. Hier, Warach, Gorelick, and Thomas (1989) found that cognitive tests were better predictors of survival in MID than in AD. Generally, both higher educational level and female sex were correlated with longer survival in MID in their sample. St. Clair and Whalley (1983) report that MID patients show greater cardiovascular abnormalities at autopsy than do AD patients.

In the behavioral area, speech and language may be differentially affected. Powell, Cummings, Hill, and Benson (1988) used a battery of tests to assess 37 elements of verbal production for both MID and AD patients. They found the multiinfarct group had more abnormalities of motor aspects of speech. Overall, they concluded that speech and language are different in the two conditions.

Semantic memory was assessed by Fischer, Gatterer, Marterer, and Danielczyk (1988). They tested MID, AD, and controls on verbal fluency and the ability to name objects. They found no differences between the demented groups, nor was severity of dementia a discriminating variable on semantic performance. In fact, Bayles and Tomoeda (1983) found that confrontation naming was not impaired in mildly demented patients; those with a moderate degree of dementia made more errors than normals but with a logic to the errors. Only the severely demented give bizarre or unrelated answers. Their sample included MID, AD, Huntington's, and Parkinson's patients. The task was to name the objects shown on 20 colored pictures. Whatever the cause of the dementia, most of the errors occurred in reference to labels that were semantically related to the stimulus. They theorize that naming errors are due primarily to impairment in the linguistic domain of cognition regardless of etiology.

Differences were found in verbal memory, using free recall, by Parlato, Carlomagno, Merla, and Bonavita (1988). In their sample, the disorder was greater for AD than for MID, primarily because Alzheimer's patients are no longer able to learn competently and rely heavily on a primary memory component. MID patients are more apt to retain learning skills and thus resemble the normal controls more in their measures.

Practical skills are adversely affected by the disease process as well. Lucas-Blaustein, Filipp, Dungan, and Tune (1988) surveyed driving habits with a 20-item questionnaire. Their sample consisted of patients in an outpatient dementia research center and included AD, MID, and mixed diagnoses. Since the symptoms had first become noticeable, 30% of the patients had had at least one accident. An additional 11% had caused accidents. Such high rates indicate the difficulty of maintaining well-rehearsed abilities as dementia progresses. Unfortunately, demented persons are not always realistic, and one of the major tasks encountered by caregivers is to persuade them to give up driving.

In the more general sense, patients may show several kinds of troublesome and disruptive behaviors. Swearer, Drachman, O'Donnell, and Mitchell (1988) used a questionnaire with caregivers to test the presence and extent of such outcomes. They found particular complaints of aggressive, ideational, and vegetative behaviors. The more severe the dementia, the more prevalent and severe the problems. There was no relation to cause of the dementia as such. Swearer et al. conclude that such behaviors are a common occurrence in dementia victims and are related to severity of symptoms. Though not determined by lack of mental competence, there is a parallel between the two.

Though without controls, Cole (1988) did a study covering 2 years with 13 persons suffering from MID. Measures were taken quarterly to indicate progression of dementia and behavioral changes. During the period of the study, almost half the patients died (46%). Among the survivors, the pattern of decline varied widely, seemingly related to the history of the fluctuating course, presence of depression, and focal neurological symptoms.

Survival has been a major theme in studies of dementia. Martin, Miller, Kapoor, Arena, and Boller (1987) compared 202 dementia patients with controls drawn from the same cohort. Over 4 years, they found that both SDAT and MID patients had the shorter survival rates. However, they found also that the prognosis was not so bleak as indicated in the literature, primarily because there were ways of intervening successfully. Agreement with longer survival than believed has been furnished by Barclay, Zemcov, Blass, and Sansone (1985). In comparing DAT, MID and mixed patients, they found a 50% survival rate *from time of diagnosis* to be 2.6 years for MID, 2.5 years for mixed diagnoses, and 3.4 years for DAT. However, the 50% survival rate *from time of onset* was 6.7 years for MID, 6.2 years for mixed, and 8.1 years for DAT. The more significant figure here is the survival in MID from onset. If estimates of onset are accurate, there may be longer development than previously proposed.

Variables important to survival, regardless of cause of dementia, have been identified by Belloni-Sonzogni, Tissot, Tettamanti, Frattura, and Spagnoli (1989) as age, type of diagnosis, and levels of autonomy on the part of the patient. Surveying 237 demented patients in a geriatric hospital in Italy over a 4-year period, they found that only 54 were survivors. The highest death rate was for DAT (87%), whereas MID patients had a death rate of 57.1%.

Over a 25-year period, Rorsman, Hagnell, and Lanke (1985) followed 3,563 persons with mental disorders. They found that mortality rates did not change significantly for those with diagnoses of MID or AD during that time. In a follow-up study (Rorsman, Hagnell, & Lanke, 1986), they report no significant changes in the prevalence or incidence of either form of dementia over the 25-year period. If the data from Sweden are typical, there was little evidence of either decreasing or increasing problems during the time covered (1947 to 1972). It is possible that such a survey updated to the present, however, would disclose greater prevalence due to greater awareness and more complete diagnostic efforts since the early 1970s.

In summary, MID would seem to present a clear clinical picture. Cause seems well agreed upon, intervention is recognized and strongly advocated, and technology allows more accurate diagnosis. Unfortunately, the literature presents an image that is more muddled than clear, and there are questions still to be answered about diagnosis, treatment, and progression. The most positive variable in this syndrome, so far as knowledge is concerned, lies in causation. If the presumption that MID comes from small strokes caused principally by hypertension (but also by other conditions that can be diagnosed and treated) is accurate, the willingness of people to avoid or control the causes should bring a dramatic reduction in MID in the next century. Certainly there is evidence that heart disease is decreasing among males, primarily because of adjustments in lifestyles. Insofar as there is a relationship between heart disease and MID, the next decade or two should show evidence of positive effects.

SUMMARY

In this chapter, we have surveyed some of the vast literature dealing with Alzheimer's disease and multiinfarct dementia, the two leading causes of demented behavior. As extensive as the publications are, there are still far more unanswered questions than answered ones. Part of the problem lies in a lack of a consistent, cooperative approach to research. Several disciplines have declared a legitimate interest in the field, and each pursues its own particular line of inquiry. Rarely is there an attempt to bring together the disparate studies for consensus. Future emphasis must be placed on coordination if maximum returns are to be achieved.

Dementia and the Patient—II

There are other causes of dementia than AD and MID, though the conditions are much less common and thus have generated less research interest. Nevertheless, each has its influence on the population, and each has investigators who are studying the syndrome and its effects. The surveys in this chapter are of necessity briefer because there is not the corpus of literature that exists for Alzheimer's and multiinfarct dementia. As a concluding section, we will examine some of the research in progress, largely in the drug field, where efforts are underway to discover chemicals that will reduce the effects of adverse symptoms found in dementia patients.

PICK'S DISEASE

Pick's disease is a rare brain condition of unknown cause (Miller, 1977, p. 5). Though the atrophy that occurs is relatively circumscribed, occurring in the frontal and temporal regions of the brain, the effects of Pick's are difficult to distinguish from Alzheimer's. The clinical symptoms illustrate why this ambiguity may occur. There are memory disturbances, accompanied by considerable apathy. Patients may become careless in their behaviors and display poor personal hygiene as though they are detached from normal human concerns. Their ability to attend is stunted so that their attention span is very short. Even though there is a distinctive finding in CT scans for Pick's patients, the only accurate confirmation of the diagnosis occurs at autopsy (Sunderland, 1990, p. 946).

An emphasis on genetic influences in dementia and research about such relationships is increasing rapidly. Heston and White (1991, pp. 62–82) have described the probability of heritability for several causes of dementia. In the case of Pick's, the data are limited, but these authors estimate that the lifetime risk is about 25% for parents, 20% for siblings, and 20% for offspring.

Prevalence in the general population has been estimated at only three to six persons per 10,000. This would mean that there are less than 150,000 cases currently in the United States compared to as many as 4,000,000 cases of Alzheimer's disease. Constantinidis (1985, p. 72) has compared symptomatology in a comparative vein: "In psychological terms, we can say that in Alzheimer disease the intellectual faculties are disturbed, while in Pick disease their utilization is faulty." In its early stages, there is often emotional blunting, altered sexual activity, hyperorality, and visual agnosias (Sunderland, 1990, p. 946), behaviors labeled as the Kluver–Bucy syndrome.

Sturt (1986) examined age of onset in relatives of patients with dementia, including Pick's. Overall, she reports that female relatives of dementia patients in her sample had a higher risk of any dementia than did male relatives. The risk in Pick's was higher for relatives than the risk in AD, though not significantly so. She proposes that the particular disease process (such as Pick's) is responsible for the pattern of risk shown by age and that individual differences in rate are under the control of genes.

Pick's occurs most often in the age range from 40 to 60 years and is rarely diagnosed in old age. By contrast, AD manifests an increasing risk with age, thereby presenting a different genetic picture. Birkett (1989) advocates that professionals should be aware of the evidence on heritability and genetics for causes, including Pick's, Huntington's, and Creutzfeldt–Jakob's diseases. Such information should be communicated to families as a part of a counseling program at the time a medical diagnosis is made. Certainly, as more knowledge accrues so that accuracy is assured, discussion of these probabilities may help reassure many relatives. Data from isolated studies are accumulating. Gustafson (1987) reports that in 20 cases of frontal lobe dementia, 4 of which were diagnosed as Pick's, there was a 50% positive heredity as compared to 30% for AD. A more extensive report by Heston, White, and Mastri (1987) used 18 families among whom there was a diagnosis of Pick's. All patients were white, and males showed earlier age of onset than females. Survival was 6.3 years for males and 8.4 years for females on average. Heston et al. say this suggests a biological effect. Among the relatives, there were 15 cases of dementia, involving 10 families. Heston et al. conclude that heritability probability is greater for Pick's than for AD, based on available data, but the total risk over one's lifetime is greater for relatives of AD patients. This is a reflection of the age-related nature of dementias cited above. Heston et al. conclude that the evidence favors a genetic contribution to the cause of Pick's.

Cause and Prognosis

As noted, the cause of Pick's is unknown. Similarities with Alzheimer's disease, both presenile and senile, have led Miller (1977, p. 5) to suggest that all three be called "primary cerebral atrophy." Yet differences are also reported. Brun (1987) performed autopsies on 158 cases of organic dementia and reported only four that conformed to Pick's criteria (thus, about 2.5% of the total). However, there were an additional 16 cases with degeneration of grey matter in the frontal or frontotemporal lobe. These he called "frontal lobe degeneration of non-Alzheimer type." Despite similarities with other causes of dementia, including Pick's, Brun proposes that there are both clinical and anatomical differences. Whether other investigators recognize a distinction or would aggregate all such cases as Pick's disease is not yet known. This reflects the lack of sophistication in defining the specific contributions that the various brain areas make to dementia. Chui (1989) has proposed that there is a certain oversimplification in classification of the causes of dementia that masks the need for precise roles of such systems as the limbic and paralimbic, the multimodal association areas, prefrontal cortices, the basal ganglia, and so on. Her comments reinforce a position that knowledge is sparse and research must continue if understanding is to occur.

Diagnosis of Pick's is increasingly using the technology developed in recent years, usually in combination with clinical data. Knopman, Christensen, Schut, Harbaugh, Reeder, Ngo, and Frey (1989) examined CT scans and psychometric data on six Pick's patients compared with seven biopsy-proven AD patients to determine the presence of distinctive features, if any, that would allow earlier diagnosis of Pick's. They report that five of the six showed marked frontal and/or temporal lobe atrophy in the scan, an outcome not observed for AD. There were also differences in the performance patterns of patients on psychometric tests, particularly with recent memory better preserved in Pick's. Nevertheless, they state that the findings are equivocal so far as using imaging and psychometrics for differential diagnosis.

> The distinctive psychometric pattern in the Pick's patients was evanescent, however. Thus, there were imaging and psychometric findings of potential diagnostic value for Pick's disease, but, for different reasons, they were imperfect (Knopman et al., 1989, p. 367)

Stigsby (1988) reports. that EEG patterns often appear normal in Pick's patients, whereas there is evidence that over a period of time the pattern changes with AD. In a case study of a 75-year-old man, Kamo, McGeer, Harrop, McGeer, Kalne, Martin, and Pate (1987) used a PET scan followed by postmortem comparison. They report that the scan pattern was sufficiently distinctive that it might be possible to differentiate Pick's in living patients. In comparison with Knopman et al., then, there may be some scan techniques better suited to given conditions than others.

Particular changes in the brain of the Pick's patient have been reported in some studies as well. Risberg (1987) examined cerebral blood flow in 18 cases, distributed as frontal lobe degeneration (non-Alzheimer's), Pick's, AD, and Creutzfeldt–Jakob. He concludes that both the extent and the location of cerebral dysfunction can be determined using blood-flow measures. Sims, Finegan, Blass, Bowen, and Neary (1987) surveyed metabolic changes in various dementia-producing conditions and found evidence that might indicate pathogenesis. Doebler, Rhoads, Anthony, and Markesbery (1989) report lower RNA (ribonucleic acid) values in Pick's disease than in AD or controls. A case study has been reported for a middle-aged male with both Pick's and AD (Smith & Lantos, 1983). At autopsy, it was found that there was no focal atrophy, but there were a number of structural changes associated with Pick's in the hippocampus and temporal lobe. Constantinidis (1985, p. 92) also reports lesions in the hippocampus, notes that they are the initial changes, and associates them with a change in the neurotransmitter glutamate.

Various tests yield some evidences of specific qualities in the brain that are unique to Pick's disease or that differ somewhat from brain features in AD at least. At present, all such findings need replication for verification. The results are suggestive rather than definitive, then.

Outcomes

As stated previously, Pick's more commonly occurs during middle age. In addition, it has a fairly rapid course. Within that context, a variety of outcomes have been reported. What is common is that these are case studies, primarily because Pick's is a rare condition and locating sizable samples to study would be very expensive and difficult. Case studies are restricted in their generalizability, even though they provide useful information about discrete elements.

An interesting example is that of a 66-year-old man who was diagnosed with Pick's and who lived to the age of 78. He kept a written record of the changes he observed in his own abilities, with the accuracy of his reports being substantiated by interviews with family members. At death, his brain was examined for pathological changes. His competencies were particularly affected in terms of language abilities. The authors of the report (Holland, McBurney, Moossy & Reinmuth, 1985) thus suggest that patients be encouraged to keep such descriptive records and that they be used to assist in our understanding of the language deterioration that occurs in dementias. They point out:

> It is interesting to speculate that the difficulty in relating Mr. E to the general literature is not that he is an unusual PD patient, but rather that since PD is relatively rare, and hard to differentiate during life from AD (or worse, 'senile dementia') patients similar to Mr. E get lost in, even washed out of, the more general data on dementia. (p. 57)

Obviously, the procedure requires a concerned and courageous patient and family members. Holland et al. make a plea for more such individual, quasi-longitudinal accounts.

A 59-year-old man who was scanned both by CT and MRI on several occasions was suffering progressive aphasia for 9 years before demonstrating rather mild behavioral problems. These tests disclosed a progressive bilateral temporal atrophy that was interpreted to be a temporal lobe form of Pick's. The only notable behavioral symptom during the progression was an aphasia. Scheltens, Hazenberg, Lindeboom, Valk, and Wolters (1990) propose that such progressive aphasia without dementia may be a presenting sign of Pick's, AD, or Creutzfeldt–Jakob, and they believe that aphasic behavior may be used as the clinical evidence until definitive demonstration of structural change is found.

Using a sample of 20 frontal lobe patients, Johanson and Hagberg (1989) compared psychometric assessments with postmortem analyses of brain tissue. They report that cognitive loss was less severe in those whose dementia began prior to age 56, with the most common finding being dysfunction of expressive speech. These cases were labeled either "frontal lobe degeneration of non-Alzheimer's type" (N = 16) or Pick's disease (N = 4).

In another study, four patients who had died with diagnoses of Pick's were examined for changes in the frontal and temporal lobes by Kamp, den Hartog-Jager, Maathuis, de Groot, de Jong, and Bolhuis (1986). They found unusual chemical changes both within and outside affected cells. Apparently, the cells are unable to deal with and remove such chemicals. There is no evidence for a relationship of these changes to cause and progression of Pick's.

In summary, there are considerable gaps in knowledge about Pick's disease, even though research data are accumulating. The lack of emphasis on this cause of dementia and the rarity with which it occurs will continue to restrict accurate diagnosis and prognosis. Definitive descriptions of the course and outcomes of Pick's are needed as well.

NORMAL PRESSURE HYDROCEPHALUS

Under normal conditions, there is a balance between the amount of tissue in the cranium and the cerebrospinal fluid that protects it. Though not the same for all persons, the relationship of fluid to tissue is usually extremely close. Under some untoward conditions, however, the increase in the amount of fluid will produce shrinkage or atrophy of tissue in the cranium. This state, hydrocephalus, occurs when there is expansion of the ventricles, enlargement of the skull (particularly the forehead), or atrophy of the brain.

During the 1960s an example of hydrocephalus was described that did not fit the conventional image. Adams, Fisher, Hakim, Ojemann, and Sweet (1965) discussed a clinical syndrome that included enlarged ventricles but *normal* cerebrospinal fluid (CSF) pressure. They reported some dementia as well. There was a reversal in the tissue/fluid balance following an operative procedure called "shunting."[1] Since that time, the surgical procedure has been used less often, whereas there has been increasing interest in the expression of the dementia. Torack (1978, p. 33) points out that the early cases of normal pressure hydrocephalus (NPH) did not show signs of atrophy or plaques and tangles. However, there were distinctive symptoms: some memory impairment accompanied by difficulty in thought processes and overt behavior, problems with gait, and urinary incontinence.

Clinically, memory loss is not noted early in the process, as it is in AD, whereas urinary incontinence appears very soon, in contrast with Alzheimer's. Further, gait disturbance is later in AD but earlier in NPH. Torack (1978, p. 33) concludes that such differences mean that NPH is not a variant of AD but a clinical condition in its own right. The primary dysfunction occurs in the reticular formation, the most primitive part of the brain (Torack, 1978, p. 34).

Raichle, Grubb, Gado, Eichling, and Hughes (1978, p. 131) comment that the cause of NPH has been proposed as reduced cerebral blood flow because of the increase in the size of the ventricles relative to total brain mass. Miller (1977, p. 122) says that there seems to be no satisfactory explanation for the condition, at least insofar as the increase in cerebro-spinal fluid is concerned. Nevertheless, the syndrome has been accepted and is described by its symptoms. Indeed, Miller points out that the enthusiasm with which the condition was accepted by some was primarily because it offered the possibility for reversal of a dementia through sur-gical intervention.

Slaby and Cullen (1987, p. 143) note that shunting has had little success; its most common positive effects are found when the patient presents symptoms of gait disturbance, dementia, and incontinence rather than dementia alone. These symptoms combined with CT-scan evidence of dilated ventricles seem to forecast greatest success for the procedure.

There may even be a connection with psychiatric conditions, ac-cording to Dewan and Bick (1985), with a possible relationship to schizo-phrenia. They also suggest that NPH may be more common than many believe. Because treatment is possible, at least for some cases, the syn-drome will probably remain an infrequent but important form of dementia.

Cause and Prognosis

As noted, there is still debate about causation; in fact, NPH has been described only in terms of its effects, not its etiology. St. Laurent (1988) laments the lack of data, particularly for aged persons, regarding the syndrome. Concern about caution in diagnosis, problems of surgical treatment, and the need for developing some alternative pharmacologic treatment is allied with that lack.

Diagnosis has been aided by the development of technology in recent years. Schroth and Klosa (1989) used MRI with 10 patients with NPH, and they point out that, even though potentially treatable, NPH is difficult to diagnose. Miller's comments about diagnostic criteria, cited earlier, re-main viable even with considerable advances in techniques. MRI has a potential that has generated optimism on the part of many diagnosticians. Thus Kunz, Heintz, Ehrenheim, Stolke, Dietz, and Hundeshagen (1989) discuss this technique's noninvasive properties as a major gain at the same time that it allows greater sophistication in the data provided by the scan.

The use of PET scans in identifying NPH also has been investigated. Jagust, Friedland, and Budinger (1985) made comparisons between NPH ($N = 3$), DAT ($N = 17$), and controls ($N = 7$) and found that the patterns of metabolic abnormality between the two causes of dementia were quite distinct. The NPH sample showed more global diminution of use of glu-cose, whereas AD patients had metabolic abnormality in the temporoparietal areas bilaterally. Such a difference, confirmed in other studies, would assist accurate differential diagnosis.

As with Pick's, part of the research reports case studies because the condition is rare and groups of patients are not available. In this respect, Newton, Pickard, and Weller (1989) describe a 66-year-old man who had received a shunt and then showed some resolution of his dementia. However, the gain was short-lived even though the shunting procedure continued to work. At his death, an autopsy disclosed numerous small infarcts, especially in white matter.

Course

There have been fewer studies following the progression of NPH than is true for other causes of dementia. The significance of abnormality in gait was investigated by Graff-Radford and Godersky (1986). They hypothesized that gait problems developing before signs of dementia would be found in patients who benefitted most from surgical intervention. In their sample of 21 persons, 16 showed improvement, whereas 5 did not. In the improved group, 11 had had gait difficulties prior to onset of dementia, whereas the others had shown the signs at about the same time as the dementia became evident. Of the 5 unimproved cases, 3 had dementia before gait problems, whereas 1 had simultaneous occurrence. The remaining case had gait abnormality prior to dementia. Overall, the hypothesis holds, although the reason for the relationship is not clear. Larger samples are needed to assure validity of the relationship.

Hartwig (1983) has demonstrated the relationship of NPH to cognitive performance in his report on a 64-year-old man. A shunt led to improvement in memory and word-finding skills for structured settings as well as a higher WAIS IQ score. However, there were continued memory problems, difficulties in dealing with verbal materials, and perplexities in spatial relationships. Hartwig advocates an extensive neuropsychological examination as a part of the diagnostic procedure. He believes that such a test will disclose specific behavioral correlates of impairment in the cortex of NPH patients.

In summary, data on NPH have been and are limited. Most emphasis has been put on the physical changes (such as gait and incontinence) and the possibility of surgical intervention. As Miller noted (1977, p.123), there needs to be a more systematic definition of the syndrome in order to allow more effective treatment. At the same time, the associated conditions (primarily reflected in the dementing process) require continued research efforts.

CREUTZFELDT–JACOB DISEASE

Among the rarest of the conditions leading to dementia, Creutzfeldt–Jacob (or Jacob–Creutzfeldt because the two made equal contributions) disease is caused by a "slow-acting virus." It is slow-acting in the sense that it has a long initial period of incubation, lasting up to several years (Gibbs, Gadjusek, & Masters, 1978, p. 117). It is viral because of its size (Torack, 1978, p. 26).[2] Once expressed, it is progressive and fatal, with death usually occurring within 2 years (Fisk, 1981, p. 49). Found in middle aged men and women (and thus presenile), it produces ataxia, muscle spasms, seizures, incontinence, psychotic behavior, and visual symptoms (Fisk, 1981, p. 49). Further, according to Fisk, an EEG will show a characteristic pattern. At autopsy, the brain shows atrophy and a degree of "sponginess."

Torack (1978, p. 26) points out that the condition has been transmitted to chimpanzees from infected human tissue so that the etiologic agent is known. However, there is no treatment. Psychologically, patients are apathetic, unkempt, and have psychomotor retardation (Sunderland, 1990, p. 947).

Gibbs and Gadjusek (1978, pp. 119–120) have detailed the major clinical signs of CJD. They include insidious onset, usually without fever or systemic illness; behavioral disturbances, expressed through confusion, emotional lability, depression, and withdrawal; progressive dementia; various physical stigmata, such as visual abnormalities, seizures, and liver dysfunction; familial occurrence; and structural brain changes identifiable by pneumoencephalopathy or CT scan.

The literature is quite limited for the same reasons as for NPH and Pick's disease. In addition, results of studies leave the issue of viral source in doubt. For example, Harries-Jones, Knight, Will, Cousens, Smith, and Matthews (1988) followed 92 cases of confirmed and probable cases of CJD during a 5-year survey in England and Wales. They were unable to identify environmental circumstances that might be etiological agents. In this regard, they examined dietary habits, including meat, liver and brain, kidney, and tripe consumption. They could find no trend of increased risk with higher consumption of such foods. Neither could they find evidence of familial transmission, although relatives of patients were more apt to display dementia than were controls. They even checked animal contact; that is, pets of various kinds, along with proximity to sheep, fur, and carcasses. None of these produced a statistically significant relationship with the occurrence of the disease.

Structurally, there is evidence of loss of the spines that extend from dendrites in several dementias, including CJD (Catala, Ferrer, Galofre, & Fabregues, 1988). However, there is no evidence that such a loss will serve as data for differential diagnosis. Using computerized tomography, Galvez and Cartier (1984) reported that the scan was normal in 12 of 15 patients with confirmed CJD. They found no relationship between the scan, severity of the clinical state, and postmortem brain examination. They reason that a normal CT scan in a demented patient may suggest CJD, with more definitive follow-up a reasonable course of action.

Although there is much less known about CJD than is needed for complete understanding, emphasis upon research probably will be limited. As it is, too little monies exist for the much better recognized syndromes that affect much larger numbers of persons. Outside of a few laboratories, the condition will continue to be neglected unless some critical finding relating the process or virus to such a syndrome as AD should occur, or if an effective treatment is discovered.

HUNTINGTON'S AND PARKINSON'S DISEASES

These diseases will be considered together because neither is the "cause" of dementia in the same sense as the others previously discussed. In those cases, the syndrome is assumed to lead inevitably to demented states; for these two the chances are less than 100%, though the incidence probably is greater than chance.

Huntington's disease (HD) is an hereditary disorder with the genetic expression occurring solely in the nervous system. As Shoulson (1978, p. 251) has noted, the genetic trait is dominant, with complete penetrance and a very small rate of mutations. Thus the prediction of probability of the occurrence of the disease is highly accurate. Yet the syndrome does express itself at different ages and with an uneven course, so that individual differences among patients will be observed. Dementia, psychiatric disturbances, and extrapyramidal dysfunction are central expressions (Shoulson, 1978, p. 251). The dementia is often expressed in loss of memory and reasoning, but language will not be affected. There are also wide differences in the amount of intellectual decline so that eventual total loss of competencies is not certain by any means. Sunderland (1990, p. 946) points out that the family history and the motor abnormalities that are the result of the disease help in clarifying the clinical picture for diagnostic purposes. Shoulson (1978, p. 252) reported almost 50% of a sample of patients (N = 30) studied by him cited problems in cognition. Estimates of the incidence of dementia in HD vary to as much as 80%. The functional disorder of depression is often found in patients also as the deleterious behavioral changes accompanying the syndrome become evident.

Parkinson's disease (PD) results in degeneration of the nervous system as well. However, the cause is not genetic but more probably some deficiency in dopamine activity in the basal ganglia. In recent years, there has been a relationship to toxic effects of drugs, at least in younger persons. Usually, Parkinson's occurs in middle age to old age with a gradual progression that may last for many years. There are no sex differences, and the incidence is approximately 1% of the population age 50 and over with some increase after age 70. Sunderland (1990, p. 945) reports that more than 25% of PD patients develop dementia but that some estimates run as high as 80%. When dementia does develop, there are severe problems because of side effects from drugs used to treat the Parkinsonism.

Recent Research on Dementia in Huntington's Disease

The occurrence of dementia with HD has become a source of major interest and research. Indeed, dementia as a characteristic of HD is widely recognized and accepted, along with the traditional inclusion of involuntary choreiform movements and psychological changes (Martin, 1984). Shoulson (1990) has discussed what he calls the "disabling consequences of gene expression on chromosome 4" plus the degeneration in the basal ganglia that leads to cognitive losses and psychiatric problems. He describes the dementia of HD as relatively circumscribed, particularly involving certain memory processes. However, there are additional behavioral disturbances that intensify the negative effects of the disease. Often there are personality change, affective disorders, and psychotic reactions. Shoulson states that the affective disorders are treatable with antidepressant therapies.

There has been proposed a concept of *subcortical* dementia in Huntington's disease (and in Parkinson's as well) that reflects the loss in mental abilities of the typical patient (see, e.g., Huber & Paulson, 1985). In this model, the syndrome leaves language and perception unaffected at the same time that it has adverse effects on memory. (This is an issue we will return to in the section on "outcomes.") There is also the division, then, into *cortical* dementia, most notably expressed in AD, where there are more extensive and comprehensive negative effects on mental competence. This distinction between "subcortical" and "cortical" has adherents on both sides of the issue.

As noted earlier, every case of HD does not necessarily lead to dementia. A case study, reported by Turner (1985), serves as an example. He describes a 54-year-old patient whose father also had been diagnosed as HD. In the case at hand, there were social and behavioral declines that were typical of the disease. However, nine siblings of the patient were unaffected, despite the hereditary nature of the condition, and he had no dementia. The description is intriguing and, to some degree, baffling, although Quarrell and Harper (1986) argue that the siblings had not outlived the major risk period and might yet develop the disease. In fact, they call for genetic counseling to clarify some of the discrepancies. This case illustrates the variance possible in HD as well as the current limited knowledge of this disorder.

Cause and Prognosis

HD is a genetic, autosomal-dominant disorder. Martin and Gusella (1986) believe that the genetic defect that causes the disease originated from a common source and that new mutations are rare, maybe even nonexistent. Such a view helps delimit the conditions under which the syndrome will be found, but it does not preclude varied manifestations among patients.

Technology is increasingly used to help diagnostic accuracy in this syndrome as it is with other dementing illnesses. Tanahashi, Meyer, Ishikawa, Kandula, Mortel, Rogers, Gandhi, and Walker (1985) used CT scans to measure brain atrophy and cerebral blood flow through gray matter to assess the degree of severity with 16 HD patients, 6 asymptomatic blood relatives at risk of HD, and 90 controls. They found that reductions in cerebral blood flow correlated directly with severity of dementia. The lack of useful results with the CT scan has been reported in other studies, but Veroff, Pearlson, and Ahn (1982) used a different analytic technique and found greater success. They report that AD and HD patients may be differentiated by analyzing numerical CT scan density information.

The locus of cell damage in HD is most frequently stated as "subcortical" as compared with AD where loss is principally in the cortex. An outcome of the location is the particular behaviors that may be affected and their expressions. Cummings and Benson (1988) maintain that both

HD and PD are due to defects in the basal ganglia. As a result, the conditions are expressed in slow thought processes (bradyphrenia), some loss of control mentally in the sense of executive functions, problems with recall, disturbances in spatial relations, and increased depression and apathy. By contrast, AD leads to aphasia, both recall and recognition problems in memory, and a certain amount of indifference about problems as the disease involves increasing numbers of cells.

The study of regional cerebral blood flow in HD patients and controls led to a somewhat different conclusion by Weinberger, Berman, Iadarola, Driesen, and Zec (1988). They had their subjects perform on two mental tasks during measurement of blood flow and took a second measure while the participants rested. Among their findings, they note that cortical blood flow was not reduced even while overt prefrontal-type activities were underway. There was a positive correlation between atrophy in the caudate nucleus (one of the four basal ganglia in each hemisphere) and regional blood flow, but only while prefrontal involvement from mental activity was occurring. Their results suggest to them that there must be a qualification of the subcortical dementia concept in HD. Apparently, there is an interaction between the pathological state located in the subcortical regions and cognitive function carried out in cortical areas. They conclude:

> The data presented here suggest that the dementia represents a loss of neocortical (particularly prefrontal) functioning and that the role of subcortical pathology is in determining the pathophysiological mechanism by which this function is lost. (p. 103)

There has been investigation of the premorbid psychiatric state of HD subjects. Mindham, Steele, Folstein, and Lucas (1985) compared AD and HD patients on this dimension and found that persons with HD had twice as many major affective disorders reported in their past lives as did AD individuals. To them, there must be a systematic relationship between psychiatric conditions and later-developing HD that should be further investigated. Perhaps the functional disorders noted in HD patients are not merely a feature of the disease process but a precursor and possible marker.

Outcomes

The principal effects of the dementia that may occur with HD will not differ for patient or caregivers from the effects due to any dementia. However, because there are some behavioral differences that have been documented, a discussion of some of the research on outcomes seems warranted.

Webb and Trzepacz (1987) investigated the psychiatric expressions of the condition with several neuropsychological measures. They found a high incidence of personality disorders, with particular occurrence of depressive, explosive, and alcohol-abuse episodes. This would accord with the research of Mindham et al., noted before. Further, Webb and Trzepacz found a strong relationship between the severity of the chorea (the muscular movements that occur due to damage to the basal ganglia) and the degree of dementia, particularly in memory. They conclude that the deterioration of the basal ganglia not only affects physical status but the mental one as well.

In the area of verbal performance, several studies have been published. Smith, Butters, White, Lyon, and Granholm (1988) compared HD patients with controls on a series of language tests. They report finding evidence of a semantic deficit in HD, along with a disruption in the lexical–semantic network. However, they note that the results are merely suggestive, particularly because there was confounding. They would place special emphasis on the dynamic nature of the seeming breakdown.

> That is, the results of the present study do not support a hypothesis that HD involves a loss per se of representation of semantic relations. Rather it appears that HD may involve disruption in a dynamic system of interactive activation (and possibly inhibition) of relations and concepts in a semantic network. (pp. 37–38)

The study of memory in HD patients has been a major concern. Brandt and Butters (1986) reviewed the literature on this variable and found reports of consistent defects in concentration, problems in spatial orientation, difficulties with visual and motor integration, memory losses, and adverse effects on using knowledge appropriately and in conceptual reasoning. The memory loss is particularly noted in poor retrieval strategies (patients have difficulty getting needed experience out of memory) along with possible deficits in skill learning. They conclude that the caudate nucleus (in the basal ganglia) must have a major role in spatial representation of knowledge, the ability to make plans and carry out actions, and the initiation of accurate retrieval processes to access memory. In a prior study, Brandt (1985) had tested HD patients against controls on the ability to recall items of general information, to make judgments about their depth of knowledge for unrecalled items, and their success in recognition of correct answers. Thus he examined both recall and recognition, the major forms of memory testing. His results are of interest, for he found deficits in recall but with the ability remaining for the patients to recognize what they could not recall. Their performance was as good as that of the controls in a prediction about the ability to recognize unrecalled items. However, the controls spent more time in searching for the information they believed they could recall than time spent on a search for data they felt they were unlikely to remember. Thus there appeared to be a discrepancy in the patients' behaviors as far as directed retrieval was concerned. Brandt speculates that the dementia of the HD person may include this defect, leading to poorer returns in retrieval.

Affective and arousal factors in memory were investigated by Granholm, Wolfe, and Butters (1985). To patients with HD and a group they labeled as "alcoholic Korsakoff" patients, plus a control group, the investigators read four types of emotionally toned stories—neutral, happy, sad, and sexual—to all subjects. Their subjects were asked to recall both immediately and after a short delay (30 seconds) with a distractor task imposed during the delay. Neither controls nor HD patients showed much forgetting between immediate and delayed recall, but the Korsakoff patients showed rapid and equivalent rates of forgetting on three types of stories. However, the one with sexual themes did not show such a result. Granholm et al. conclude that their data are consistent with a retrieval-deficit hypothesis for persons with HD.

This difference in memory function between Korsakoff's and HD patients has been reviewed further by Butters (1984). He notes that the commonly used memory tests that are included in neuropsychological batteries often do not disclose important differences in memory between amnesiacs and demented persons. For this reason, he surveyed the literature to find evidence in previously published studies of both anterograde amnesia (loss of memory for events *preceding* the incident causing the amnesia) and retrograde amnesia (loss of memory for events *following* the incident). The studies frequently report small or no differences between the groups on memory quotients and scores but highly significant differences on both recall and recognition. Moreover, the ability to acquire information based on rules is affected. Korsakoff patients showed losses in both recognition and recall but could follow rules to acquire information better than those with HD. By contrast, the latter group consistently did better in recognition than Korsakoff's patients. Using test scores alone, the psychologist would report no differences between the two in memory function. However, comparison on specific types of memory alter that position considerably. Butters has made a significant point at the same time that we are reminded again of the lack of depth in our knowledge of how dementias express themselves.

Further evidence on memory has been reported by Martone, Butters, Payne, Becker, and Sax (1984). HD and Korsakoff's patients were compared with each other and with a control group on skill learning and verbal recognition. The Korsakoff's group performed like the controls on the skill learning task but were greatly impaired in word recognition. HD patients had greater difficulty in acquiring the skill (a mirror reading task) but were able to recognize the words used. Martone et al. accord the differences to anterograde factors, favoring the persons with HD. They explain the memory problems of the HD group as being much more severe when recall is the measure rather than recognition.

Huber and Paulson (1987) examined memory in HD patients as a function of the degree to which dementia had progressed. They found that, early in the process, there is slowed cognition but relatively intact memory acquisition and retrieval. As the dementia progresses, cognition shows greater slowing, and the processing of verbal information is increasingly impaired. They maintain that memory impairment in HD changes qualitatively as the dementia progresses. As a result, memory acquisition and retrieval are cumulatively affected but become severe only in later stages of the disease. Studies controlling for the principal element of time since onset or diagnosis are needed to test this hypothesis.

Comparison of memory functions (associative encoding and retrieval processes) for AD and HD patients, compared with controls, has been studied by Granholm and Butters (1988). Both types of dementias showed severe impairment compared with controls on memory for word lists. However, HD subjects were more like controls when semantic retrieval cues were provided during input. AD patients were unable to encode semantic relationships between the cues and words to be recalled. As a result, they demonstrated more free associations to cue words during the retrieval test. Comparison of the same types of dementia, plus controls, on a figural memory task was done by Jacobs, Salmon, Troster, and Butters (1990). They required immediate recall of figures from a subtest on the Wechsler Memory Scale as their measure. The type of error they looked for was the inclusion of a characteristic of one figure in the reproduction of a subsequent figure (prior-figure intrusion errors). Both dementias were more likely to show intrusions than normals, and AD patients made significantly more intrusion errors than HD ones.

Recent Studies on Dementia in Parkinson's Disease

For our purposes, PD must be accompanied by dementia to be of interest. As with HD, the assumption that all PD patients develop demented

behavior is false. The literature surveyed here is restricted to the combination of PD with dementia or to the combination as compared with
cases of PD without dementia.

Medically, PD is a disease of the basal ganglia that leads to specific
motor disability. There are various cognitive losses that are often found,
losses that are more often associated with damage in the cortex than
the subcortex. There must, then, be more complex physical relationships
than some models have proposed. At the same time, cognitive losses
that occur uniquely in the presence of PD have not been demonstrated
(Knight, Godfrey, & Shelton, 1988) so that comparisons with other causes
of dementia, and particularly AD, are inevitable. Dieudonne (1984) believes that the psychological problems found in the PD patient (including
not only dementia but depression as well) may be the result of diffuse
lesions that interfere with dopamine (a neurotransmitter) activity in neurons. Dopamine deficiency appears to be necessary to PD, but it may
not be a sufficient explanation of intellectual decrements.

The issue may be extended to the comparison of PD and AD. Hofman, Schulte, Tanja, Van Duijn, Haaxma, Lameris, Otten, and Saan (1989)
point to a possible joint etiology for the two. They traced the family
histories of 198 patients who had been diagnosed as AD prior to age
70. These histories were compared to those of 198 age- and sex-matched
controls. Almost half the AD patients had close relatives with dementia,
and there were also more occurrences of PD in these families. They
state the findings are evidence of a familial aggregration of both diseases.
There is, then, some possibility of a statistical relationship that has no
explanation as yet. By contrast, Stern, Gur, Saykin, and Hurtig (1986),
in a review of the literature, maintain that there may be coexistence of
the two conditions in some individuals but that PD has its own distinctive
chemical disequilibrium (the dopamine connection) that will ultimately
differentiate both its pathophysiological qualities and appropriate treatment. As yet another possible dimension, Passafiume and Boller (1984)
propose that there are two *forms* of PD. One of these leads to rapid
development of dementia; the other expresses itself only in specific visuospatial deficits. Calne (1989) says that there is sufficient evidence to
presume that PD has multiple causes and calls for a term, such as *idiopathic Parkinsonism*, that indicates the fact that the cause is unknown.

At present, the prevalence of dementia in combination with PD is
unknown. Mayeux, Stern, Rosenstein, Marder, Hauser, Cote, and Fahn
(1988) reviewed the records of 339 patients with a diagnosis they describe
as "idiopathic PD" and applied DSM-III criteria to determine evidence of
dementia. Only 11% met the latter criteria. Other studies have reported
much higher occurrence, so that there may have been some overestima-

tion in such cases or underestimations by Mayeux et al., due to using DSM criteria. There are other possible explanations, of course. One concerns the stringency of the criteria set in the DSM-III, as these may have been more restrictive than those used by some authors. Another may be somewhat related in that Mayeux et al. identified the subsample that was severely demented only. It is interesting that those PD patients who developed dementia also had a later onset of motor effects with more rapid progression of physical disability. They were more likely to show adverse effects to levodopa as well: "Where PD began after age 70 years, dementia was noted three times more frequently than when the disease began at an earlier age" (p. 260). Whatever the reason, such results indicate the probability of disagreement and inaccuracy in the assignment of the label of dementia. This position is reinforced by a study reported by Girotti, Soliveri, Carella, Piccolo, Caffarra, and Musicco (1988). They investigated the clinical characteristics and types of cognitive impairments in 147 cases of PD. The DSM-III criteria for dementia were used. They found only 21 persons (14%) to meet the specifications, a figure that compares favorably with that of Mayeux et al. This suggests that the percentages are more closely related to the standards imposed by the American Psychiatric Association than to other sources.

Cause and Prognosis

As mentioned earlier, the cause of PD is assumed to be a lack of dopamine or the use of certain drugs, especially neuroleptics. The dopamine connection has led to a "treatment" that helps to relieve some of the intensity of muscle tremor but has no effect on the progress of the disease. This intervention is a chemical substitute for dopamine called "L-dopa" or "levodopa" that may be prepared synthetically. Sometimes treatment involves other chemicals. For example, de Smet, Ruberg, Sedaru, Dubois, Lhermitte, and Agid (1982) surveyed patients in a hospital who were receiving anticholinergic therapy. A side effect was created, confusional states, in 93% of those PD patients who were demented. By contrast, less than half the demented cases not on anticholinergic drugs suffered confusion. The authors propose that such medications should not be used when there is intellectual impairment because there is already a cholinergic deficiency present in the cortex and hippocampus of PD patients. Using the chemical merely intensifies a problem already present.

Even L-dopa may have negative effects. Rinne (1983) believes that it may contribute to increased intellectual decline and dementia as well as allow greater sensitivity to side effects. Benefits from a reduction of tremors, then, may come at a high cost, particularly if there are larger doses of L-dopa.

Technology is an increasingly important element in attempting to define the meaning of dementia that accompanies PD. Neufeld, Inzelberg, and Korczyn (1988) did EEG readings on 128 patients with PD. They then examined relationships of the patterns to age, mental status, and motor disability. The findings focused on the fact that slowing in the pattern of occipital background activity most commonly occurred in the patients with dementia but that those without dementia displayed an association between the frequency of occipital slowing and the degree of motor disability as well. The relationship suggests to them that the subcortical structures that are involved in motor control may influence occipital background activity also. It is worthwhile to note that in patients under 60 years of age, they found no instances of EEG abnormalities. Because the older patients are the only ones involved, there is a suggestion as well of an age-related factor that is not disclosed as yet.

Corthesy, Hungerbuhler, Assal, and Regli (1985) compared the amount of motor deficit and of cerebral atrophy, determined by CT scan, with mental impairment for PD patients. Men showed the greater intellectual impairments, and there was a strong relationship to cortical and subcortical atrophies. MRI was used by Besson, Mutch, Smith, and Corrigan (1985) with both demented and nondemented cases of PD, and the scans were compared for both groups to normal controls. They found a correlation between the severity of the dementia and the effects in the basal ganglia and cerebral white matter for both groups of patients. Also with MRI, comparisons were made on 68 patients and 28 controls for mental deterioration (Huber, Shuttleworth, Christy, Chakeres, Curtin, & Paulson, 1989). About one-third (N = 23) met criteria for dementia established by them with neuropsychological tests. Half had mild to moderate intellectual disturbances, and the remainder (N = 11) were not impaired. They then compared 10 persons with and 20 without dementia, matched for severity of PD, with 10 normal controls. This sample was used because 10 patients with dementia volunteered for the MRI scan, and they then sought volunteers from the other two groups to have roughly proportional numbers to the original sample. The scans on MRI did not disclose any particular pattern or abnormalities such as generalized cerebral atrophy or ventricular enlargement. If these studies are representative, technological advances do not make any special contribution to understanding PD, although they may assist in the exclusionary process in diagnosis.

There are a number of changes that may occur in or be associated with the structure of the brain. Globus, Mildworf, and Melamed (1985), for example, examined regional blood flow in the cerebrum to determine a correlation, if any, with dementia. They also had results of a neuropsychological test battery as their measure of cognitive loss. Blood flows were reduced for PD patients as compared with controls, and there was greater cognitive impairment. However, they found no relationship between the amount of blood-flow reduction and the type and degree of intellectual losses. They assume that the two must be independent, as least so far as causative factors are concerned. The neurochemical features of PD and AD as related to hemispheric damage were included in a study by Direnfeld, Albert, Volicer, Langlais, Marquis, and Kaplan (1984). They report that PD patients with greater disease involvement of the left side of the body had different chemical levels than those with principal disease involvement on the right side of the body. The left-sided group also had greater loss of neuropsychological abilities. There is the possibility, they say, that there are functional or anatomic asymmetries in the dopaminergic systems of the central nervous system.

Rinne, Rummukainen, Paljarvi, and Rinne (1989) found neuronal loss in the gray matter of the midbrain (substantia nigra) that was correlated with dementia. Dopamine-producing nerve cells are located in the substantia nigra, and their production tends to be deficient when the person suffers PD. These results indicate a relationship between the lack of cells yielding dopamine and mental competence. Rinne et al. conclude that intact projections from the nigra to the caudate nucleus and limbic and cortical areas is necessary for normal cognition. When these projections are lost, there may be the result of dementia. Cell loss in the substantia nigra has been reported by Sudarsky, Morris, Romero, and Walshe (1989) as well. Using four cases of PD for their analysis, they discovered no senile plaques or neurofibrillary tangles (associated with AD) in the neocortex. They conclude the possibility of subcortical pathology because there is no evidence of AD as an accompanying condition. The presence of depression and dementia often found with PD may be due to the neural substrate of the Parkinson's syndrome, according to Rabins (1982).

Effects on cognitive behavior may occur even when there is no overt dementia. Cummings (1988), for example, reviewed 27 studies in the literature on PD. In the more than 4,000 individuals who were subjects in these studies, about 40% were reported as having dementia. Of the remaining 60%, there were deficits reported in memory, visuospatial skills, language function, the ability to abstract, and performance on motor programming tasks even though the patients were judged to be normal on mental status examinations. The difference in the percentages would seem to be one of degree because the types of deficiencies reported are characteristic of those reported as evidence of dementia in such individuals.

Perhaps, in part, the scores obtained on the mental status tests mask the nature of the mental incompetence of the patient. This would be true where the content of the mental status examination is limited to more specific recent memories. It is possible for a dementia patient to recall certain recent events but not others, particularly in the earlier stages of development of the dementia. As the process continues, these tests become more precise in their identification of mental deficits.

Rogers (1986) has discussed the concept of bradyphrenia, which he defines as slowing of cognition, impairment of concentration, and apathy. The term has a 60-year history and has been linked with the dementia of Parkinsonism. Psychological loss of motor control and sub-cortical source for the dementia are more recent synonyms for the term, according to him. One would expect that the concept is applicable to most, if not all, cases of PD where dementia occurs, but there is dis-sension even here. Mindham, Ahmed, and Clough (1982) report on a group of 40 PD patients and matched controls. All were administered tests of cognitive abilities, and the tests were readministered after 3 years. They report no differences between the groups, either pre- or posttest. However, there were differences in measured intellectual abili-ties between patients and controls, with those who had greatest deficits at the beginning of the study showing a higher death rate. (There was a loss of 10 persons: 7 had died, 2 were not formally assessed because of behavioral limitations, and 1 could not be found.) There was also an increase in the prevalence and severity of dementia that was greater in the patients, yet the differences were not significant statistically. This implies an artifactual presence in the cognitive outcomes that may be explained by the death rate in more impaired subjects. There is the implication that bradyphrenia, as defined, is more pronounced in ad-vanced degrees of PD. Mindham et al. point out the need for appropriate methodologies in such studies. Their point should apply to the entire field as well as experiments with PD.

> Our experience underlines the importance of an appropriately se-lected control group, the use of standardized and appropriate methods of assessment which can be successfully carried out in patients with PD, the study of patients over a suitable period of time with measures which allow for the loss of patients from relevant causes, and num-bers of subjects and controls which would allow full statistical evalu-ation of the results. (p. 973)

The relation of severity in PD symptoms to cognitive loss has been substantiated by Oyebode, Barker, Blessed, Dick, and Britton (1986). Al-though there were deficits usually found in AD in a small proportion of their sample (7%), most of the Parkinson's patients showed a different psychological pattern. The more severe the symptoms of PD, the more likely the cognitive impairment. The prevalence of such deficits is not clear at this time, and they point out that the incidence is above that of the age group but not so high as reported in other studies. Again, the use of DSM-III criteria may be an important component.

The degree of cognitive impairment may be a function of other variables. Age of onset is one such possibility investigated by Hietanen and Teravainen (1988). They studied a group of PD patients whose disease process began before age 60 and compared them with a group with later onset. Although the early group had a variety of cognitive problems, only 1 (of 49) was classified as demented using DSM-III criteria. By contrast, late onset was more often associated with meeting these criteria, a fact that agrees with findings in other studies. Another possible variable concerns the particular functions involved. Caltagirone, Carlesimo, Nocentini, and Vicari (1989) looked at mental functions controlled from the frontal lobe for a group of PD patients subdivided by presence or absence of dementia and compared them to a group of normal controls. They found that nondemented patients did not differ from controls on several intellectual functions (including linguistic and general abilities). There was evidence of deficits in concept formation, maintaining a coherent thought pattern, and being able to shift thought appropriately that was independent of the dementia normally found in the syndrome of PD. As reported in other studies, the Wisconsin Card Sorting Test was the only measure to show such pathological performances. They agree with Weinberger et al. (1988) on the selective nature of impairment. The explanation, they believe, may lie in the afferent pathways from the basal ganglia and midbrain to the frontal cortex. They hypothesize that the reduction in the dopaminergic activity of the caudate nucleus disrupts the normal patterning.

Still another source of cognitive impairment, if not of degree, is a function of the condition itself as compared with other causes of dementias. A number of studies have made such comparisons, as alluded to earlier. Huber, Shuttleworth, and Freidenberg (1989) compared AD to PD and found that there were differences in the abilities affected. Alzheimer patients show greater losses both qualitatively and quantitatively in memory, language, and orientation, whereas persons with PD are more deteriorated in verbal fluency, partially because of retrieval difficulties. With the same groupings, Freedman and Oscar-Berman (1989) compared performance on a learning task with controls. There were two aspects to problems in visual and spatial learning—original learning and reversal learning. They found the AD subjects had greater difficulty on original learning and reversal learning in the visual mode as compared to PD. Using the spatial task, both groups showed impairment on reversal learning but not original learning. They suggest that the differences on the visual task may help differentiate the two diagnoses.

For the different types of memory functions, there may be differences in performance as well. Huber, Shuttleworth, and Paulson (1986) report that sensory register[3] was relatively intact in a sample studied by them and compared to normal controls. Short-term memory, however, seemed impaired in all their subjects. Only as there was significant overall mental decline was remote memory affected in PD. Another reflection of memory function is the type of error made on specific tasks. Intrusions in stories were studied by Helkala, Laulumaa, Soininen, and Riekkinen (1989). They had samples of AD, PD, and normal controls. With stories told to subjects, they found that the patient groups had more intrusion errors, both from prior stories and extralist (i.e., unrelated terms) than controls. AD subjects exceeded PD ones in extrastory errors, exceeded the PD group in extralist errors, and identified more false positive instances in a recognition task. Helkala et al. conclude that there are different patterns of memory dysfunctions. The PD patients show sensitivity to proactive interference, whereas AD ones are sensitive to any interference. Further, the AD persons seemed unable to inhibit irrelevant information as well as PD ones.

> The AD patients perform poorly because of their inability to inhibit irrelevant information and increased sensitivity to interference, whereas the deficits of PD patients solely reflect a sensitivity to proactive interference of perseveration, but not, however, an inability to inhibit irrelevant information. (p. 1247)

An outcome not so often considered but one that has great meaning for patient and spouse or partner has been discussed by Mayeux (1987). He maintains that depression and dementia are impediments to the emotional and psychic well-being of PD patients. One result is sexual dysfunction, and the PD treatment may be part of the problem. Thus dopamine improves motor function but may interfere with normal sexuality. He cites frequent complaints by male patients of the detrimental effects of medications on erectile maintenance and delay of ejaculation. Whether one sees such matters as a concern, Mayeux has succeeded in bringing attention to a personal variable that is important to quality of life. The point may be well taken that there is an overabundance of attention on variables such as memory function, where redundancy does not necessarily bring greater knowledge, and a lack of focus on the meanings and outcomes of well-being for patients and caregivers.

As with other conditions, there is a sizable and rapidly accumulating corpus of literature on HD and PD where dementia occurs. Several aspects of the relationship between syndrome and dementia have been investigated but with little effort at synthesis. The result is a rather amorphous set of data that sometimes conflict, sometimes agree, but are more often difficult to compare. With time and continuing study, the mosaic may be clearer.

CURRENT RESEARCH IN DRUG THERAPY

The point has been made previously that the great need for controlling dementia is first to find the causes of the syndromes associated with the decline. Once a cause (or causes) is specified, research can seek means to prevent its occurrence. Prevention is worth at least a pound of cure, as has been demonstrated in such diseases as measles (rubella). The development of a vaccine that effectively produced a low-grade infection in the body allowed the immune system to develop the appropriate antibodies. There is no reason for persons to have measles today, and certainly no reason for epidemics to occur that kill large numbers, a phenomenon that occurred episodically before the vaccine was developed. When society finally decides that the cost of an answer is worth the investment, it seems likely that a solution will be achieved.

Basic research is ongoing in several areas. Among the efforts, briefly described, are the following ones.

Genetics

In some cases, there does appear to be a familial type of syndrome that is predictable with high accuracy. Huntington's disease has been identified as due to a single dominant autosomal gene, for example, with about 50% of all offspring affected. Alzheimer's disease has been found present in a fairly large percentage of Down's syndrome patients who live past the age of 35. Although the occurrence may be due to error on Chromosome 21 (the source of Down's), the exact connection between the two conditions is not yet certain. There may be a familial type of Alzheimer's due to genetic error on Chromosome 19, and this research is ongoing. There is even speculation that the factors associated with stroke, principally hypertension, are heritable. A resulting multiinfarct dementia would have a genetic cause in that case. As answers are reached, there may be at least some explanation of the dementia caused, even if correction for genetic error is not possible. However, it would seem that a genetic basis will not explain all sources of dementias.

Environmental Toxins

A structural change noted in many Alzheimer's disease patients is the increased amount of aluminum, a trace mineral that is stored in body cells. As the storage occurs in brain cells, the effects are destructive to normal functioning. The source of the aluminum has not been detected, though the mineral is prevalent in many products in common use, such as antiperspirants and antacids. Even aluminum cookware has been indicted in some quarters, but such origins do not seem reasonable as the explanation for the disease and dementia. Nevertheless, the need to determine why aluminum collects in cells is a legitimate basis of exploration whether or not it turns out to be the significant factor in the development of AD. Indeed, other possible sources of toxicity in the environment may become candidates eventually as investigation of toxins, hazardous wastes, pollution, and the like, continues.

Neurotransmitter Deficits

The neurotransmitters serve essential roles in the transmission of signals that allow us to function in a complex environment. Located at the axonal terminal of the nerve cell, the neurotransmitters assist the conduction of the electrical impulse across the synapse to an adjacent cell. If there is insufficiency of the chemical, the "message" may be interrupted before the signal reaches the appropriate portion of the brain. When this happens, the person will be unable to interpret and respond to stimuli in the affected neuronal areas.

Dopamine is one of the neurotransmitters, and it has been implicated in Parkinson's disease. Because of the lack of dopamine, there is loss of control of motor systems, apparently, so that patients will show tremors and poor motor coordination. It is now known that a chemical substitute (called L-dopa or levodopa) will cross the blood–brain barrier and simulate the action of dopamine, thereby reducing some of the motor effects for the patient. This approach influenced the attempts to reduce symptoms in Alzheimer's patients. That is, there is an insufficiency of another neurotransmitter in this case—acetylcholine—so the reasoning went that a chemical substitute for it might be tried. Efforts have proved relatively fruitless, however, not because the logic is incorrect but because the brain will not take up the substitute. Still, ways to encourage increased production of acetylcholine remain primary in research activity. Drug companies, in particular, are working on possible stimulators, as we shall see later in this section.

Beta Amyloid

A more recent finding that has caused considerable interest is the presence of a form of protein, called amyloid, which, when present in the chemical form called beta amyloid, is associated with plaques in Alzheimer's-diseased cells. There is a current position that beta amyloid leads to the plaques associated with nerve cell degeneration for the patient. Research is underway, particularly with a natural substance called Substance P, which offers considerable promise that nerve cell degeneration may not only be stopped but perhaps even reversed. If the hypothesis is accepted with sufficient scientific proof, a major intervention may become available. That promise seems some years yet in the future, however.

Slow-Acting Virus

The cause of Creutzfeldt–Jakob disease is known; it is a slow-acting virus. It is "slow" in the sense that it takes time to express itself, sometimes months, other times years. Unfortunately, knowing the cause is not sufficient because scientists have not been able to isolate the virus, discover its nature, or prepare appropriate interventions. Once present, the course is always certain, terminating in death usually within 2 years.

There has been some speculation that other causes of dementia may be due to a virus also. Although there is some effort in this direction with Alzheimer's, the results have not been encouraging. Many scientists believe that this avenue will not be fruitful, primarily because AD is not transmissible as is CJD. In the latter, for example, transfer of tissue from an infected human to a chimpanzee led to a later expression of the disease in the animal. Other transfers have proven successful also. To date, there has been no successful transplantation of AD to animals. Indeed, this condition appears to be uniquely human, perhaps because the locus of diseased cells is largely cortical.

Immune System Decline

Though this approach has not found adherents to the degree that others have, there is nevertheless research being conducted to assess a possible connection between immune system function and conditions producing dementia. The immune system is our protection against invasion by harmful substances. The reasoning is that certain dementia-producing syndromes may be the result of a cell or germ or virus that is not recognized by the immune system or for which no antibody is available or can be created. This returns us to the issue of causation again and in the basic sense that some better understanding is necessary to support the logic of this argument. Conversely, there may be a case made for inducing the immune system to create an antibody that will overcome the effects of beta amyloid, say, or neurofibrillary tangles and plaques. The greatest return may lie in the concept of autoimmunity, based upon the changes occurring in the competence of the system. With age, the immune system develops a tendency to assist rather than repel invasive units. Thus over time the body works against its own welfare.

The dedication to many areas of research is exciting and has been applauded by scientists and by agencies. Yet, progress has been slower than one would hope, considering the ravages on human lives from dementia. The central factor is lack of money for research. Although federal funding is in the hundreds of millions of dollars today, and there is support from a number of foundations and corporations, there are fewer studies pursuing fewer alternatives than are necessary to assure answers for today's generations. It is true, of course, that research in the area of dementia is recent, with major efforts beginning only in the last two or three decades. Other conditions have a longer history without having established answers to the basic questions raised; unfortunately, many of these syndromes also have had much more money invested in their behalf. Society determines priorities; as society decides that the threats are greater from dementing conditions than from others, the shift in emphasis will occur.

Meantime, drug companies are investing in a variety of studies intended to develop an intervention that will control or reverse the process leading to dementia. There are three possibilities in the use of any medication. First, there is the chance that whatever is being treated will be stabilized in its progression so that things do not become worse, even if they don't become better. In effect, the disease process will be halted, or the behavioral outcomes will be improved. In the latter case, this would mean amelioration of memory loss so that the patient can more effectively deal with the everyday problems and demands of life. Such an outcome would be welcomed by caregivers as well because it would offer some relief in the burdens imposed. The disease process would continue, though perhaps at a slower pace, so that the ultimate degeneration would be unchanged. Intervention in this direction is evident in some of the drugs currently being developed and tried.

Second, and perhaps ideally, there might be a kind of "magic bullet" that would in fact reverse the disease process so that the patient recovers at least partially. This would bring major positive behavioral changes as well. Essentially, such a drug would have to be able to restore cell function for those neurons that have been altered or destroyed. Realistically, such a medication would be viable only where cell bodies and nuclei are still healthy. If there could be a restoration and proliferation of dendritic spines, the effects would be positive, and the outcomes would be dramatic. This, also, is an endeavor already under investigation.

Finally, it would be marvelous indeed if a drug could be compounded that cures the disease and returns the patient to normal status. Few drugs are in fact curative, of course, and at the present stage of knowledge, to find such a medication seems improbable if not impossible. More sensible, as mentioned earlier, would be identification of cause and institution of prevention. Never to experience a condition at all is even better than to find a cure when the syndrome is already active.

The attempts to find an intervention are based on a number of theories about causation. This has led to a "clutter of ideas surrounding what might be setting off or feeding the disease [in this case, Alzheimer's]" (Starr, 1990, 41). There is consequent focus and interdependence within strategies by particular drug companies, but without coordination in efforts due to the desire to patent and exclusively market profit-making products. Companies are developing and testing drugs depending on "whether you want a compound that slows or arrests the degeneration process, one that allows nerve cells to regenerate, or one that alleviates symptoms, helping patients to live as normal a life as possible" (Starr, 1990, 41). Each is a commendable goal, and perhaps all will be accomplished.

A principal candidate for intervention is the development of a drug that will increase acetylcholine (ACh) because this neurotransmitter results from cells more often damaged by the disease process. Some of the attempts are directed at increasing production of the chemical and others at ways to prevent the destruction of the available chemical. There have been prior attempts to employ a substance that would combine with the receptor on a neuron so that the binding activity would be initiated. Choline is an example of such a substance, but it has not proven effective for the purpose.

Already, an application for a new drug to be made available has been filed with the Food and Drug Administration. Called Cognex, its scientific name is tetrahydroaminoacridine (THA). Its action is to inhibit cholinesterase, an enzyme that breaks down ACh. Unfortunately, THA appears most helpful to those in the earlier development of dementia and is not universal in its effects even there. It also is short-lived, so that benefits are time limited. As must be expected, it has no effect on the course of the disease (Alzheimer's), and there is some evidence of adverse side effects, principally liver toxicity (Starr, 1990). Though caregivers have heard about this drug because of drug industry support provided for its development and the selection of subjects from current cases, it may have higher visibility and greater expectations than it deserves. For cases where it brings even temporary reversal of symptoms, it will be most welcome. Prescriptions, even if it is made available, are apt to be limited to selected individuals.

In early 1991, after reviewing the evidence from studies presented by the drug manufacturers, an advisory committee to the Food and Drug Administration recommended that Cognex not be approved. There was insufficient evidence to support the position that it offered substantial relief for symptoms for AD while assuring no adverse side effects. Though a disappointing outcome to many caregivers, the Alzheimer's Association (ADRDA) has accepted and supported the decision because "over the long term . . . the scientific approach to drug review will best serve patients and caregivers" (Truschke, 1991, p. 2). The drug company producing Cognex has implemented a new national study (on-going during 1992) designed to yield data which might lead the FDA to grant approval.

A similar drug is physostigmine, which also blocks cholinesterase. The results have been problematic. Positive effects, when found, are short-lived as a result of the dosage and its rapid utilization. A form has been prepared that will permit controlled release over a longer time period, and this will permit more sustained action and positive results. There is a belief that this compound will prove more successful than THA and that memory improvement may be more substantial. The characteristics of patients who benefit may be limited as they are for THA, however, and there is a definite diminishing return due to its action. That is, with increasing severity of dementia, there is less ACh produced so that blocking its destruction may no longer be an effective strategy (Starr, 1990).

An alternative approach is based on the observation that some agency (Starr mentions trauma, genetics, or age as possibilities) causes the amino acid glutamate to become toxic. If so, then a drug that would reduce its release or cause the nerve cell receptor to be less receptive to it would benefit the patient. Several companies are researching this avenue in conjunction with conditions that lead to short-term degeneration. If successful here, the compound may be tried with diseases having long-term effects.

Efforts are also directed at the nerve growth factor (a protein that helps development of the sensory and sympathetic nervous systems) on the assumption that it could help prevent cell death or lead to the regeneration of dendritic spines. Should this course prove viable, it would probably lead to implantation of a pump in the chest cavity to disperse the chemical (Starr, 1990). On another tack, other companies are examining the nature of amyloid, considering how it is assimilated and its nature in AD. There is especial emphasis on the plaques and their inhibition as the assumption is that plaques are the central element both in cell death and decreases in neurotransmitter production.

Mitochondria are the power plants of the cell, and one direction pursued in drug development is based on the possibility that lesions occur that reduce this ability to produce energy for the cell. If so, there will be dysfunction in the neuron and probable death, according to this view. A drug has already been tested in Europe that seems beneficial for mitochondrial lesions (Starr, 1990). This compound, called acetyl-l-carnitine, is a natural substance in the body that is involved in energy production in the cell. *How* the substance works is unknown, but scientists studying it believe that influencing energy production in the cell may retard neuronal damage, perhaps even reverse it (Alzheimer's Association, 1991c). If ever to be used in this country, the drug would have to meet the relatively rigid standards of the Food and Drug Administration. Called Alcar, the medication is now being tested in this country. There are 27 sites involved, and around 400 patients will participate in the trials over a year's period (Alzheimer's Association). Results have not yet been reported. The concept of metabolic enhancement has encouraged other efforts as well. Just what the mechanisms of cell energy may be is not so clear, but some scientists assume that glucose and oxygen utilization are increased, thereby increasing the source of energy available to the cell.

There is a drug already approved for some stroke patients that is being used with patients with age-related dementia to determine if it has positive effects on behaviors resulting from dementia. This drug, Nimodipine, was designed to prevent cells from accumulating calcium in excess amounts, as too much calcium is toxic to nerve cells. The testing is designed to see if the chemical can reduce the rate or number of cells that are dying from calcium poisoning. If so, then it may help stabilize AD, and thus act as a treatment. On another tack, another drug that at one time was thought to offer promise, Hydergine, has proved to be ineffective. The benefits that were hoped for in terms of mental competences have not been realized so the drug probably will be rarely used for treatment in the future. Perhaps this will be the eventual resolution for a number of the chemicals discussed in this section. Certainly, there must be care exercised so that patients and caregivers are not allowed to establish expectations that cannot and will not be met.

Although other developments are underway, it should be clear that drug corporations are investing heavily in ways to overcome some of the handicaps associated with dementia. Admittedly, these focus on reducing behavioral effects, and there are too many medications being tested to judge which may be most promising. There may be a breakthrough as a result of these efforts in the near future. Certainly, some drugs for AD will become available and will be prescribed even though they are limited in their effects and the patients who may benefit. If costs are not prohibitive, the results will offer some hope to all and some benefits to a portion of the affected group, at the very least.

SUMMARY

Although they occur in many fewer cases than AD or even MID, there are several causes of dementia that need to be recognized and understood. In this chapter, I have surveyed these in terms of cause, prognosis, and outcomes. A review of some of the progress being attempted by drug companies in this country offers promise but with considerable reservation due to the limited nature of research results at present.

CHAPTER NINE

Dementia and the Family

Any devastating illness has effects on members of a family as well as the patient. Though there may be evidences of sympathy and empathy, there are also different effects and degrees among the involved parties. In the case of dementia, there is a ripple effect that has been described for several years now. Usually, there is a primary caregiver, most often a spouse or middle-aged child, who becomes responsible for the care of the patient as the process moves slowly but inexorably to its termination. Increasing physical and mental demands accompany the changes, with physical illness and stress as potential outcomes for the caregiver. Even if the demands are handled successfully, there will be a need to consider legal and economic factors, including the eventual placement of the patient in a long-term care facility. The complex of such events has led to the awareness of multiple and severe "burdens" that must be faced and adjusted to by the primary caregiver. The challenge may be met, or it may become overwhelming.

In most cases, there are other family members, children especially, but also close relatives. These persons may represent a resource because they can be supports to the primary caregiver even if they are not so directly involved with the daily problems. Social scientists have been especially aware of both the caregiver and family members and have studied roles, relationships, interventions, supports, and outcomes in recent years. The primary emphasis has been on sociopsychological variables with the production of a large body of literature exploring various aspects of the dimensions of caregiving. A survey of this research and its findings is the purpose of this chapter.

STRESS AND BURDEN

A model or theory allows speculation about conditions or causes of events that do not yet have an explanation. Systematic investigation may follow to gather evidence about the accuracy of the speculation. More often than not, the result is some change in the model to accommodate the actual data, with subsequent further study. The process is neither simple nor successful always. However, it does allow the implementation of the scientific method with problems that need solution.

Unfortunately, such a systematized approach to the study of human involvement and suffering has not been the rule. More often than not, a problem is posed, and investigations begin based upon personal judgments about the relevant variables and their consequences. Among investigators, labels may differ for the same intended manifestations. The measures used, differing at the same time that there is overlap, lead to conclusions that seem at variance. The outcome may be confusion and restrictions in generalizations. These comments are pertinent to the varied literature that has been published in journals and books concerning the effects of dementia on family members and primary caregivers. Yet the need to understand and assist caregivers and patients is so important that a survey of research and an attempt at synthesis is essential.

At present, there is no model of caregiver effects from dementia that is either widely accepted or that has received adequate experimental proof. Nevertheless, there have been studies that specify possible effects and test interventions. Mace (1986), for example, has described needs of Alzheimer's patients and families. For "therapeutic" purposes, she suggests day care, recreation programs in long-term care facilities, home assistance, and outpatient services as ways to help the patient deal with stress. She also cites needs of family members that may be met by services such as respite and residential care. Perhaps the specific listing is less important than the reason for their presence—stress reduction, both for patient and caregiver.

The matter of stress, or burden, is a recurring one in the literature. Morycz (1985, p. 333) says that "burden" is a result of the subjective viewpoint of the caregiver and that it gives an indication of the levels and types of care that is given to the patient. Citations about burden range from discussion and description in media, to empirical studies in journals, and eventually to books that combine the two (see, e.g., Zarit, Orr, & Zarit, 1985).

Zarit and Zarit (1982) have proposed three specific forms of intervention: education, particularly about the disease and its consequences; problem solution, as a technique that will have general utility for the caregiver and patient; and support, both of a formal and informal nature. These interventions have been advocated by Pratt, Wright, and Schmall as well (1987, p. 111). Marples (1986) has described how such resources may be used along with their specific characteristics. The patient, she says, suffers anxiety early, and with increasing regression shows denial and depression. Family members develop confusion and grief. She agrees with Zarit and Zarit and with Pratt et al. that education and support are essential to help overcome such traits and must coexist with clinical interventions. From her discussion we may add a second variable—depression.

McNew (1987) has presented a more systematic model, intended to contribute to the ability of the caregiver to develop competence. There are three major components. First, there must be a "transactional" unit, involving support. Here competence is influenced by the ability of the caregiver to expand the environment beyond the caregiver–patient relationship while adapting to environmental demands. Second, there is the "personal" capacity component that she calls interpersonal effectiveness. The competence affected by this realm is based on interpersonal relationships. Finally, McNew speaks of a "cognitive" element, expressed as perceived personal control. Thus the ways in which the caregiver interprets events and their influences affects her or his competence. She advocates that professionals may use this schema to develop practices to use with caregivers once their competencies have been assessed.

The caregiving process itself may be subdivided, as Hogan (1990) has done. She cites five behaviors—anticipatory, preventive, supervisory, instrumental, and protective—that the caregiver must serve. The "anticipatory" phase includes those events that impact on the caregiver's actions due to considerations external to the caregiving setting. She mentions, as an example, the opportunity for the caregiver to move to a better job somewhere else. This offer is kept secret (she speaks of "intentionally invisible") from the patient because the caregiver feels a responsibility to remain in the present setting. "Preventive" behaviors are things done to assure maximum health in the patient. Included are questioning of the patient about symptoms and medications as well as making changes in the physical environment to provide more protection for the patient. "Supervisory" demands extend to the caregiving act itself with its many components. "Instrumental" actions are the hands-on functions that maintain the patient's health status. Hogan says this is the type of caregiving most often studied but the least important of the roles in the perception of the caregiver. Finally, "protective" efforts are described by Hogan as the most difficult but the most important type. Here the caregiver wishes to protect the patient from consequences that *cannot be prevented* regardless of one's attempts. These include the threats to the self-concept of the patient by trying to disguise an awareness of being cared for. Obviously, this is a no-win situation.

By contrast, Pilisuk and Parks (1988) consider caregiver burden in terms of resources needed to meet the challenges involved. They see a problem so large in scope that a national policy on caregiving is needed with a shift in national priorities to permit necessary funding.

Thus there are numerous views and priorities, all of which may be appealing but few of which accord with system and direction. Though intended for medical labeling, Maletta (1990) has illustrated the problem succinctly. He points out that, at least in some areas, the literature lacks clarity and rigor in terminology. He refers to definitions of dementia as an example, but his position can be applied to caregiver/patient behaviors also. Clarity and rigor are imperfect in the vocabulary of social scientists as well. Too often we are faced with the dilemma of individual preferences, custom, and jargon.

The "social construction of dementia" (a term coined by Lyman, 1989) is muddled at present. Lyman believes reliance upon the biomedical model has interfered with the development of a coherent construction. As a result, there is a negative impact on the understanding of treatment contexts and caregiving relationships as they interact with disease progression. Whether that position explains the dilemma is problematic, but Lyman has focused on an issue needing clarification. For example, she applies her criticism to the need to make a decision about institutionalization of the dementia patient. The medical model reduces uncertainty about the best interests of the patient because it predicts progression of the disease in some stages that lead to deterioration. This outcome permits the caregiver to exercise a certain strategy, such as institutionalization, believing it to be the most appropriate. After all, if a "disease" forces this outcome, there can be no blame The certainty presented by the model may help relieve stress, at least in certain directions and even though it may produce stress in other directions. Lyman makes a cogent point that is worth repeating.

> However, the biomedical model includes disease typifications that limit the self-identity of demented persons, . . . Research in family caregiver groups . . . finds a similar pattern of overgeneralization about dementia: once the family member has been diagnosed, people see "impairment" everywhere! (p. 602)

Research on Caregiver Burden

In an attempt to clarify the sources and outcomes of burden, there are studies that consider conditions under which burden occurs and its effects. George and Gwyther (1986), for example, proposed four possible dimensions involved in feelings of well-being. Results indicated that, as compared to noncaregivers in the community, two of these dimensions (mental health and social participation) were more likely to represent problems for feelings of well-being than were physical health and financial resources. The mental status of the patient was less likely to interfere with well-being than was the caregiving situation. Thus some caregivers are apt to find themselves overwhelmed with the tasks with which they must deal, without being able to find relief through acceptable outlets. George and Gwyther make a point that reinforces the quote from Lyman: There is a common belief that caregiving over time brings deterioration of the caregiver. However, their data showed no relationship between the duration of patient illness and well-being of the caregiver.

> Our findings thus suggest that it is the characteristics of the caregiving situation and the resources available to the caregiver, rather than the condition of the patient, that most directly affect caregiver well-being. (p. 259)

The intensity involved in caregiving is demonstrated in a study by Birkel and Jones (1989). They examined caregiving of patients still mentally lucid with those who were demented. They report that members of the immediate household are more likely to have to care for dementia patients, whereas caregivers of patients without dementia often are provided with assistance. It would appear that the problems *are* more intensive for caregivers of dementia patients, although the reasons why this is so are not clear. Certainly, the intensity of caregiving is related to factors more complex than the severity of the disease alone. In many communities, multiple services and agencies are present to assist with caregiving tasks. It may be that cost and/or preference are the major reasons why such services are not used in the majority of cases. Houlihan (1987) inspected available data and concluded that caregivers of dementia patients receive greater effects from emotional support, whereas those who care for the frail elderly (without dementia) benefit more from learning skills used in nursing a patient. The attitudes of the two must differ greatly if Houlihan is correct, with greater feelings of stress present in those who must deal with demented individuals. In a study described in an earlier chapter, DeBettignies et al. (1990) reported that inaccurate reports by dementia patients about their competencies was a significant influence in the degree of burden felt by the caregiver. This variable reintroduces one of the effects of loss of mental competence—the discrepancy between capability and perception of that capability by the patient. When the person makes claims about competencies that are at variance with the actual abilities still available, conflict occurs. Resolution of the patient/caregiver conflict may be difficult to achieve. This adverse relationship is extended and expanded when a third party (such as a relative or friend) is told by the patient that competency still is present but expression is forbidden. For example, the demented person may claim that driving skills are still intact. The statement *sounds* reasonable, and there may be a known history of success in driving, so why is driving forbidden? The caregiver is placed in a position that intensifies feelings of burden under such circumstances.

Further, reality is altered, perhaps lost, in the patient at the same time that verbal skills may remain relatively intact. The demands of the patient may cause severe difficulties for the caregiver because communication is no longer possible. The result is a person who talks and appears to be "normal" but who is unable to understand the discrepancy between reality and unreality. As an example, the patient may say that a prized possession has been stolen and that the caregiver must have taken it. There is a demand that it be returned at once! Explanations about misplacing the article, denials of having taken it, reference to other instances where the caregiver has been accused wrongly—all are rejected by the patient and the anger intensifies. Such a situation increasingly puts the caregiver at risk when there are no skills or supports to bring relief.

Under conditions producing such stress, the appearance of depression would seem understandable. In this regard, a study comparing caregivers to controls (Haley, Levine, Brown, Berry, & Hughes, 1987) reported significantly higher levels of depression for the caregivers. They also had more negative feelings about their relatives, whether deserved or not, and low satisfaction with life. Either as a consequence or accompanying this personal pattern, social interactions were less satisfactory, even though there were no differences in contacts. Health care was adversely affected as well, both in terms of self-reported health status and in terms of usage of the health care system, including drug use. Haley et al. state that clinical observation indicates that, as a group, caregivers are "selected" for the role "largely by virtue of their psychological strength" (p. 410). Where true, it is obvious that that strength may erode in several directions and with severe damage.

The declines in the patient are factors related to stress and depression. However, these declines are not uniform in appearance, degree, or severity

(Haley & Pardo, 1989). Early in the process, instrumental self-care deficits begin, for example, whereas the more basic self-care deficits do not come until greater dementia is achieved. In fact, many of the more stressful symptoms begin to fade with progression and eventually are lost altogether. For these reasons, Haley and Pardo advocate the need for an assessment of patient impairment at different points in time to assist in understanding what the particular stressor operating for the caregiver may be. This position is reinforced by results of a study by Montgomery, Gonyea, and Hooyman (1985). They subdivided burden into two types: subjective and objective. The former was primarily related to age and income of the caregiver, whereas the latter involved tasks that demanded time and/or space, thereby confining the caregiver. Patient impairment would lead to restriction in freedom for the caregiver and consequent stress. Montgomery et al. conclude that objective burden can be reduced through services: personal aid, equipment permitting more self-care, and respite. Considering the research reviewed, the accessibility of such aids would not necessarily lead to their acceptance and use. For the caregivers of dementia patients, the relationship seems not to be so direct as it is for frail, nondemented elderly.

A study by Scott, Roberto, and Hutton (1986) reports data about respite effects on caregivers. They hypothesized that, where adequate support was provided by family members, there would be less burden and better coping with problems on the part of the primary caregiver. There were differing styles of family support among their sample members, but overall Scott et al. found assistance benefitted the caregiver. Principally, the assists included efforts that allowed respite from the heavy demands, either through personal visits or by relief for a period of time. The hypothesis seemed supported because those who received the most beneficial support were better able to cope with problems. Also, caregivers who did not receive adequate support were the most burdened. Surprisingly, however, the group that received the *most* support (noted as "more than enough" by the authors) reported very nearly the same level of burden as those receiving inadequate support. Those who received "enough support" in the caregivers' judgment (neither too much nor too little) had significantly less burden than the other two groups. Scott et al. speculate that the group with "more than enough" respite were at-risk for dysfunction and thus received increased efforts by the family. They may be correct, though one might wonder if "too much" of a good thing may not be about as disruptive as "not enough." Whatever the reason, there is an obvious challenge to sorting out the interventions that overcome the disruptive elements in stress and using them appropriately for effective intervention.

Research on Sources of Burden

The context of caregiving inclines many (though not all) to stress and increasing feelings of burden (though not in the same directions or degrees). It would be helpful to know what the sources of such feelings may be because this knowledge would delimit the components and suggest a focus for interventions. The research in this direction is limited at the same time that it is confusing.

For the general case of caregiving, Stoller and Pugliese (1989) surveyed informal helpers of 173 elderly persons (not necessarily demented) for the various roles they, as helpers, must play. Through personal interviews, Stoller and Pugliese determined that the feelings of burden of their subjects involved additional roles they needed to fulfill as well as those that were related to caregiving demands. This was particularly true when the time demands for the care of the elderly patient were heavy. This suggests a source of stress that lies outside the boundaries of caregiving; if the helper has such demands that are difficult or impossible to meet due to contingencies of caregiving, there will be greater burden. This is most true, Stoller and Pugliese say, when the needs of the patient demand high levels of assistance. At the same time, outside roles contributed to feelings of well-being, Stoller and Pugliese found. This was true when the "other roles" served as buffers against stressors. There may be the Catch-22 of the imbalance needed to provide balance. There is also the implication of the need for respite, however it may be defined. They found that neither instrumental nor emotional support directly affected burden or feelings of well-being. However, emotional support did help to alleviate the burden that results from the summation of large time demands and care responses.

This position is supported by research by Killeen (1990). She also surveyed caregivers ($N = 120$) to determine the presence of stress and ways of dealing with it. She found that *younger* caregivers expressed greater feelings of stress, particularly when they had to serve multiple roles. Their coping strategies involved both problem solution (as suggested by Zarit & Zarit, 1982) and emotion focusing (which might imply a less orderly and potentially defeating effort). Most often, they simply gave up their own personal time, thereby sacrificing opportunities for respite. Killeen (1990) found a relationship between the time sacrifices and negative feelings of personal health status.

These two studies (Stoller & Pugliese, and Killeen) suggest that caregiving should permit the assumption of roles that are separated from the context of service to the patient. In and of themselves, these external roles may bring feelings of burden. Thus the concept of respite is probably not an accurate one to use in relation to such involvement outside the caregiving situation. It may be that a kind of "partialing" of sources of burden leads to less intense negative results than concentration into narrower channels. Not only are the parts different, but the sums may be different as well. Research is needed to pinpoint such dynamics.

Within the situational context, there has been effort to delineate the components leading to stress. Pruchno and Resch (1989) examined well-being of caregivers in terms of certain demanding behaviors found in their AD patients. They report direct relationships between burden levels and the disorientation found in patients as well as asocial behaviors that conflicted with norms and with past competencies. As the behaviors were considered by caregivers to be more burdensome, there were greater mental health problems expressed by caregivers. The disruptive behaviors required more sacrifices of social life by caregivers. Pruchno and Resch speak of some support for a "wear and tear" hypothesis. "As the frequency of behaviors increases, so does the level of caregiver stress" (p. S181). The most commonly cited result of dementia—memory loss—was related in a nonlinear fashion to burden, perceived mental health problems, and social adaptations. As memory loss increases, there is an increase in burden. However, the relationship reverses with higher levels of forgetful behaviors. As patients show memory loss "often" and "most of the time," caregivers experience less stress. In fact, the authors state that stress levels of caregivers who report little or no memory loss are similar to those where the patient is severely impaired. Pruchno and Resch interpret their results as due to the course of the disease and role expectations for caregivers.

In the spirit of the discussion to this point, the latter (role expectations) may be more profound than the former (disease progression). In this regard, Dunkle and Nevin (1987) examined management problems experienced by both medical and family caregivers. They report that professional assessment assisted in providing better care in the home, but it did little or nothing to improve the coping of the caregiver. This would accord with Lyman's (1989) criticism of such strong dependence on the medical model, whereas the dynamics of caregiving are relatively ignored. Directly to the issue, Novak and Guest (1989) found that duration of caregiving and feelings of burden were not related (in accord with other research already cited), and only a moderate, though statistically significant, correlation obtained between burden and the functional status of the patient. What *was* significant were the subjective feelings and needs of the caregiver (admittedly a dimension that may include a myriad of possibilities). Novak and Guest suggest that programs and services should not be designed by professionals but be based upon the expressed feelings of the caregivers. Interviews and discussion sessions will help define the more appropriate content for such efforts. There are, of course, such approaches used in many settings, though it is not uncommon to expect the caregivers to adapt to the professional situation rather than the other way around.

In most instances, females more commonly serve as caregivers than do males. A few studies have examined sex differences as they apply to the role. Among women, Staight and Harvey (1990) have compared primary to secondary caregiving. They found both types of caregivers were susceptible to the burdens that come with the role. However, there were differences in time demands, with secondary caregivers receiving more respite in this regard. The symptoms of the role—loneliness, depression, financial difficulties, and low life satisfaction—were areas of vulnerability found in both groups.

Differences in stress and stressors between sexes were investigated by Barusch and Spaid (1989). They report (contrary to some research referred to earlier) that the difficulties associated with the patient's cognition and behavior predicted burden most reliably. Other factors of significance were caregiver age, unpleasant social situations, caregiver sex, and ability to cope with difficult situations. Their findings diverge from others in some interesting ways. For example, there was a gender difference in cognitive problems but not in the expected direction. Men, in this case, were caring for more disabled persons and were therefore subject to greater burden. The authors state that women were found to express greater stress particularly because they were younger. Further, the belief that men are more difficult to care for than women as patients was not supported by the data. Finally, the belief that men receive more formal and informal supports than women caregivers was true only for home-delivered meals. Perhaps these unexpected findings result from the characteristics of their sample and thus need further verification.

Gregory, Peters, and Cameron (1990), in a survey of the literature on male spousal caregivers, found several variables that influenced the meaning of caregiving. Included were sex-role socialization, previous experience in domestic chores, work-role behaviors, personality, and the cultural background of the caregiver. Gregory et al. note that men are more likely to seek out formal supports and to benefit from informal ones than are women. Yet males do not involve themselves often in the traditional support sources such as support groups.

The picture of the effects of caregiving is complex indeed. The search for a global meaning for burden may not yield useful information (Reed, Stone, and Neale, 1990), even though caregivers explicitly see their lives in a negative light. Reed et al. could find only 2 areas of life (out of

11 measured) where caregivers were significantly different from controls. (These were the number of negative events reported during a week and the undesirability of such events.) At the same time, the caregiving group gave more frequent and intense reactions of a negative kind in all the areas. Overall, Reed et al. found no support for a position that caregiving demands tend to disrupt and restrict activities in general; at the same time, they point out it would be premature to conclude the obverse. Kosberg, Cairl, and Keller (1990) also report that more global scores and measures do not give information of the specific type needed to identify components of burden. This would require intensive measurement to predict problems, anticipate adverse consequences and allow preventive intervention. Yet they say that

> The analysis of data . . . leads to the conclusion that certain variables are related to components of burden. For example, female gender is related to several components of burden. . . . Further, living with a patient increases the probability of caregiving burden. Also correlated . . . are behavior problems of patients and self-reported health problems of caregivers. (p. 241)

The concept of burden or stress has been widely used among professionals who work with caregivers and patients in the field of dementia. There is the assumption that the demands of caregiving predispose to burden that may increasingly affect the caregiver adversely. More current thinking does not reject the basic assumption but is directed toward more precise definition and segmentation of the concept. The dynamics involved may be better understood by charting a new and different approach to study than has been the traditional one—the biomedical model. If there is some unique aspect of burden in caregiving for dementia patients, the characteristics must be designated, and their contribution made explicit. A beginning in that direction has shown some evidence that factors such as duration of dementia may be less important than previously thought, whereas access to different roles, even when stressful, outside the caregiving setting may be more important than previously thought. Stress may be more common in females, for whatever reasons, whereas supports, both formal and informal, may be beneficial in terms of their relation to felt burden more than in terms of their context.

INSTITUTIONALIZATION

The prevailing norm in this society, at least in terms of expectations, is that the dementia patient will remain at home as long as conditions will permit. These "conditions" include a number of contingencies from economics to physical status and mental well-being. Thus, in most instances, the patient will stay in the home setting under the care of a primary caregiver, usually the spouse or older daughter, for a period of years. Even so, should both patient and caregiver survive long enough, institutional placement is expected and accepted socially. The decision is usually not an easy one, even when it occurs earlier in the process. Marriage partners of 40 or more years duration may not have had the happiest of relationships, but some kind of dependency that is comfortable has often developed. Particularly if the marriage has been a rewarding one for both partners, it takes more than realism and objectivity to allow what appears to be abandonment of one who deserves better from one's partner, if not from life. And this is not an issue related to the patient alone. Even in the face of a seemingly irreversible dementing illness, there is the question of what happens when the partner is committed. After all, life and its patterns have been well established. One cannot easily go back and begin again, and especially if one is already 70 or 80 years old. What is to fill the void left by the demented spouse? It should not be surprising that many caregivers, even after placement, spend as much or more time at the facility with the partner than they do in pursuing some remnants of an active and satisfying life.

There must be quite severe burdens, then, when institutionalization is used. Indeed, as Moak (1990) reports, the conditions that lead to the decision are most often difficult ones. He found that aggressive behavior and wandering were the most common reasons offered by caregivers of AD patients, rather than some need for custodial care. Interestingly, he also reports that the stay was a fairly short one in the psychiatric hospital where the study was done. This may be more the result of the institutional characteristics than the placement one, however.

Colerick and George (1986) surveyed 209 caregivers of AD patients and found that placement decisions depended more on the characteristics of the caregiver, including feelings of well-being, than on patient traits and behaviors. They suggest the need of professionals to consider factors other than duration of illness and cognitive competence when counseling families about placement. More germane in the consideration would be assessment of the support system available to the caregiver. They surveyed their sample over a 1-year period, comparing those who kept the patient at home ($N = 136$) with those who institutionalized during the year ($N = 63$). At the time of the first measure, those who had institutionalized the relative were apt to be female, employed, and among the youngest in the sample. A year later, the pattern remained: female, younger, employed plus being a child of the patient. They report two factors that significantly reduce the probability of placement: relation of the caregiver to the patient and the caregiver's need for caregiving assistance. A spouse who is receiving some forms of assistance is less likely to institutionalize. There is the factor, also, that children frequently have their own families and, often, jobs, so that there is the danger of "role overload" that disposes to placement.

Related factors involved in the decision for placement have been specified by Lund, Pett, and Caserta (1987). Anticipation for commitment was greater where the patient was older and dementing rapidly and where the patient was not a spouse of the decision maker. If the relationship of caregiver to patient was not a close one and the role was perceived as burdensome, the likelihood of institutional placement was greater. This study introduces the factor of distancing in the emotional sense between patient and caregiver as a major factor.

Teresi, Toner, Bennett, and Wilder (1988–1989) found the central element in planning for placement was task inconvenience. In an indirect way, the patient contributed to the task inconvenience because he or she now had limitations that reduced personal activity and they showed behaviors that were disturbing to the caregiver. In a unique but direct way, the kind and extent of informal supports available to the caregiver also influenced the planning for placement. These elements may well be part of the emotional distancing proposed, regardless of the causative agents.

Morycz (1985) approached the decision about institutionalization in terms of the strain felt by the caregiver. Strain is defined as "cognitive, affective, and physiological changes induced by stress. The degree of strain therefore is moderated by the individual's perception of the stressor" (p. 331). As he points out, the amount of strain may not be related to the degree of disability of the patient but may be related to the caregiver's perception of any actual stressor as a problem. He reports that the desire to institutionalize was increased under two conditions of relationship. First, when the caregiver felt greater strain and when the demands of caregiving involve more physical labor. Second, when the patient was widowed and when living alone. The former buttresses the argument for emotional distancing. The latter would seem more related to personal distancing. Morycz makes no such division; instead, he lists the groups for which strain was a strong and significant predictor: whites, females, daughters, spouses, white daughters, and wives. Males and all black caregivers are not so influenced by strain in predicting the desire to institutionalize. On follow-up, he determined that there is a significant relationship between desire and later commitment, though the correlation is only moderate in size ($r = .53$).

The decision for placement may be worthwhile according to a study by Brown, Potter, and Foster (1990). They found that burden decreased over a 12-month period for caregivers who sought assessment of the patient. The greatest reduction came for caregivers who had placed the relative in a nursing home. Pratt, Wright, and Schmall (1987) report data that do not agree with the latter statement, however. Their measure of burden showed virtually identical scores for caregivers of community dwelling patients and those with institutionalized relatives. However, the two groups did show significant differences on several variables. The "community" group said they had less time for themselves, more inter- ferences with social life and friendships, and a lack of privacy. The "in- stitutional" group members were more concerned about money to pay costs, being able to continue the care being provided, wishing there were someone else to assume the care burden, and feeling that they were not doing enough for the patient. Either way, there is burden.

So far as coping is concerned, Pratt et al. report that strategies did not differ between the groups. In contrast to Brown et al., Pratt et al. conclude that the assumption that institutionalization relieves stress does not have much foundation. They propose that education and training in problem solving will be helpful to all caregivers and help reduce the level of burden.

It would seem that placement of a patient in a setting such as a nursing home depends primarily on caregiver characteristics and needs. Whether or not the effect benefits the caregiver is not yet clear. The nursing home industry is predicting significant placements in the twenty- first century with more older persons and a consequent increase in the diagnosis of diseases leading to dementia. There are increasing adjust- ments to the perceived needs of the patients, including the development of so-called "special care units" where only dementia patients are housed. At this point, the predictions do not seem unlikely, though whether the outcomes will be beneficial to patients and caregivers needs to be studied.

COPING STRATEGIES

In the current generation of caregivers, there are probably few in- stances where preparation has been made for the problems to be en- countered. The change in the statistics for the elderly in this country indicates to us that many conditions are more common now than ever before and require decisions that did not need to be made in the past. Perhaps grandchildren of today's demented patients will have had more contact and awareness that will benefit them; even so, it seems unlikely that one can be adequately prepared.

The question arises, then: How do caregivers cope with a situation that is increasingly demanding? Are there discrete skills that make the tasks of caregiving easier or more successful? Are there tools that have been tested and found successful and that can be taught to caregivers? Though far from complete, we do have evidence of caregiver coping strategies that help answer such questions. Some of these study specific techniques, others compare various strategies, and still others are directed at success and failure rates.

A comparative study has been reported by Sistler (1989). She surveyed spouses of SDAT patients and compared them with spouses of the physically impaired and a control group. She reports that caregivers of SDAT patients sought more social supports and tended toward wishful thinking about the positive effects that might be obtained. Though some of the caregivers in this group were problem-solution oriented and used coping strategies reflecting this approach, they had no higher feelings of well-being than those who did not. In fact, Sistler questions whether either social supports or problem-solving strategies accomplish much for the well-being of the caregivers. The gist of the problem may be in the differentiation she describes between the *process* and the *product* of supports. "Perhaps social workers should focus more on the product of social supports, rather than on simply encouraging the caregiver to seek social support" (p. 419). Sistler also finds the importance of problem solving as a coping technique to be problematic, particularly for situations involving interpersonal contacts. But Pratt, Schmall, Wright, and Cleland (1985) found that scores on a burden scale were affected by coping strategies used. They report that three "internal" strategies—confidence in the ability to solve problems, being able to reframe the problem to achieve some workable solution, and degree of passivity—were related to the burden felt. In addition, two "external" strategies—spiritual support and extended family—also were influential on the amount of burden perceived by the caregiver. Pratt et al. report that the two positive internal approaches, confidence in problem solution and reframing, may make the problems more understandable and manageable. Passivity, by contrast, means avoiding responding to the problem and thereby actually increasing the burden. The external approaches may help to displace some of the burden felt because seeking spiritual support and interacting with others than family members widens the field of supports.

Discrepancies between conclusions of studies may be explained by the particular strategies investigated or the outcome variables identified in the behavior of the caregiver. In this light, Haley, Levine, Brown, and

Bartolucci (1987) found that effects on the individual were a complex of the pattern of stressors perceived, how these were appraised, and the coping skills available to apply to them. In addition, the social supports and activities available to and utilized by the caregiver were significant varibles. Their results have led to the development of a stress and coping model that they believe will assist in clinical intervention with families.

Levine, Dastoor, and Gendron (1983) have approached the problem from a different direction. They hypothesized that the ability to tolerate the behaviors leading to stress is partially related to the complex of patient problems but also to the availability and quality of coping skills possessed by the caregiver. They developed a skills training program to increase the number and quality of such skills. They included efforts at increasing motivation and assertiveness along with ways to reduce stress and solve problems. Zarit and Zarit (1986) have used a similar approach based upon their belief that caregivers need to learn effective ways to manage behavior and receive more assistance in the caregiving role. They propose this may be accomplished through three strategies—provision of accurate information to the caregiver, assistance in determining possible solutions for perceived problem behaviors, and identification of supports that will sustain the caregiver. The model is as apt for caregivers with relatives in institutions as for those still at home. They point out that placement may do nothing more than shift the burdens felt by the family, without giving relief.

> Thus, families are caught in a dilemma. While home care may be more desirable for personal and/or economic reasons, it can take a toll on the caregiver. Although nursing home care can relieve that strain, it places a different set of emotional and economic pressures on the family. (p. 103)

Their approach has been tested to some degree as well (Zarit, Anthony, & Boutselis, 1987). The authors compared family counseling and support groups as they affect feelings of stress and burden. Each of the interventions (counseling or support groups) utilized the Zarit and Zarit (1982) model that includes the three approaches of information giving, teaching behavioral problem solutions, and identifying sources of support. Zarit et al. found gains for both treatment groups; unfortunately, they did not differ from others on a waiting list who also showed improvement. The gains made were maintained over a 1-year period. Though the results are not as positive for the effects of these interventions as one might wish, one study seems hardly sufficient to draw a conclusion about the effectiveness of assisting caregivers with coping strategies. Both the Zarits' approach and alternatives need much more research.

The principal need to be able to cope seems to involve negative choices, often where all alternatives seem undesirable, according to Wilson (1989). She conducted interviews with family members and found evidence that this generalization is reflected in the fact that "choice" may center on institutionalization *or* perseverance of an intolerable situation in the home. Obviously, neither of these is desirable, and the family must decide which is the least reprehensible. She found variation in the ways in which caregivers behaved in the decision-making process. According to her, there are three stages of coping (taking it on, going through it, and turning it over), each showing its influence in the resolution finally adopted. She describes the strategies used in each stage (e.g., taking it on would include self-dialogue, finding solace, and unburdening, whereas going through it encompasses the elements of facing up to the problems and dealing with them).

> Each stage had characteristic properties, problems, and coping strategies; however, *the overall process is a consciously examined, self-reflective, strategic, and difficult means of surviving on a day-to-day, if not moment-to-moment basis under conditions of initial uncertainty and unpredictability, pressing demands with a paucity of support, and a dreaded future.* (p. 95, italics added)

The study of coping strategies available, the ones used, and the success of each is a relatively new area. It has been enlarged by attempts to intervene through education and training to assist caregivers in becoming more proficient and satisfied. The goal of such research is to relieve burden and stress. To date, the data are not definitive. The general thesis is compelling and appealing and so should continue to instigate investigation.

SUPPORT GROUPS

The notion of the support group is not new and has been applied to a variety of conditions where patients and/or family members are experiencing psychological distress. Support groups for families and primary caregivers of dementia patients are no exception, though groups for patients as such are less commonly found. The group may serve one or more of several purposes: catharsis, education, social contact, respite, and the like. Leadership may vary from professional to volunteer to none at all. Composition may be from two to any number, with the membership and attendance changing from meeting to meeting. The group may assemble weekly, biweekly, or monthly—or may even be more occasional.

Obviously, there is no "model" of the support group. Regardless of these matters, the essential question becomes: What does the group, under whatever conditions, accomplish? What are the goals, and how well are they met? Do support groups bring change in the attendants?

Simank and Strickland (1985–1986) define the purposes of such groups as giving information, providing referral sources, furnishing an accepting environment, sharing emotional burdens, and allowing support and empathy from others who have experienced the difficulties of caregiving. The first two items in the list would seem to be educational, whereas the others are rather explicit means to help achieve catharsis. The approach described by Zarit and Zarit (1982) and echoed by other investigators may provide a more useful structure for experimental purposes. Such contrasts do indicate that "support" has wide meaning.

When there are specific goals established for the support group, they may be tested over time. Hamlet and Reed (1990) report on such a test. They followed a support group of some 26 members where the intent was to provide emotional support, develop social contacts and networks, give appropriate information about normal aging, and teach the participants problem-solving skills. These outcomes combine possibilities from both Simank and Strickland (1985–1986) and Zarit and Zarit (1982). At 3-month intervals, the members were assessed for their attitudes about the success of the program with the eventual outcome that the group became a part of a network in the community.

Structure was the focus of a study by Steuer and Clark (1982). They had three groups: One was structured but open-ended; the other two were closed and time-limited. Success was correlated with relationship of caregiver and patient as well as a setting that was unstructured and time limited. The first group met every 2 weeks for an hour and a half. No one was committed to attend a session, and each session featured an "expert" who talked about a topic chosen by the group, followed by a question and answer period. Attendance ranged from 3 to 10 persons, depending on interest in the topic, apparently. The group developed no cohesion as a result.

Groups 2 and 3 were asked to commit to attendance for each meeting. They met weekly for $1\frac{1}{2}$ hours, without a designated topic, though the group members were surveyed in order to focus the meetings on interest areas. Group 2 consisted of spouses, whereas Group 3 was a mixture of spouses and children.

Among their findings, Steuer and Clark report that the didactic meetings did not seem very successful. Most caregivers did not care for a "lecture" because they most often wanted short, direct answers to specific questions. The most successful approach was with closed groups having only moderate structure and focus, seemingly allowing the airing of feelings and receiving of direct information requested. Here, group cohesion was high. The spousal group developed most cohesiveness and member support.

Effects of support group participation on caregivers show variable results. Greene and Monahan (1989) assessed 34 groups over a 14-month period. Interviews were conducted prior to the initiation of intervention, at the end of the intervention period (2 months after baseline), and 6 months after baseline. They report that the support group efforts brought significant reductions in anxiety and depression for the members, even though they had been highly stressed before entering the groups. The benefits were greatest at the end of the intervention and then became attenuated.

Kahan, Kemp, Staples, and Brummel-Smith (1985) also report positive effects from support group efforts. Their focus was principally educational, using a cognitive–behavioral model. A group of 22 relatives of AD patients met for eight sessions and was compared with 18 controls who were on a waiting list. Their experimental group expressed somewhat higher levels of burden at the beginning of the study than did the controls, but the difference was not statistically significant. There were no mean differences on measures of depression and knowledge about dementia. At the conclusion of the sessions, the members of the experimental group on average expressed less burden, whereas the members of the control group expressed more burden. The sessions did not produce changes in depression scores, though the authors maintain that there was some evidence that the treatment was effective in reducing the overall level of depression for the experimental group. This is based on the fact that these family members had a higher proportion who showed improvement with fewer numbers with increased depression. Those who participated scored higher on a test of knowledge about dementia at the end of the sessions, whereas the controls had no change in mean score. Kahan et al. point out the possibility of a Hawthorne effect because there was no control over relationships between patient and caregiver prior to the experiment. In addition, "Overburdened families respond well to professional care that is concerned and interested in dealing with their problems" (p. 668). They suggest the need to compare different means of intervention rather than intervention versus no intervention. Nevertheless, "the program was helpful in aiding participants to feel more useful, less downhearted, and less like crying." Whether such outcomes were maintained over time was not determined in this study.

Other studies have reported less positive results. Haley, Brown, and Levine (1987a) looked at effects of support group participation on depression, life satisfaction, and increased social activity. Presumably, those involved might benefit by less depression at the same time that they have improved feelings of well-being and become more socially active. Assessments were made at the initial point, at the conclusion of the study (10 sessions of $1\frac{1}{2}$ hours each) and in a later follow-up. The comparison group consisted of those on a waiting list. Haley et al. report that there were positive reactions to the efforts, with caregivers citing the groups as being "quite helpful." Empirically, however, there were no improvements on measures of depression or life satisfaction. Social supports were not increased or even bettered, and coping skills remained unchanged. Jenkins, Parham, and Jenkins (1985) found that support group impact was correlated with burden but that belief in help from such sources decreased over time.

Support group functions seem better defined than do their effects. The intention to improve the lives of caregivers by providing the opportunity to participate in regular sessions has not been proved or disproved. The surest thing that may be said at present is that caregivers who attend support groups, even if irregularly, usually state that the sessions are "helpful" but are not greatly influenced in ways that can be measured systematically.

CAREGIVER DEPRESSION

It would seem reasonable to expect depression where a spouse or parent is deteriorating slowly but surely. Because there seems to be no hope for reversal and because there are few techniques to relieve the pressures associated with caregiving, the expectation seems even more reasonable. The literature substantiates this position by including depression as a variable in many studies, demonstrating its presence, and often showing increases with time (see, e.g., Dura, Haywood-Niler, & Kiecolt-Glaser, 1990). Intervention for depression is a viable alternative that should be considered and used.

Variables that are associated with depression and its effects have been identified in several studies of dementia caregivers. Morris, Morris, and Britton (1988) investigated marital relationships between dementia patients and their spouses prior to the identification of the effect of the disease and at the time of their study. They found that those who had lower levels of intimacy, both before dementia and at the present time, showed more strain and depression. Where intimacy had been high but declined in the face of dementia, greater depression was reported but not increased strain. Morris et al. wonder if a poor or strained relationship between marriage partners before the occurrence of dementia may not make it more difficult for the spouse to perform successfully in the caregiving role. The possibility is supported by data gathered by Motenko (1989). She found that wives who thought marital closeness was maintained despite the dementia felt greater gratification associated with well-being and less frustration. As life plans were disrupted, usually greatest as the symptoms first expressed themselves, there was increased frustration. However, as routines were established that helped in handling the relationships, frustration tended to decrease, even though the demands of caregiving increased. Motenko agrees with others that the *meaning* of caregiving is more important than the amount of care needed.

The process of giving care (including such elements as supports available or degree of involvement with a patient) may affect feelings of burden in several different ways, but Stommel, Given, and Given (1990) report that depression dominated perceived burden in caregivers across all dimensions. Its pervasiveness influenced the evaluations of caregiving that were expressed as burdens. Indeed, there is evidence that patient depression may significantly influence caregiver depression and burden (Drinka, Smith, & Drinka, 1987). Expectations influence depression as well. Where caregivers perceived that the stress they felt currently would continue and eventually affect all parts of their lives, there was an increase in depression and strain (Morris, Morris, & Britton, 1989), though the relationship is dependent on the disabilities and disturbances that the caregiver perceives in the patient. Nevertheless, as the caregiver recognizes a lack of control over his or her own emotional reactions and the behaviors of the patient, there is significantly greater depression and strain.

The personal interpretation of the caregiver seems to be the prime determiner of adjustment. Thompson, Bundek, and Sobolew-Shubin (1990) found depression in caregivers of stroke victims to be related to the functional level of the patient, the perceptions of an increase in work and burden directly due to the stroke, the quality of the relationship between the patient and caregiver, and how the caregiver interpreted the situation. Specifically, Thompson et al. say that depression is greater when there is greater physical impairment, disharmony in the family, and loss of hope. In cases of dementia, one might extrapolate that the complex is greater mental impairment along with the other two. Of course, many caregivers would probably agree with William of Orange that "it is not necessary to have hope in order to persevere." The quality of life may be poor indeed when there is only perseverance because there is no other option.

This theme is exemplified further in a study by Pratt, Schmall, and Wright (1986). They found morale scores to be correlated negatively to burden. (Thus the lower the morale score, the higher the burden felt.) Burden was much higher in caregivers who reported the mental status of the patient to be poor. Where the emotional relationship between caregiver and patient had been poor prior to the dementia, there was greater burden than if the relationship had been close. This outcome relates to findings about burden and marital status reported earlier.

The extension of affect to more general states than depression yields similar results. Thus Gilhooly and Whittick (1989) found significant correlations between "expressed emotion" and caregiver sex, psychological well-being, social contacts, and quality of relationship to the patient. Whittick (1988) has evidence of greater "emotional distress" in daughters caring for a demented parent than that found in mothers who are caring for a mentally handicapped child or adult. As is to be expected, both groups exhibit more distress than that found in the general population. These findings accord with the spousal/child differences in institutional placement reported earlier.

As predicated, depression is a common disorder in caregivers and perhaps particularly in those caring for a demented person. The presence of the disorder does not indicate the effects of treatment or even if treatment was attempted. Given the success of interventions, one would expect improvement in the depressive levels of caregivers where treatment occurs.

SELF-EFFICACY

Within recent years, concepts have been suggested, defined, and tested that offer alternative ways of analyzing caregiver burden and efforts. Among these, one that seems very promising is the proposal of "self-efficacy" by Albert Bandura (1977, 1982, 1986a,b). Essentially, the concept centers on the perception or belief that one has about her or his own competencies in the face of particular tasks. One's belief that one can or cannot succeed and that one can or cannot achieve certain goals are mediators of behavior. The perception may lead one to attempt a task or avoid it. Even with an attempt, the self-efficacy perceived by the individual will influence effort and persistence. One strength of the approach is that consideration is given only to the circumstances and events immediately involved. This is in contrast to other concepts (locus of control or stress, for example) that include the particular but also posit a *generalized* state influencing many aspects of behavior.

Bandura (1977) has proposed that there are four informational sources upon which we base our perceptions of efficacy. The first of these is a kind of historical review, including how well or poorly we have done on a task or one similar to it in the past. As we are cognizant of past mastery, we have greater expectations of continued mastery and success. Effectively, our history of successes leads us to expect even more success. The second source of information reflects modeling. As we observe the success with which others, and particularly persons important to us, deal with events and experiences, there is some integration into our own mental experience. What we have observed may have a positive influence on our own behavior in future circumstances. Third, Bandura leaves a place for verbal reinforcers, though he believes these to be relatively weak as a source of information to add to our mental fund. Such reinforcers may at times and in a limited degree have some effect in changing our efficacy attitudes; they can never replace the actual experience of personal success. Fourth, our emotions may become a factor as they are aroused; particularly if they are negative ones, the usual role of such emotions is to induce *in*efficacy. After all, the emotional reaction may most often signify that we are *not* successful, and failure never tells us what the better response may be. Indeed, as we are emotional in our reactions, we provide ourselves with evidence of ineptitude.

There are two experiential sources that are positive in their effects, then. One is performance based: we prove to ourselves that we can accomplish. This is also the most influential on our feelings of self-efficacy. A second is based on vicarious experience but evidence nevertheless of what actually works. Such observations become a part of our potential for future actions. The other two are less positive in their influence and perhaps may actually lead to reduced self-efficacy. These include the feedback provided by others that we have done something well. At best, this operates only weakly, and if it conflicts with our own perception of our performance, it may serve negative purposes. Emotional reaction, particularly if in the form of anxiety or fear or similar feelings, may be quite detrimental to our self-assessment and reduce our belief that we can succeed at a task.

The model was developed further and described, along with some research, in 1982 (Bandura, 1982). At this point, the theory conceived that our belief and our expectation concerning an event may express themselves separately. Thus I may *believe* that I have the competency, and I may *expect* to succeed at whatever task demands are impinging on me. In another setting, however, I may *not believe* that I have the

Relationships	Effects on Personality
Category 1: The Positive Effect a. I <u>can</u> perform (+) **and** b. I <u>will</u> succeed (+)	Bringing positive, probably successful effort
Category 2: The Negative Effect a. I <u>can't</u> perform (–) **and** b. I <u>won't</u> succeed (–)	Bringing lack of interest and surrender to defeat

Category 3: The Mixed Effects
a. I <u>can</u> perform (+)
   but
b. I <u>won't</u> succeed (–)
   or
a. I <u>can't</u> perform (–)
   but
b. I <u>will</u> succeed (+)
	Bringing remonstrance
	and complaint
	Bringing dejection
	and personal
	devaluation

FIGURE 9.1. The self-efficacy hierarchy. Developed from Bandura, 1982.

competency, and I may *not expect* to succeed. These extremes offer two intermediary possibilities also. I may *believe* that I have the competency, but I may *not expect* to succeed, for whatever reasons. By contrast, I may *not believe* that I have the competency but I may *expect* to succeed anyway, for whatever reasons. Figure 9.1 illustrates these possibilities.

These four attitudes may be related to personality effects as well, influencing the efforts one may attempt (Bandura, 1982). If one perceives one's efficacy in terms of the two positive elements (Category 1 in the figure), there will be positive, assured, and probably successful effort in the given circumstance, adding to the mental fund about one's efficaciousness (Bandura, 1982). This, of course, is the ultimate behavioral goal, though none of us probably maintains it consistently. More likely, we experience more positive instances than negative ones, so that, on balance, we feel self-efficacious. In contrast, one may encounter settings where the two forces are negative (Category 2 in the figure). Whenever this occurs, we are most apt to feel apathetic and resigned to failure (Bandura, 1982). We may give in and refuse to face the "problem" that is inherent in the event. The intermediate stages will occur, also, on occasions. Where we feel adequate but do not expect to succeed (Category 3), we may express more protest and grievance (Bandura, 1982). We may become activists in the social sense. Instead of facing and resolving the "problem," we express a type of aggression, against society or against self. Admittedly, social activists are not necessarily in this category. If, however, their perceptions of self-efficacy accord with the dichotomy of belief and expectation expressed here, their actions will demonstrate this category. The other combination in Category 3 may lead to self-devaluation and despondency (Bandura, 1982). Even though success is achieved, it will be discounted because of the lack of belief in one's own competencies. The result did not occur *because* of self but *in spite of* self. There will be little or no increase in feelings of self-efficacy in this case.

In a further extension of the theory, Bandura (1986a) points out that, as a person perceives inefficacy in coping with a circumstance, there may result both fearful expectations ("I cannot succeed") and avoidance of action ("I will not try").

> If people judge themselves as inefficacious in exercising control over potential threats, they view threats anxiously, conjure up possible calamities were they to have any commerce with them, and avoid them. (Bandura, 1986a, p. 1390)

(For a more complete description of the model and research, see Bandura, 1986b.)

The implications of self-efficacy theory would seem appropriate for application to caregivers, both in the observational and the research sense. Individual events and reactions become the basis of analysis rather than a generalized, comprehensive state that may or may not be present. Yet little effort has been published to date using this perspective. Haley, Brown, and Levine (1987b) included the concept in a study of specific behavioral problems that occur while the patient remains in the home. They found that certain specific behavioral problems caused greater stress to caregivers than did self-care deficits and disorientation. Among the particularly difficult behaviors reported by the caregivers were agitation, hallucinations, and dangerous or embarrassing behaviors. Their estimate of self-efficacy was based on an inquiry where caregivers reported problems.

Inclusion of self-efficacy theory in other studies is needed to assess its relation to an understanding of the burdens affecting caregivers as well as its utility as a source for intervention; specifically, change in perceived self-efficacy in those settings that cause the greatest trauma.

RESPITE

Respite is a term used to indicate the availability of diversion or relief from the varied and demanding tasks of caregiving. The assumption is that those providers who manage to become involved in activities outside the caregiving setting will be better able to contend with demands than those who find themselves isolated to the tasks of caring. Gruetzner (1988, p. 131) points out that such relief prevents earlier institutionalization of the patient. Improving the ability to cope is an outcome cited by Heston and White (1991, p. 125). *How* respite is provided depends on circumstances. Thus family members may relieve the primary caregiver for a period of time, from hours to days. Volunteers may take over the supervision of the patient, usually for a shorter period of time. Professionals may be employed to attend to the patient if economic conditions permit. Whatever the means used, the object is to reduce the burden felt by the caregiver, to give a chance for that person to experience other aspects of life. Earlier in this chapter, research by Montgomery et al. (1985) was described. They spoke of "objective burden," a type that makes demands on the time and space of the cargiver and are thus confining. One means of reducing the feelings of burden in this case was to provide respite services. Scott et al. (1986) agreed with this position, providing evidence that respite does help to reduce the level of burden felt by the caregiver.

Lawton, Brody, and Saperstein (1989) compared respite and non-respite conditions for a large sample of caregivers of AD patients ($N = 632$). They measured attitudes toward caregiving, health, and psychological well-being in both groups. A year later, they found that those individuals who had received respite care kept the patient in the home significantly longer than those without respite. (This was a difference of 22 days, which has statistical importance, though it seems relatively unimportant in a practical sense.) However, respite was not helpful in terms of level of burden felt or mental health status as measured. Caregivers did express satisfaction about the help received, another indication that efforts are appreciated even if they are not very effective behaviorally. Lawton et al. conclude that respite can provide some added quality to the life of the caregiver, though it is not a strong intervention.

A variety of respite or educational services was part of a study by Montgomery and Borgatta (1989). Compared to a control group, they found that burden for caregivers was lower after a year where the patient remained in the community. Providing services seemed to delay nursing home placement where the caregiver was an adult child but accelerated it when the caregiver was a spouse. These two studies, then, seem to have found opposing results though the latter one did not compare only respite and nonrespite. Perhaps part of the reason for differences is in the statement that,

> One of the most important findings of the project is the fact that families who are caring for elderly people in the community are difficult to reach and to serve. These families are fiercely independent, have little contact with formal service providers, are reluctant to accept help, and are difficult to find or serve until they reach a crisis point. (Montgomery & Borgatta, p. 463)

Using a sample of only three caregivers and a single control, Lundervold and Lewin (1987) provided in-home respite for a period of 4 to 6 hours per week. They measured health, depression, stress and burden. After 6 months, they found no change in depression, stress, or burden as compared with the person receiving no respite. There seemed to be slight improvement in health. Social support remained unchanged in frequency, type, or persons providing support. This may indicate that the time in respite did not generate new support possibilities.

Burdz, Eaton, and Bond (1988) considered respite from the standpoint of the patient and the consequent effects on burden felt by the caregiver. Within a 5-week interval, one group of patients was placed in a nursing home for a 2-week respite period. Another group remained in the home with care provided during the period. Interviews with caregivers were done at the beginning of the 5-week period and at the end. Because part of the patient group was demented and part not, Burdz et al. hypothesized that the diagnosis would interact with respite exposure so that more improvement would be found in the nondemented group. However, caregivers in both groups (demented vs. nondemented) reported that the patient's memory and behavior were improved regardless of the respite condition experienced.

Respite is a frequently advocated procedure to assist in handling the burdens of caregiving. Evidence that it accomplishes its goals is less certain than the positive attitudes about it. With such conflicting evidence as is present, the concept needs further study. Whether "real" changes occur or not, the idea has face validity and will probably remain as a strongly accepted principle. Indeed, the Alzheimer's Association (1991b) has taken a strong stance favoring the concept. There is an effort to have Congress enact legislation and funding for caregiver support. Further, the association has proposed a set of "broad" principles to be used by state and federal policymakers in developing policy (Alzheimer's Association, 1991b, pp. 1–2). Apparently this advocacy group has set a high priority on achieving funding that will permit caregivers to have respite opportunities.

THERAPEUTIC INTERVENTION

There have been various attempts to intervene with caregivers with what may be termed *therapeutic* efforts. The outcomes are influenced not only by the techniques employed but by the point in the process at which the intervention occurs and the characteristics of the persons with whom it is used. Chenoweth and Spencer (1986) have noted that new and different stresses occur at each progression of dementia with the consequent increase in demands for care. They maintain that professional assistance, when appropriate, can help ameliorate the stress incurred. A part of this "appropriate professional assistance" would be represented in interventions devised and applied for the purpose.

One such technique is to provide counseling directly to caregivers. Sutcliffe and Larner (1988) used two different counseling methods where patients remained at home. They found that where emotional support was a part of the procedure, there was greater reduction of stress. If only information was provided, stress was not reduced, even though knowledge was increased. From a different point of view, ours is a society that has placed emphasis traditionally on the role of religious belief and spiritual support. Wright, Pratt, and Schmall (1985) espouse such efforts as a form of coping by caregivers. They had found previously that burden scores were correlated with spiritual support, suggesting that the religious community may be helpful as a source of assistance. The reliance on religious faith has been demonstrated as a means of coping by black caregivers (Segall & Wykle, 1988–1989). Stress is more tolerable when faith is strong enough. It is interesting to note, however, that these authors also found that black caregivers felt the need for affordable respite services, counseling for themselves and family members to reduce conflicts, and information about the cause of dementia. Further, they requested greater access to available community resources.

Quayhagen and Quayhagen (1989) have reported on the effects of strategies involving cognitive stimulation with AD patients. Using conversation, memory exercises, and problem-solving techniques, they found that patients did not show cognitive decline or increased behavioral problems during an 8-month program. Further, the patients showed some improvement emotionally. By contrast, a comparison group showed negative changes on these measures. The caregivers also benefitted, maintaining their sense of well-being and enhancing their coping resources. However, there was a significant decline in cognitive function by patients during a 6-month program in a day hospital (Winogrond, Fisk, Kirsling, & Keyes, 1987). Yet behavior problems did not increase. Caregivers perceived less stress, implying that an offshoot of the program was some enhancement in coping. Winogrond et al. believe such a therapeutic program may lead to less behavior deterioration in patients and increased coping ability in caregivers. They propose intolerance in the caregiver as a significant factor in burden and morale.

> It appears that as the caregivers learned more about the disease process and gained skills in patient management (problem-solving coping), and as they shared with others their stress and gained acceptance of their negative feelings (emotion-focused coping), they became better able to separate feelings of burden and low morale from intolerance toward the patient's behavior. (p. 338)

Mobily and Hoeft (1985) make a case for recreation and activity, not only for respite but also for enhancement of quality of life by both patient and caregiver. Panella, Lilliston, Brush, and McDowell (1984) used structured activities on a daily basis with dementia patients in a day care center. The study was continued for 3 years. A spinoff was respite for caregivers, an outcome that they report was well received and appreciated. They point out that cognitive decline continued but that patients could be kept at home longer without hiring additional help. Thus the intervention seems cost-effective as well. Day care is an expanding concept in this country and generally receives acceptance as an appropriate source for patient involvement and caregiver respite. Though too costly for some, Panella et al. point out that it is less expensive than nursing home placement.

Various interventions and techniques have been proposed, some of which have been tested. There is probably no end to the possibilities so long as professionals conceive of ideas and so long as caregivers seek assistance. The general aura about such interventions is positive, though frequently the reaction is based on less than compelling evidence of outcomes. No doubt the literature will continue to expand with descriptions of such programs and attempts.

SUMMARY

The family of a dementia patient becomes increasingly involved in the effects of the process. Typically, there will be a primary caregiver, usually a spouse or adult child. In the latter case, the individual is more apt to be an older daughter, whereas in the former it is the wife. Whoever bears the responsibility will be faced with demands that eventually may bring feelings of burden and that may be associated increasingly with stress and depression. Concern for the caregiver has led to attempts to devise and provide means of reducing the burden. Some of these efforts have been tested empirically, though not always with rigor. Because professionals involved with caregivers wish to relieve stress and depression, they are apt to employ recognized procedures, like support groups and counseling, in the belief that these efforts will bring positive results. In this chapter, we examined some of the dynamics of caregiving and their effects. Several recognized and accepted means of intervention are surveyed, particularly where research has been done to determine their effects.

CHAPTER TEN

Intervention Techniques

Rational for Intervention

The point has been stressed in this book that dementia exerts its effects on both patient and family. The consequences are not equally destructive, because the patient gradually but certainly deteriorates mentally and becomes increasingly dependent, whereas family finds increasing devastation in loss of personal liberty, financial credibility, emotional resourcefulness, and physical stamina. The specifics of the changes are not well documented or understood for either party. General trends and patterns have been proposed and, to a degree, demonstrated in the literature. The result is an awareness among professionals that severe problems exist at all times in the progression of the dementia at the same time that precision is lacking on several dimensions. It is apparent that individuals in either category suffer, and it is understandable that those dedicated to human service want to ameliorate the suffering as much as possible. For this reason, there have been attempts to develop interventions—not to change the circumstances of disease and consequence, which presently is felt to be impossible, but to assist the parties to adapt to and manage the realities of day to day problems.

Assumptions

Whenever we try to intervene with some other person(s), no matter the reason or technique, there must be some implicit or explicit rationale for doing so. The more explicit the reasons underlying the intervention, the more likely that they may be tested experimentally and justified (or not justified) empirically. This requires both time to allow deployment and practice of the intervention and use in various settings or conditions to test generalizability. If a mediation is restricted to few persons and/or situations, it may not receive general acceptance and adoption. As it is demonstrated to be applicable to a variety of different cases and conditions, the intervention may attain acceptance as an efficacious procedure. *A basic assumption that must be met by such an intercession is that it has been tested appropriately and has withstood rigorous examination.* The worth of the approach has been demonstrated under the circumstances, and its utility may be accepted. No matter how logical the arguments presented for the technique, no matter how much "face validity" is obvious, no matter how badly some course of action is needed, one must not assume that an intervention is successful unless that success has been proven. This basic assumption has been violated more often than proven with current methodologies that are employed in human service fields, as will be demonstrated later in this chapter.

As overriding as that basic assumption may appear, there are others that need to be met also, even though they are more or less related to the basic one. A second assumption that needs to be met is that *the intervention is appropriate to the specific group or client with whom it will be used.* This might seem so obvious as to be trite, but that does not mean that the premise is not violated in human service efforts. What is implied here is that it is possible to describe instances where the process is both appropriate and inappropriate. Certainly, the appropriate nature of the intervention is found when the implementor can demonstrate close similarity of conditions described in the model and shown through empirical test. The closer the relationship of persons with whom the technique has proved viable to the individuals in the setting where it will now be applied, the more certainly this assumption will be met. That relationship includes the kinds of problems involved, the setting where the procedure will be used, and the goals to be accomplished. For example, if Technique A has been shown to work with older individuals who are caregivers for dementia patients in their own homes, where demands are greater than the caregiver can tolerate, then the professional may reasonably apply the intervention with an expectation of success. That expectation may not be met, of course, for any of a number of reasons. The most critical element may lie in the statement "has been shown to work" because it is important to know the conditions of development and testing for the technique and to assure that the situations' elements are comparable. Even when these conditions are met, there are numerous uncontrolled variables in the best of efforts in the social–psychological field. Where all else seems adequate, the professional must be alert to possible failure and be willing to consider alternative explanations for the lack of success.

At the opposite extreme are the instances where the technique would seem clearly inappropriate. Here there would be a violation of the similarity of conditions, in part or in whole. Because an approach will work for a given group or client does not mean that it will work in any situation. Differences in persons, problems, settings, and goals must be considered and described before trying an intervention. If the comparison is done carefully, time and effort that would otherwise have been wasted may be put to better use. There is always the possibility to be considered that doing nothing may be less harmful than doing something which is inappropriate.

Assumption 3 applies to conditions where there may be divergence. *The intervention allows adaptation in details without destroying its basic efficacy.* There must be some latitude in administration at the same time that the procedure assures appropriate outcomes. If the model is too rigid, it becomes restrictive and restricting. At the same time, the intervention must be clear enough that it allows description of the details where latitude is permissible and the limits of those departures. Under these circumstances, the outcomes may still be achieved and demonstrated. There will be clear specifications of adaptations that were applied, where and how used, and subsequent effects.

The purpose of any intervention is to reach some particular goal or goals. A fourth assumption, then, is that the model *allows demonstration of the effects and outcomes of its use.* To do so, the procedure must be clear in its purposes and techniques. If the process offers only personal reactions and feelings of the agent implementing it, the validity of the outcomes will be in doubt. There must be components that meet the criteria for "testing." This means a "process" that has some structure permitting internal evaluation and ongoing testing.

The fifth assumption emanates from the fourth. The intervention must *allow demonstration that goals, objectively set before implementation, have (or have not) been met.* Effectively, the program must be so structured that there can be perception of the relation of the implementation to what is accomplished for the client. It is necessary that one can recognize if and when the goals have been met.

Before beginning the use of any procedure, the professional who is making the decision needs to examine its details to assure that the assumptions noted are met. If they cannot be accepted, at least there should be a description of the shortcomings and the set of limitations that exists and will deter the effectiveness of the intercession. Some procedures will meet more of the assumptions than others, given the development of such efforts, but all should be subject to examination and critique, rather than being accepted as valid without some proof.

Testing the Intervention

Once the decision has been made to use a given program, regardless of the basis for that decision, it is necessary to have a means to evaluate the outcomes. Essentially, this requires employing as precisely as possible the procedures of experimentation. Although it may be satisfying to believe that one has "helped" someone by doing something, the attitude is not proof of accomplishment. If change has occurred, either positive or negative, that change should be measurable and accounted for by the intervention itself. In any setting, it is possible to arrange conditions to give evidence, even though the rigor of laboratory experimentation may not be achieved. There are some steps that will assist in this task.

1. *What is to be achieved by this endeavor?* There are several elements involved in this step. One, as already mentioned, is to decide on the procedure to be employed. Another is to decide the individuals who will participate. Still another is to determine what behavior changes are desired. These are not independent steps but closely interrelated ones. *Where* one begins will depend on the circumstances, the problems perceived in the setting. Is the effort intended for dementia patients or for caregivers? Will the procedure be employed in an institutional setting or the home or both? Are the outcomes to be specific, as in remembering the date, or more general, as in handling stress? As such questions are listed and answered, the choices of outcomes to be met will be reduced to a manageable level.

2. *Who should be used as subjects?* Once the question of outcome has been decided, the next step will be to decide who will be appropriate individuals with whom to use the intervention. If one wants to improve memory status of nursing home residents, the answer would seem self-evident. To some degree, that is true. But there are other considerations. In order to demonstrate change, there must be at least two groups: one to whom the program is applied and one to whom it is not. The latter group, the "controls," will provide data to indicate whether or not change occurs in the absence of some systematic intervention. The members of both groups should be chosen on some basis. One possibility is to take the total available population and divide it randomly; for example, using an alphabetical list, numbers 1, 3, 5, and so on become members of the experimental group, whereas numbers 2, 4, 6, and so on are assigned to the control group. Better yet, the samples will be chosen on the basis

of matching characteristics, particularly if the entire population cannot be used. Thus significant variables like age, sex, diagnosis, severity of condition, time in institution, and the like will be used to assure that there are not variables that will influence results that would be misleading. This means that for each 75-year-old woman with a diagnosis of Alzheimer's disease, with moderate impairment, who has been in the nursing home for 6 months, there must be as close a match as possible. *Exact* matching may not be achievable, though it should be attempted, but the group means, at least, must be equated. Above all, one must not pair the woman described with a 53-year-old man with a head injury who has been institutionalized for 9 years, even though both are described as "demented." A cardinal rule is: The more exact the match between experimental and control groups, the more probability that outcomes may be credited to the use of the intervention.

3. *What assures that a change has occurred?* This brings us to the issue of testing. There must be at least a pretest and a posttest. These measures must be derived in terms of the goals to be attained. If the program is to help a patient remember the date, there must be a demonstration that the members of both control and experimental groups are unable to remember this fact before instituting the procedure. Once the intervention is over, another measure is taken to see if the experimental group remembers the date better than the control group. Differences may be statistically tested, but often the issue is the practical one of demonstrating the outcome behavior. One might even plan a follow-up after a period of time to see if the behavior persists without further training (if the outcome was favorable, of course).

Whatever the outcomes to be achieved, the measures used must be *reliable*. Reliability means consistency, that is, the person measured should show the same test behavior when remeasured unless there has been a change through intervention from some source. Before either the pre- or posttest is accepted, they should be checked for reliability. Here, a group of persons like those to be used in the experiment (and as controls) will be administered the measures, at least once but it is better to do so on two separate occasions. If the tests are administered only once, a correlation coefficient may be computed by comparing internally (a so-called split-half coefficient). If administered on two occasions, performance on Day 1 will be correlated with performance on Day 2. In the case of the subjects who are to be "trained" in remembering the date, there might be a reliability check on 6 different days, say, and one can examine the data to see if there is a consistent and reliable outcome. This would not require statistical computation but would indicate that the procedure ("test") is valid. The principle observed here is that without reliability, there cannot possibly be validity. Unfortunately, reliability does not assure validity so that we have a condition of necessity without sufficiency.

The procedure can be summarized as: State the problem, decide the appropriate methods to find a solution to the problem, apply the intervention, measure the changes that occur, and determine the adequacy of the procedure. Simple as this may sound and valuable as it would seem to be, it has not been well-enforced in human services efforts. This will be more apparent as we survey the research on some of the commonly used procedures employed by professionals working with patients and caregivers.

INTERVENTION METHODS

Because dementia resulting from the various disease entities described in this book are considered to be irreversible, direct intervention on behalf of the patient is not yet possible. At the same time, there are problems demonstrated by patients that may be ameliorated, controlled, or even improved under appropriate conditions. For example, depression in the early development of dementia is treatable; memory loss may be modified by cuing techniques; disturbed sleep patterns may be altered by exercise programs and involvement in activities during daylight hours. For the caregiver, an opportunity to vent feelings and share experiences can be provided by support groups; in-home respite may relieve burden; depression is treatable. Such applications have been done on an individual basis, with varying degrees of acceptance and success. What would be most useful would be some techniques or methods that can be taught or applied systematically to groups of persons and assure a relatively permanent, positive change in behavior.

Of the several possible themes that may be found in therapeutic approaches, Busch (1984) has proposed four from his survey of the literature. These general modes include social interaction, orientation of group participants to reality, the life review process, and remotivation. These are more commonly referred to as resocialization, reality orientation, reminiscence, and remotivation. Each represents a potential method of intervention, given definition and structure that describe their components in a way that allows systematic application.

That Busch has cited elements that are generally accepted is demonstrated from other citations. Capuzzi, Gross, and Friel (1990) list reality orientation, remotivation therapy, reminiscing, psychotherapy, and support groups as categories of group therapy. Levy (1987), in yet another literature review, includes sensory stimulation, activity stimulation, milieu modifications, reality orientation, group therapy, and behavioral techniques as conventional approaches. Zimpfer (1987), assessing the effectiveness of group therapy in 19 studies, cites both comprehensive and specific approaches. His conclusions include the position that when clients' needs are diagnosed accurately, the treatment efforts are equally effective. Indeed, he says that some treatments that are otherwise successful produce poor results because the participants were inappropriately selected. (This possibility ties in with the discussion on assumptions and procedures at the beginning of this chapter.)

There seems to be some general agreement, then, that intervention by those who work with the aged is not only a distinct possibility but that there is a common body of such procedures as well. Sometimes these will be used in combination for some specific outcome. Maloney and Daily (1986), for example, wished to increase sensory awareness in a group with a diagnosis of dementia or organic brain syndrome. To effect such a change, they utilized reality orientation, reminiscing, remotivation therapy, and sensory stimulation. Here, the interest was less on which technique might be best than it was on whether or not in some systematic way, sensory awareness can be improved. Similarly, Rosin, Abramowicz, Diamond, and Jesselson (1985) designed a community project that involved demented and cognitively impaired elderly over a 2-year period. They focused on reality orientation but also included social interaction, physical activity, dance therapy, and crafts. Support groups were available for spouses, and educational programs were offered to staff, professionals, and the public. This project is obviously so extensive that it would be difficult to partial out what elements are accomplishing whatever results were obtained, but it does indicate the strong efforts that may be made to assist in ameliorating problems of patients and caregivers.

The *need* is manifest even if the *proper procedure* is not so clear. Garland (1985) has noted that such interventions as reality orientation, behavior modification, memory and reminiscence training, counseling, even bibliotherapy, and psychotherapy have been used often with elderly persons. Yet rarely have any of these been evaluated thoroughly. In fact, there may be implicit difficulties present in any attempt to improve functioning of the elderly. Bledsoe and Lutz-Ponder (1986) list the goals of group counseling in nursing homes as developing alternative coping styles, sharing both personally and supportively, discussing common experiences and redeveloping social interaction. Such goals might be achieved through reality orientation, resocialization, remotivation, reminiscing, or psychotherapy. However, there are potential pitfalls. Positive

outcomes will not be achieved where there is staff resistance about perceived intrusion and increased work load. Even establishing the condition
for the therapy may decrease the possibilities for success. Screening group
members is essential but may involve considerable difficulties. Finding
an effective location for meetings, and establishing a time that will fit
the schedules of participants is often a problem. Such factors confound
the attempts to assist older persons in a meaningful way.

Yet efforts continue, and procedures have been proposed, are being
employed, and should be tested. There are four such interventions of
some popularity, and there is some literature where an attempt has been
made to assess the effects of each. These interventions include reality
orientation, reminiscence therapy, validation therapy, and remotivation.

REALITY ORIENTATION

Reality orientation is a technique that has been used for almost 30
years. Usually credited to the efforts of J. C. Folsom, it is based upon
the belief that certain portions of the brain remain intact and may be
used for reeducation purposes (e.g., Taulbee & Folsom, 1966; Kohut,
Kohut, & Fleishman, 1983, p. 79). The rationale has been explained by
Taulbee and Folson (1966) as

> The attitude adopted is one of active or passive friendliness; it is
> supportive and makes the patient feel that he is worth something
> after all, that he can still accomplish something, that life has not
> passed him by, and that there are still people in the world who
> care about him. The therapeutic atmosphere is quiet and calm. The
> demands are minimal; the patient progresses slowly in the treatment
> program. (p. 134)

Kohut et al. (1983) state that the premise is that an individual can
continue to function adequately in an environment so long as she or
he is oriented within that environment. (The role of orientation as it
affects our ability to relate to the environment was discussed in Chapter
One.) Orientation comes from awareness of time and place and the person's relationship to such elements. In conditions of confusion and disorientation, such awareness is lost. The technique is intended to help
ameliorate conditions due to lack of social interaction and loss of positive
stimuli (Kohut et al., p. 73). This role is accomplished by supplying the
individual with the information needed to reconstruct the environment
in a meaningful way. To be effective, the procedure must be used in
the same positive manner by all persons who come in contact with the

disoriented person during the entire 24-hour period. Symptoms of confusion lead immediately to information about who the individual is, where he or she is, why she or he is in this place, who is speaking to him or her, and the time of day. This is always done in a positive and supportive fashion, *never a corrective one*. Repetition is continued in all settings as the need arises. Kohut et al. (pp. 78–80) have detailed the procedures and given an example of their use.

The intervention has proved popular in a variety of settings and with varied age groups. Folsom (1986) describes reality orientation (RO) as a psychological approach for treating the problems of confused elderly persons. Lloyd (1985) says that it stimulates the patient by repeatedly presenting basic information and creating social contact in order to overcome the adverse effects of isolation. Thus it is a treatment modality that may bring a healthier environment for institutionalized older persons. The effectiveness of the therapy is not wholly within the structure itself, however. Buckholdt and Gubrium (1983) used the technique and observed the effects on the work of staff in a nursing home. They propose from their results that the problems of patients must be separated from the work of caregivers. In the setting they used, at least, the staff did more than provide care; they also contributed to the problems.

Reviews of the literature have not been supportive of the technique in most cases. Godfrey and Knight (1987), in their review of the literature, included reality orientation as one of the attempts to rehabilitate those with memory loss. Though they found that patients could be taught some rather specific information and memory skills, there was little or no generalization and virtually no maintenance. Only if there were clearly defined behavioral goals and definitive efforts to assure maintenance and generalization were treatment gains effective at all. Gropper-Katz (1987) reviewed five studies where the emphasis was on RO as a technique to help the confused elderly. She found both methodological and theoretical weaknesses that led to discrepancies in results.

> Few research studies are to be found; most work is descriptive in nature, attesting to the promotion of this therapy. Actual research currently published in this area is weak in the research process. . . . Commonly, theoretical frameworks are lacking or poorly developed. (p. 17)

The intervention has been reported to produce deleterious effects in some cases (Dietch, Hewett, & Jones, 1989). *Why* it may do so perhaps is less a function of the process than bias on the part of those responsible for the conduct of the RO. Dietch et al., for example, report that nursing home staff are often cynical about the value of the technique and use it at all only because of an institutional requirement as part of their jobs. Techniques are frequently applied in a rote fashion, and there is often an emphasis on communicating information and giving instructions rather than on the positive, supportive approach described in Taulbee and Folsom (1966). Dietch et al. advocate a more humanistic approach (as in Validation Therapy) because the constant relearning of RO necessary to current orientation is difficult and may lead to frustration, anxiety, depression and loss of self-esteem.

> Living in the past may bring the psychological rewards of reexperiencing times when the subject felt a sense of belonging and competency. Seen in this context, RO may attempt to bring unwilling subjects back to an intolerable reality—only to provoke anger, misery, or both. (p. 974)

They then describe three case studies where adverse effects were found, though their description might as easily be inferred to reflect inept application of RO as a deficiency in the technique. They do extend the case studies to demonstrate Validation Therapy and to show its superiority in their estimation.

Outcomes

There have been a number of studies conducted to determine the effectiveness of RO. Though there are methodological differences between them, all are focused on outcomes of the application of the technique. A review of several of these studies will not only provide us with some information on success and failure but also offer the opportunity to observe variations in the conduct of the research.

One means of judging the effectiveness of a technique is to use it in the accepted form with one group and in a modified form with another. This does not test the efficacy of the intervention so much as it discloses its power. Hart and Fleming (1985) used "traditional" RO with one group of psychogeriatric women patients in a hospital, emphasizing the repetition of current and relevant information visually shown on a board (e.g., "Today is Monday," etc.). The other group of women received the "modified" treatment that used behavior modification techniques (shaping, reinforcement) as well as a game strategy to encourage social participation. The procedures were used for 8 weeks. On the pre- and posttests (a measure of psychiatric orientation), the modified group showed more significant improvement than the traditional group. However, there was no generalization effect, indicating that positive outcomes were limited to the precise setting and circumstances of use. A follow-up measure (after 8 weeks) disclosed that both groups had returned to the pretest level; thus the gains had been lost when the program was no longer being conducted. Such results would seem to indicate that changes in behavior are possible using RO or an enhanced form of RO but that such changes are transitory and situation-specific. So far as this is a general finding, it indicates a limitation. How severe that limitation is considered to be depends upon whether it is worthwhile to institute *and continue* RO intervention. Further, the extent of the applications will be a factor in how widely the procedures are applied by subjects. Such issues have been considered in other studies to determine their presence and effects (see, e.g., Cunliffe, 1984).

One means of determining the efficacy of a technique is to compare the procedure with experimental and control groups. Wallis, Baldwin, and Higginbotham (1983) randomly divided a sample of 60 middle-aged and older individuals who had been diagnosed as demented or withdrawn or both. The experimental group received RO for 30 minutes a day, 5 days a week, over a 3-week period. The other group was broken into three subgroups, each receiving a form of occupational therapy but not RO. Unfortunately for the rigor of the study, only 19 subjects remained in each subgroup for analysis at the end of the test period, though the authors report that the characteristics of the remaining persons were not different from those who were dropped. For the experimental subjects, those who had received RO showed more improvement than those not, but the differences were not statistically significant. There were positive effects on the cognitive functioning of patients in both groups, but behavioral changes were not found for either. The authors believe this was due to the "classroom" atmosphere and practice effects. Again, we have mixed results, supporting the use of the technique at the same time that there are limitations that may be disappointing.

In this regard, a study by Parker and Somers (1983) is relevant. They implemented 24-hour RO in a psychogeriatric unit after training the staff in the principles involved, the role of staff members in RO, and the rationale for undertaking the endeavor. Six patients, diagnosed as major depressive disorder, were given a pretest, several weeks of RO, and a posttest. The results showed improvement for two, no change for two, and a decrease for the remaining two on the test measure. Yet they do report that, by observation, there were positive changes in behavior. These were disclosed by the use of the RO board and daily activities schedule over the course of the intervention. Further, there seemed to be more group interaction. They observed less wandering and agitation. These findings would, of course, assume greater significance if they had been anticipated and actual measures taken both before and at the end of the training period. Parker and Somers felt that the technique would have been more beneficial had it been used for a longer period. In fact, the intervention was maintained (though not with the same patients) over a 3-year period, with some positive outcomes reported. Among these was an improvement in staff morale. *Why* they achieved such results is not disclosed from the study itself. Because the patients suffered depression, and presumably were under treatment, some or all of the gains observed may reflect the effects of treatment for depression, not RO. A control group would have been helpful in determining the effect. Staff morale may have improved under almost any alteration in routine that involved patients more consistently and directly. Such issues are typical in studies of every intervention and reflect the position of Gropper-Katz (1987) described earlier.

A more positive outcome has been reported by Paire and Karney (1984). They had 12 weeks of treatment (sensory stimulation, staff attention, or standard hospital treatment) with 30 elderly patients, about 20% of whom had a diagnosis of organic brain syndrome, whereas nearly all the remainder were schizophrenic. They hypothesized that including sensory stimulation in the RO would yield better results than RO accompanied by increased staff attention or orientation with the usual hospital routine for patients. In fact, all three groups showed increased RO at the end of the treatment period. However, the sensory stimulation did not produce the added effect they had hypothesized. Maintenance of gains for another 6 weeks was found. Similar positive results for RO have been reported by Quattrochi-Tubin and Jason (1987–88) for cognitive behaviors. Less than compelling results were found by Gotestam (1987) for time and room orientation and orientation to person and by Johnson and Frederiksen (1983) for process behaviors and feedback.

Such outcome studies present a conflicting picture that may represent methodological differences more than viability of technique. There seems to be fairly consistent agreement that carefully controlled and prescribed procedures that are documented and supervised bring behavioral change. The length of the program and its specificity then assumes importance for the degree to which change is maintained. It is essential that the technique be employed in the same way by all persons at all times if success is to be attained.

A limited generalization phenomenon has been reported by Woods (1983) also. In a single case study, a 68-year-old woman with Korsakoff's psychosis was trained on lists of verbal orientation items. There was virtually no generalization to any other list, a result that is discouraging even though this is a case study. Woods advocates that treatment programs (not restricted just to RO) need to focus on particular target areas of functioning.

The strength of RO would seem to be limited to very particular circumstances and content. It has been shown to be useful under such conditions. To train individuals or groups and expect to find effects on other, even similar, behaviors seems unlikely from the studies currently available. The general conditions imposed in experimental studies, described early in this chapter, would seem essential to assuring description of strengths and limitations of RO.

REMINISCENCE THERAPY

Butler introduced the intervention of reminiscence, or life review, in 1963. As a psychiatrist, his rationale and explanation fit the therapeutic mold more than the behavioral one. He took the position that life review is a process that occurs naturally in all of us. It is expressed in a mental process that allows the progressive return to our consciousness of various past experiences but particularly by those events that represent unresolved conflicts. Once we have allowed them into the conscious, it becomes possible to examine them and integrate them as part of the self. The most basic reason for reminiscence during old age is that it permits the realization of impending death, though it may also reflect the inability to continue maintenance of our personal invulnerability. When present, reminiscing is shaped further by ongoing, current experiences.

Reviewing one's life, Butler says, is a general response whenever crises occur, with imminent death being only one example. Of course, impending death is more crisis-laden for some persons than for others. In fact, many older persons seem to have accepted and adapted to the finality of life as a natural occurrence. What Butler intends to convey here, then, is that " the biological fact of approaching death, independent of—although possibly reinforced by—personality and environmental circumstances, prompts the life review" (Butler, 1963, p. 67).

The life review is more comprehensive than reminiscence, but includes that process certainly. Nor is life review some unexpected or unwanted awareness of repressed memories, or purposely trying to achieve them, though both contingencies may occur as the process continues.

> In its mild form, the life review is reflected in increased reminiscence, mild nostalgia, mild regret; in severe form, in anxiety, guilt, despair, and depression. In the extreme, it may involve the obsessive pre-

occupation of the older person with his past, and may proceed to a state approximating terror and result in suicide. (Butler, 1963, p. 68)

Obviously, reminiscence and life review are complex and potentially dangerous conditions when they are induced in the lives of the elderly. If Butler's description is accepted, the professional will need to assist many, perhaps all, elderly to realize the necessity to conduct life review, to be able to deal with the process therapeutically, and to assist the elderly individual to resolve the conflicts now realized. Such a procedure requires a skilled, empathic, sophisticated professional; otherwise, considerable harm may result to the older person. Given such a professional, the role of reminiscence/life review may benefit the individual.

The distinction between reminiscence and life review has been clarified further by Burnside (1990). She sees reminiscence as supportive, with some rather clear dynamics. First, the process does not increase anxiety; instead, it acts, second, to reinforce life decisions. At the same time, it reinforces the lifestyle of the elder as a third dimension. Fourth, in the process, one does not dwell on losses. Where reminiscence is employed as an intervention, there is the fifth outcome that the group leader uses strategies that are ego supportive. By contrast, life review is intended to bring insight, a reworking of recovered memories, and working through them. An outcome of the therapy will be tolerance of anxiety, with the occurrence of transference to the therapist and eventual countertransference. Life review, then, is more psychoanalytic, requiring a highly specialized professional. Reminiscence, Burnside says, focuses on the psychosocial, although it requires clinical skills and judgment. It would seem, then, that life review is a technique of the psychiatrist, and particularly one who is trained in psychoanalytic therapy. Reminiscence, by contrast, may be employed by trained and skilled clinicians as a supportive and reinforcing intervention. There are constraints on the use of the technique that are closely correlated with skills and education, so that either will be used only under restricted circumstances. This caveat should delimit the application of the procedure.

Within this context, there have been reviews and studies published about the application and results of reminiscence therapy. Hughston and Cooledge (1989) believe that it has been underutilized—and too little investigated as a strategy for the elderly as well. They contend that family therapy should use the process of reflection on past events in order to develop positive understanding of the role that experience has in avoiding repetition of mistakes. As an outcome, there should be creation of future success for those who are involved in reminiscence. Moody (1988) concurs in the opinion of the positive role of reminiscence and speaks of a "collective myth" that produces a hopeful view about old age. Poulton and Strassberg (1986) state that reminiscence can lead to resolution of previously unresolved conflicts, maintaining goal-directed behavior, and prolonging feelings of self-esteem and personal significance. Though they also acknowledge some potential maladaptive results, the overall picture is one of considerable positive potential. Buechel (1986) expands these effects to the professional, speaking of enhancement of skills and effectiveness as clinicians in working with the aged.

The method may even be subject to enhancement. Sherman (1985), for example, developed a procedure that went beyond experiencing memories in terms of recall of external details. He used what he calls "experiential focusing" wherein the client is taught to gradually allow a review of the current quality of life. If there are problems as a part of this review, one may be selected for some eventual analysis. Such an approach is phenomenological, reflecting the subjectively felt meaning of experiences. Sherman says that it is benign and nonintrusive, allowing a person to deal with conflict and stress at a personal pace and in a unique fashion. He feels that its phenomenological and experiential basis makes reminiscence more vivid and meaningful. The result will be enhancement of the subjective quality of life for the older individual in the present.

This intervention, whether called life review or reminiscence, differs markedly from RO. The psychological character of reminiscence emphasizes very different dynamics and functions and requires expert supervision. Only as such competence is available should the technique be used.

Outcomes

Given the rationale of reminiscence, it might be expected that few studies have been conducted using the criteria described earlier. Instead, the literature contains a number of articles where a recall of experiences has been the technique. Whether the project in any given case met the standards for reminiscence is problematic, but in every instance the title has been used. Thus Baker (1985) held a 6-week program that she called "reminiscence group therapy" with eight elderly women. She stated the goals of her approach to be an increase in feelings of self-worth, a promotion of personal role identity, provision of opportunity for physical contact, and assistance in validating past experience. The subjects were significantly impaired, being unable to remember much beyond their own names. A mental status examination was the pretest measure, but the posttest evaluation was observational. She reports evidence of improvement for all subjects in verbal interaction, eye contact, touching others, smiling, participation in activities, and accepting leadership responsibilities.

Baines, Saxby, and Ehlert (1987) used reality orientation and reminiscence therapy in a residential setting. They report that both approaches were enjoyed by staff and subjects and both helped the staff to become more knowledgeable about moderately and severely confused residents. The condition that provided RO first, followed by reminiscence therapy, led to improvement in cognition and behavior where either alone and the control condition did not. Baines et al. suggest that RO may be beneficial for confused persons before attempting group reminiscence. Smith (1986) reports that, with AD patients, reminiscence, whether cued verbally or musically, significantly improved language scores on the Mini-Mental State Examination (Folstein et al., 1975) but had no effects on orientation or attention scores. Mixed outcomes are cited by Goldwasser, Auerbach, and Harkins (1987) as well. They found that self-reported depression levels were decreased after the use of reminiscence therapy, but cognitive and behavioral functioning were not changed. When one considers that the reminiscence group showed greater depression than the other groups initially, the finding is less convincing. In addition, at follow-up the reminiscence group showed a return toward their original higher levels of depression. Holland (1987) linked present semantic realities (time, place, and people) with past memories for language-impaired patients. She concluded that an intervention that included autobiography, daily treatment topics, and training in questioning skills increased verbal appropriateness and time orientation.

A comparison between a reminiscence group and one that discussed current events was conducted by Lappe (1987). Self-esteem was measured both pre- and postintervention. She found that scores increased more for those who reminisced than for the discussion group. Habegger and Blieszner (1990) examined relationships between personal and social aspects of reminiscence using either oral or silent recall. There were 50 older adults in the community in their sample. They found components of the technique to include the fact that early life exposure to the process was significantly correlated with total reminiscence frequency. Interestingly, the correlation between enjoyment and silent reminiscence was negative. The content of the silent process may be a factor here, perhaps in the directions indicated by Butler (1963).

A study by Orten, Allen, and Cook (1989) serves to indicate some of the methodological problems that may arise in studies of an intervention. They established three experimental groups, all receiving a

16-week course of reminiscence group therapy, and three control groups who were provided "milieu therapy," that is to say, routine activities of daily living and physical and medical care. They hypothesized that those in the experimental groups would achieve higher levels of social behavior than would the controls. They also thought that there would be a direct relationship between participation in reminiscence groups and levels of social behaviors. They felt reminiscence would be effective because remote memory is usually much later to decline and deteriorate. Further, they reasoned that there is a certain "redundance" in facilities, reflected in restricted living space, absence of opportunities for new learning, and sameness of daily routines. These elements make decrements cognitively appear greater than they really are or should be.

Their results were mixed and inconsistent. There were no differences between experimental and control groups on the social behavior scale at the beginning of the intervention. After 8 weeks, two experimental groups differed significantly from controls, but one group did not. After 16 weeks, the one group that was not different previously now was, and one of the two that were different at midpoint no longer was. When groups were combined, no differences were found at either Week 8 or 16. The hypotheses were not accepted as a result. The variability in outcomes led them to suggest that they were unable to produce unqualified support for the procedure, though successes occurred that made it seem probable that it is useful when properly conducted.

Orten et al. make a cogent comment that may have considerable generalizability.

> Perhaps an indirect value of the study is that it can help dispel the attitude that reminiscence is a simple technique. When initially introduced to the procedure, the reaction of many individuals, especially nonprofessionals, is that it can be used by anyone and with little training. But there are few therapeutic processes that are powerful enough to help that can be used without training and skill. This study suggests that reminiscence therapy is not an exception to that rule. (pp. 85–86)

The disclaimer is well taken. Indeed, there is some basis for suspecting that, among the studies surveyed here, in certain instances the procedures were not reminiscence therapy at all, at least as described by Butler (1963) and qualified by Burnside (1990). It is difficult to draw conclusions about outcome and effectiveness under these conditions. No doubt a case may be made for therapeutic results when the intervention is employed appropriately by competent professionals. Whether or not the approach has received testing is debatable at this point. Life review and its component, reminiscence, is more than rehearsing memories of past events, at least if it is to have therapeutic value. There must be a facing of the suppressed content so that a resolution is achieved. Though one may ultimately "feel good" as a result, the frequently extolled virtue of reliving happy days is not life review. Potentially, reminiscence and life review are usable with both patients and caregivers.

VALIDATION THERAPY

The intervention titled "validation therapy" (VT) was proposed by Feil (1982) during the 1960s. She defines validation as the acknowledgment of the feelings of an individual (Feil, 1982, p. 1) through accepting what the person feels as truth, regardless of what others may consider to be reality. This procedure is not an analytic technique; instead it utilizes empathic understanding. Feil (1982, p. 3) states that empathy accepts whatever feelings are expressed without attempting to examine feelings that the individual chooses not to express. Where employed, the intervention is intended to lead to a decrease of mental deterioration along with increased control and interaction with others (Feil, 1982, p. 11).

As one becomes very old, a new life task is encountered, called "resolution versus vegetation" (Feil, 1985). This task is defined as a stage where resolution must occur or vegetation results (Feil, 1982, pp. 20–22) based upon a belief that much of the behavior among the disoriented elderly is the result of conflict resulting from unsatisfactory management during previous life stages (Feil, 1985). If this task is recognized and accepted, there can be more accurate diagnosis and appropriate therapy. The elderly individual may be able to face aging more satisfactorily through dealing with earlier life tasks in a better way. The process combines empathy with the use of touch, eye contact, mirroring body movements, matching voice rhythms of the elderly person, attending to cues concerning feelings and translating these into verbal form, acceptance without judgment, and listening. These procedures lead to validation of the feelings of the person with a consequent feeling of happiness and the potential for a return to the present and its reality (Feil, 1985). All old people are not disoriented because some of them are more realistic about losses as they age. As a result they live in present time successfully. For those few who do become disoriented, the history includes denial of their losses with an attempt to hold on to past lifestyles and meanings. Because this effort cannot be successful, they panic in order to avoid pain and fear (Feil, 1982, p. 98). What results is emotional thinking, attempting to restore the past and amend old conflicts never resolved. Unless there is resolution, achieved through VT if at all, they will continue to vegetate.

Dietch et al. (1989), in a study described as part of the discussion of RO, report greater success for VT in three cases where RO had had adverse effects. They state that VT is a viable alternative for some demented patients. Babins (1986, 1988) speaks of validating the "uniqueness" of the old-old so that they regain their sense of dignity and self-worth. This is accomplished without being judgmental. Two principles seem to be involved. First, early emotional learning is retained in the very old, even when there has begun to be cognitive loss. Second, there are stages of life that may be described, and one of which is Feil's (1982) "resolution versus vegetation."

From the conceptual perspective, Babins (1988) describes VT as a humanistic approach that allows the very old and disoriented an opportunity to resolve conflicts from the past through expressing their feelings. Compared to life review (Butler, 1963), VT would seem to apply more to the acknowledgment and acceptance of past problems in order to achieve resolution for the present than to the facing of imminent death. According to Babins, the focus is on empathy, acceptance, and acknowledgment. He has described four stages of disorientation (malorientation, when RO will be more effective than VT, time confusion and repetitive motion, when VT will be more successful than RO, and vegetation). He points out that VT is intended for those who do not have psychiatric disorders, and it should not be used with those who have a diagnosis of primary dementia or other medical illness known to cause disorientation. This not only avoids problems of therapeutic training and education but restricts the application only to persons with the discrete characteristics described by Feil. Babins says that the groups must be small (no more than five or six persons) and deal with issues like death, family relations, loneliness, and disappointments with vocations.

Babins, Dillion, and Merovitz (1988) studied the effectiveness of VT with 12 disoriented, institutionalized elderly women (ages 80 to 91). Five of the women received VT over an 11-week period, meeting twice weekly. The other 7 were part of a control group that received no treatment. Measures were taken pre- and postintervention on cognitive abilities, social competencies, and behavioral adjustments. The therapy did not produce cognitive improvement over the nearly 3-month period, but there were some changes in social competence. Observation indicated to Babins et al. that the women expressed themselves more during the last 3 weeks than in the first 3. The results are mixed in the sense that there were some gains in expected areas but not in others. Whether 11 weeks, and

22 sessions, are sufficient to bring change is not certain. Feil (1982, p. 53) has pointed out that drastic changes in behavior are not possible and should not be expected among the very old. Further, behavioral change will be slow and fluctuating (Feil, 1982, p. 11). Given the characteristics of the sample, almost any positive movement may represent a major accomplishment.

A study of VT over a 9-month period has been reported by Robb, Stegman, and Wolanin (1986). They used the method with moderately to severely disoriented elderly who were age 60 and over. The sample selection alone may have introduced some bias, at least as far as the expected application of VT is concerned. In any event, the 21 subjects involved were randomly assigned to a no-treatment control group or a VT group that met twice a week for the 9-month period. Robb et al. hypothesized that the therapy group would show less decline cognitively, would have higher morale, and more adjusted social behavior than the controls. Pre- and posttreatment measures were used. Interestingly, the authors report that the study was seriously flawed, so that results were compromised and could not be properly evaluated. However, they believe that VT must be tested and encourage that other studies be done to produce some empirical evidence either supporting or rejecting the approach.

The need for research is manifest. At present it is not possible to evaluate the quality of VT simply because the evidence is not available. Given the very limiting circumstances, particularly subject qualities, under which the intervention was developed and is currently used, it may be that such documentation will be minuscule. Without empirical test, one uses a technique such as this based on belief or faith that it is worthwhile and beneficial. The only comment that can be made is that there is little evidence either supporting or rejecting that position. What is essential to bear in mind is that the therapy is intended *only* for those over 80 who are struggling with losses and unresolved conflicts. Participants must not suffer from psychiatric and medical illnesses that lead to disorientation. These conditions may well have been set as a consequence of rationale proposed by Feil prior to developing the technique. Whether or not that is true, the disclaimers separate the procedure from others, particularly Butler's life review, which require highly educated and trained personnel.

REMOTIVATION THERAPY

Remotivation therapy (ReT, to separate it from reminiscence therapy) is related in several ways to reality orientation and uses some of the same techniques. However, there are some distinctions as well. Kohut et al. (1983, pp. 91–95) have pointed out that the principal goal is to renew motivation in an individual who has effectively discontinued interaction with life. Utilized in group settings, ReT attempts to attain three goals. First, the technique allows mental stimulation and may produce greater involvement with other people and the environment. The withdrawn personality is changed as a result of this effort. Second, the involvement with the real world may produce a better perspective of the personal problems experienced by the patient. His or her world is not only expanded within the institution but may generalize to the outside world as well. Third, the therapy permits the patient to practice interacting with other people in a supportive and accepting atmosphere.

ReT also may benefit staff because it brings greater understanding of patients and their problems. Where an individual is withdrawn and passive, the assumption may be that this person may be ignored. The more disruptive and abrasive patients are apt to dominate staff time. By interacting with those who are not seen as problems, staff members may discover needs that were unrealized and help achieve adaptation and growth that otherwise may not have occurred. The motivation principle works in both directions under these conditions.

There have been several descriptions of ReT as one intervention that represents group therapy (see, e.g., Capuzzi, Gross, & Friel, 1990; Forsythe, 1988–1989; Zimpfer, 1987; Maloney & Daily, 1986). There has been little research directed toward testing the outcomes from the use of RT. There is a national organization that certifies remotivation therapists and documents settings where ReT is being used (National Remotivation Technique Organization). There is insufficient evidence to assess the efficacy of the procedure and to describe its limitations.

In summary, there are four intervention techniques that have been described and that are used in various settings. Of these, RO seems clearly intended for patients who have memory loss and disorientation. It encourages continued use of cognitive abilities even though the disease progresses and dementia increases. The assumption is that some parts of the mind continue to be functional and should be utilized to prevent the patient from deteriorating as rapidly as will occur without intervention. The procedure requires implementation by all who deal with the patient and throughout the 24-hour period. A popular technique, the research done to date has produced mixed results, in part because of methodological problems.

Reminiscence therapy is more closely allied to psychoanalytic techniques and requires educated and experienced professionals to accomplish its goals. Through life review, the individual allows repressed experiences to reach consciousness in order to deal effectively with them. Part of this experience is directed toward acceptance and compromise with impending death in the elderly. The technique may be used either with patients, at least in earlier stages of dementia, or with caregivers. Research has produced inconclusive results, but there is the possibility that life review has not really been used or tested. In some instances, it appears that the technique is interpreted to mean rehearsal of events from earlier life that have been pleasurable and are worth reliving. Such a procedure may be enjoyable and may be worthwhile but would represent something other than reminiscence in the sense proposed by Butler.

Validation therapy has been reserved to the very old and disoriented. Using empathic reactions to the elderly, it permits feelings to be expressed and accepted by the therapist so that the patient feels validated. Only a few research efforts have been reported, with mixed results. The premises have not really been tested to this point. Seemingly, the intervention is intended for patients and would not be applied to caregivers unless they were very old and disoriented also.

Finally, remotivation therapy is an attempt to help the withdrawn, passive personality become reengaged with life. The procedures are clearly described and controlled, but there is little evidence about its efficacy. Given the principles involved, ReT might be used with caregivers as well as with patients.

The overall assessment of such interventions is less than compelling. Well-intentioned, often clearly described and defended, with rationales that seem worthwhile, there simply is no basis for assuming that any of them work effectively. At the same time, there is no basis for rejecting them either so that we must restate the dictum of human services: Further research is needed.

PSYCHOTHERAPY

Though historically there has been an attitude that elderly persons cannot benefit from psychotherapeutic intervention, more recent attempts have given evidence that they can. There may be individual differences in the willingness or ability to respond to therapy among older patients, and there may be differences in the willingness to undertake intervention among therapists, but success can and has been obtained when conditions are appropriate (Zarit, 1980, p. 17). Soloman (1990, p. 257) points to the motivation for help found in older persons, with a consequent reduction in resistance. Both individual and group psychotherapy are pertinent for the elderly.

Generally, this form of intervention is reserved for more serious maladaptive cases. This is in part due to the fact that highly skilled professionals are required, persons who themselves have been properly educated and have had internships where they apply their skills under supervision. When used, the technique is applicable to patient or caregiver in most instances. Most depression, as one example, may occur in either or both and should be identified and treated as soon as possible. The particular modality that may be used depends upon the maladjustment and patient characteristics so that referral becomes a major element.

REASONS FOR INTERVENTION

Whatever particular form of intervention may be used, and whether undertaken with patient or caregiver, there are some assumptions underlying the process.

1. In the case of patients, there is the belief that the condition producing the dementia is irreversible or incurable. Because the option of recovery is not present but because there are other problems that *may* be ameliorated, the decision is made to help the patient become as self-sufficient and productive as possible. The treatable problems will need to be identified and the appropriate interventions decided upon. The outcome is less than ideal but better than a benign neglect that simply permits the patient to deteriorate.

For caregivers, the rationale is related but somewhat different. Here, there are maladaptive behaviors emanating from the patient's condition that interfere with adequate adjustment and optimal caregiving. These maladaptive behaviors must be identified and appropriate means used to change them to adaptive ones. The interventions, then, are intended to assist the caregiver to perform more adequately under conditions predisposing to burden and failure.

2. Even in the worst of conditions, there may be competencies remaining. As a patient shows deterioration, there will certainly be more difficulty in discovering mental states that remain usable. However, if the professional is involved with and for the patient, there is the possibility that adaptive behaviors remain available. Permitting their expression and channeling their energies insofar as possible may allow the patient to continue a more realistic life.

The caregiver will retain many behavioral potentials that may be disguised by the effects of the demands of caregiving. Competencies are suppressed, not lost, and intervention techniques may be devised and applied that recover them. Instead of decline into apathy and self-deprecation, the caregiver can be encouraged to become more self-efficacious.

3. For the patient, there is the possibility that the use of competencies that remain may slow disease progression. There is no evidence of the truth of this assumption, but it does encourage an attitude that the patient has the right to continue functioning at as high a level as possible for as long as possible.

4. As competencies are expressed, the patient controls self and the environment in a more direct and positive manner. Interaction with others is a sign to oneself that orientation is still possible and evident. Intervention, of whatever type, is a mode that will permit such evidence. For the caregiver, this principle is reflected in the attitude that one still controls the elements of one's life. One is not so helpless as previously appeared.

5. Though beneficial to the patient in many ways, there is the possibility that intervention benefits caregivers even more. When applied to patients and especially when some results can be seen, the message to the caregiver is a positive note of resistance to a hopeless situation. Even small gains in the patient are reinforcing in the face of what had seemed only decrement.

The caregiver who receives intervention can note not only that others are concerned and caring but also that control is still possible. The effect can be a change in attitude that leads to an increase of effort. Humans tend to resist giving up, though conditions in life may push them in that direction. Even in the negative state, evidence of more positive outcomes can lead to abandonment of hopelessness and increased attempts to experience life.

SUMMARY

There have been several modes of intervention proposed and described by those who are involved with the elderly, including dementia patients and their caregivers. In choosing a technique, it is important that the professional understand the assumptions underlying intervention and seek evidence of the adequacy of the procedure. When making applications, once a technique has been chosen, it is equally important to be able to demonstrate the results. Conditions to be met that satisfy this condition are described.

The more commonly used interventions are detailed, and the literature attesting to their natures and demonstrating their effectiveness is surveyed. Reality orientation, reminiscence therapy, validation therapy, and remotivation therapy are the specific procedures that are included along with a discussion of psychotherapy as an alternative approach. Finally, reasons for using intervention techniques are described.

CHAPTER ELEVEN

Dementia and the Future

Clearly, there have been major efforts in the past quarter-century to understand the nature and meaning of syndromes leading to dementia as well as to disclose the course of significance of the dementing process. The literature is increasing with each decade. Indeed, in a book such as this one, it is impossible to review all of the published material even of the past *decade*. Such activity should indicate that our knowledge and competencies have increased just as much. Unfortunately, the increase in publication rate does not guarantee equal increases in usable results. There has certainly been an accumulation of helpful data, but it seems disproportionate to the volume. Because it is probable that the amount of research—of whatever value—will increase in the future, it would seem well to summarize where we currently are on several dimensions.

DEMENTIA IN THE PRESENT

Based upon the content presented in the preceding 10 chapters, it is possible to draw some conclusions about the present state of knowledge and application available to the professional community.

The Status of Diagnosis

There have been major developments that have brought greater precision to the diagnostic process. Many of these have involved the invention and manufacture of technological devices, not solely intended to assist in diagnosing conditions leading to dementia but certainly having a positive influence on that procedure. Though the use of these devices (particularly computerized axial tomography, positron emission tomography, and magnetic resonance imaging) is expensive, they provide data that are unchallenged in their quality. Further, there is no need to use surgical procedures to obtain these data so that the process is nonintrusive to the body. There is some belief that the newest of these technologies—magnetic resonance imaging—has capabilities even greater than those realized thus far (see Heston & White, 1991, p. 155).

However, when we consider why diagnosis is needed, the gains are limited as compared to what is desirable. These procedures offer detail and precision of brain *structures* superior to any other tools and allow the diagnostician to rule out (or rule in, as the case may be) physical signs that may have been missed with less sophisticated instrumentation. Unfortunately, it is not possible with present expertise to produce images of nerve cells so that the status of neurons in a patient is not known. By using the information provided from several sources (the medical examination, case and personal history, and psychological testing as well as technology), the clinician will be able to make a judgment about the cause of demented behavior that is more likely correct. If, or when, the ability to scan neuronal integrity becomes available, many questions surrounding diagnosis will have been answered.

Certain conditions that may be treatable can mask as dementia. The most commonly recognized is major depression that, in the older person, can present symptoms similar to those in demented patients. There is increasing awareness of this possibility, and this should lead to fewer misidentified cases. Depression is treatable and should receive appropriate intervention when it occurs so that the individual may resume an active life. This principle applies not only to those without dementia but to persons who present signs of demented behavior as well. Treatment for depression will not affect the dementia process, but it may increase the quality of life for the dementia victim. Other conditions that may produce behaviors mimicking dementia are AIDS and vascular disease (Heston & White, 1991, pp. 36–37). Even infections in other parts of the body may influence brain functioning in such a way that there may be a presumption of dementia, and the deleterious effects of some drugs on behavior has received wide notice.

Diagnostic precision has greater importance than to assure accuracy only. Once a label has been decided upon, certain consequences normally follow. One of these concerns *progression* of the condition. There is the assumption, for example, that Alzheimer's disease is incurable and irreversible. The patient is expected to show increasing deterioration, though the pattern may not be consistent, and the course may take months to years. Professionals are increasingly urging that such an assumption is unfair to the patient. There are interventions that may be tried and that may allow more quality to life than if the patient is abandoned. This positive attitude is expanding among all disciplines. Though proof of the efficacy of interventions is unavailable and would be difficult to achieve, the position is commendable.

Patient Characteristics

It would seem plausible that every case that is labeled "dementia" has a developmental history. The details of that history are often poorly recognized and reported, both by patient and caregiver. This outcome is due, in no small measure, to the fact that elderly persons who become demented have been productive, competent individuals throughout their adult lives. Stereotypes exist about aging that include the decline, even loss, of faculties, including mental abilities. As behaviors contrasting with the usual competence of the person begin to occur, it may be easy to dismiss them as "normal" or unimportant. Probably the early behavioral symptoms of a developing dementia are short-lived and circumscribed, so that it will be easier to misinterpret them. The period when signs of a developing disorder are present serves as a gap in our knowledge and competencies that needs definition and recognition. Research will help to provide the definition; for example, there need to be some studies of groups of middle-aged persons who are measured on a series of relevant tasks at periodic intervals to describe behavioral changes and correlate these with later diagnoses of dementia. This would yield systematic data about the nature of the "early signs" and permit education of citizens about the meaning of certain behavioral changes.[1] Because current knowledge about the precursors to diagnosis is suspect, the investment of effort and money in such a study would seem warranted. At present, the more likely sequence is to ignore "warning signs" until the number and extent of adverse behavioral changes forces admission of a major problem. A physician usually is consulted and asked to identify the cause and treat the condition. Unfortunately, the dementia may have reached a level too severe to allow effective medical intervention.

Research about the characteristics of persons after diagnosis has been extensive. It is clear that there is a developmental pattern, probably continuing from the period before diagnosis, that is consistent with the syndrome. For example, multiinfarct patients typically show a "stepwise" decline, whereas Alzheimer's patients demonstrate an irregular pattern of deterioration. There is a loss in memory that seems to be shared by the various causes of dementia, but some research indicates that, on the more specific level of semantic and episodic memories, there may be differences among the several causes. Confusion and disorientation are frequently described as attributes of a developing dementia. However, it is not clear how these states may manifest themselves, the conditions under which they progress, or whether interventions may reduce their strength and effects. There may or may not be personality changes with the traits intensifying, decreasing, or being replaced by other traits. The overall picture is clouded and, consequently, difficult to explain to patients and caregivers. Most frequently, the studies are descriptive and of limited generalization. There are few models or theories that are tested by a series of studies where results permit modification, alteration, or substantiation. Each discipline, and subdiscipline, has its own research focus, and the results are sometimes difficult to compare across disciplines. As a consequence, the large number of published studies becomes overwhelming and is difficult to assimilate. Professionals in the field complain that there is little from research that is practical in working with patients or advising caregivers.

The need for a "model" that may apply to efforts in various disciplines has been cited in this book on several occasions. As an example, Bowlby (1990, p. 466) has described a physiological model that classifies causes for disorders into four types. Two of these are essential, though neither alone is sufficient. The first deals with *predisposing* factors that have their influence on the organism, particularly during development. Where present, these predisposing factors will determine significantly the degree to which the organism is vulnerable to a *provoking* factor. Thus if one is susceptible to a particular outcome (predisposed), being exposed (provoked) to the conditions associated with the outcome may lead to its expression.

The last two types of causes describe conditions under which the outcome may assume greater probability. There are several kinds of *contributing* factors. Among those mentioned by Bowlby are ones that increase vulnerability, others that are associated with the probability of encountering a provoking factor, and still others that exacerbate a prevailing condition. Finally, *symptom-specifying* elements are related to the form that the outcome may take in a given individual. These are more often obscure than one would like, resulting in diverse and confusing symptoms from one person to another (see Table 11.1).

The application of this model to physical diseases seems straightforward and relatively precise. For conditions that produce dementia, such an application may not be so obvious, however. In Alzheimer's disease (AD), for example, there may be predisposing factors, but they have not been clearly defined or empirically verified. It may be that aging nerve cells are more "at risk" than when one is younger, as Pfeiffer (1978, p. 171) has suggested. Perhaps there is a predisposition associated with

TABLE 11.1.
A Classification of Causes for Disorders

Type	Period	Influencing	Function
1. Predisposing	Developmental	Organismic	Essential, but not sufficient
2. Provoking	Developmental	Organismic	Essential, but not sufficient/ dependent on predisposition
3. Contributing	When Type 1 and 2 are present	Probability of occurrence	Sufficient/increase vulnerability, encountering provocation, exacerbation
4. Symptom specifying	When Type 1 and 2 are present	Outcome form on individual	Sufficient/diverse, and confusing

Source. Based on Bowlby, 1990.

systemic disease that has a "delayed effect" in certain persons but not others. Perhaps there is a familial basis for the occurrence of the disease. Whatever the predisposing factor(s) may be is not yet known, which is a major reason why so many avenues are being investigated. Once such predisposition is clarified, there can be efforts to define precisely what provokes the expression. Until *both* of these elements are specified, the cause of Alzheimer's remains a mystery. Research should and is being focused on these issues.

Data relating to predisposition and provocation are clearer in other syndromes leading to dementia, however. Creutzfeldt–Jakob disease (CJD) is known to be caused by a virus, though the nature of that virus is unknown. Although predisposing factors have not been isolated, there is the assumption that some individuals are more susceptible to the virus than others. Given this assumption, there have been attempts to specify some of the provocational factors involved. For example, Harries-Jones et al. (1988) investigated the relationships of diet, familial transmission, and animal contact as possible etiologies of CJD. Their search, done with 92 cases, was inconclusive. Obviously, this outcome merely excludes some possible provoking factors without proving or disproving the case.

So long as Factors 1 and 2 are in doubt, evidence relating to Factors 3 and 4 is problematic. Overall, there is a case to be made for employing the model in application with research already published as well as in the design of future research. More meaning would certainly accrue to what is known and what needs yet to be learned. This would require analyzing and categorizing already accumulated research in medicine, psychology, and sociology/social work in terms of the factor(s) reflected in the problem investigated. This would permit viewing what is currently known in a more systematic framework and suggest the direction that future research should take in order to provide needed data. Of course, a more pertinent and useful model might be developed than this one, but the issue should be faced in order to avoid a morass of independent findings that confounds and confuses rather than enlightens.

Caregiver Characteristics

Much the same confusing picture of characteristics is found for caregivers that exists for patients (with the same need for model-directed efforts). However, there is even greater need for some consistent applications because the caregiver must live with the increasing problems as the patient becomes less aware and more dependent. Several variables have been identified as outcomes of caregiving: increased burden (which may continue to increase so long as the patient is alive, whether remaining at home or in an institution), stress that is induced by the perceptions of problems rather than by the demands of caregiving, loss of control over ordinary aspects of life (such as sleeping, respite, and sexual intercourse), and so on. In some instances, interventions have been proposed and tested by research. Though by no means comprehensive, the results have not been encouraging for use of the interventions. Either the procedures advocated are inadequate, or they are focused on the wrong problems. In either event, they don't seem to work effectively. There needs to be a model developed from the mass of literature that generates more systematic research. This may help to clear up some of the confusion.

The one clear finding is that caregivers suffer psychological distress. The source, the meaning, and the assists needed are not clear at this time.

Interventions

Medically, there is no treatment for the sources of dementia that are irreversible. Currently, the major drug companies are involved in efforts to develop a chemical that will relieve, at least partially, some of the behavioral symptoms of the dementia. To this time, several have been tried and found to be largely failures; among these are lecithin, choline, hydergine, physostigmine, and tetrahydroaminoacridine (THA). Although for each of these drugs, a few persons will receive temporary relief of symptoms such as memory loss, most individuals do not benefit. Other drugs are now being developed and tested by the drug laboratories in hopes of finding a chemical that will be consistent, long-term, and effective.

The emphasis still is upon the memory loss that is increasingly prominent in the dementia patient because this is a problem of central concern to caregivers. Results will be reported over the next several years, and one or more may be shown to be effective for the purposes intended. Even if this happens, there will still be no treatment for any of the conditions leading to dementia; the drugs will treat symptoms, not causes.

Nondrug interventions to benefit patients behaviorally have been devised and employed in several directions. Among the first of these was reality orientation, intended to keep the patient in contact with reality to the greatest degree possible for as long as possible. More therapeutic in their intent if not in their outcomes have been remotivation, validation, and reminiscence therapies. Though popular in some institutional settings, there is little or no evidence that they are particularly effective. Unfortunately, few controlled studies have been conducted with any of them. Claims of their success are unsubstantiated in most instances and placed in doubt in the few instances where rigorous research has been employed.

For caregivers, the most popular intervention has been the support group. Here, too, the variations on a theme are so many and so common that it is difficult to get a clear picture. Support groups may be small (at least 2 persons), large (more than 10), or anything in between. They may have professional leaders with or without training in group techniques, volunteer leaders, or no leader at all. Most are cathartic in their emphasis, but many include education by specialists, others are social in their focus, whereas still others operate on a "nothing planned" basis. Participants come and go as they find their needs met by the group, so that noncoherence is more common than coherence. Under such circumstances, it is no wonder that research demonstrating the effectiveness of the support group is absent. Even if successful, only a modest percentage of the caregivers for whom the support is intended take advantage of the opportunity.

Respite, defined as some relief from the demands of caregiving, is often cited as a major need for caregivers. Providing such respite is difficult because the patient must be left with someone who has at least minimal competencies and understanding about dementia and its effects. Using volunteers has not been very successful because many persons will not volunteer for such a role, and there may be legal implications as well. Most caregivers cannot afford to hire a professional for respite, and funds for assistance are rarely available from public or private agencies. Medicare and private insurance programs do not cover costs associated with mental disorders, and causes of dementia are excluded from coverage as a result. Where there has been some systematic test of the effectiveness of respite, the results have been disappointing. What the caregiver considers to be "respite" may not fit the definition used by the researcher. In this, as in other areas, then, the picture is obscured. Though efforts to help caregivers cannot be said to be failures, neither can they be pronounced successful.

Research

A brief statement about research on dementia can apply to medical and scientific, psychological, and social efforts together. The use of controlled experimentation is increasing and will eventually provide more reliable and valid conclusions. There is little communication between the disciplines, however, that leads to fragmented and sometimes confusing results. Obviously, some research will necessarily be discipline-specific, but other research might be cross-disciplinary. This is true particularly where effects for patients or caregivers is the major concern.

A model for such cross-disciplinary research is the Baltimore Longitudinal Study of Aging (see Shock, 1984). Not only has data-collection been ongoing since 1958, but there has been extension of age-cohorts to include those as young as 20. All participants are volunteers, with an impressive retention rate.

Many caregivers cooperate in efforts to identify psychological and social variables in dementia—and particularly in drug research—so that it seems likely that a coordinated, longitudinal, multidisciplinary study would be feasible.

DEMENTIA IN THE TWENTY-FIRST CENTURY

The final decade of the twentieth century began with some tacit recognition by the government and many social agencies of the extremity of unfaced problems that accompany increases in dementia. Funding for research into causes increased slightly but at a rate still far below the annual costs attributed to care for those suffering the diseases leading to dementia. Drug companies were investing in efforts to find a chemical that might ameliorate some of the symptoms—notably memory loss— found most vexing to patients and caregivers. Foundations and agencies continued to raise funds to support research conducted in medicine, psychology, and sociology to allow adjustment and support for the many difficulties faced by patients and caregivers. Still, the total (estimated, with federal funding, to be around $300 million annually) was insufficient to bring much return for the myriad of questions still unanswered.

There are, of course, legitimate concerns that need recognition and solution about many other conditions than dementia. All the major medical and behavioral problems that make up the complex need to be the focus of financial support during the 1990s and on into the twenty-first century. Presently, it does not appear likely that such an effort will be forthcoming with the possible exception of AIDS. The political atmosphere must change rather dramatically before it will do so. Because politicians are responsible to an electorate, the focus of endeavors must be to educate the public about the extent and destructiveness of physical and mental conditions. One factor that may contribute is the current concern about the cost of the health care system in this country, along with the recognition that millions of Americans have little or no health care coverage. The current discussion in Congress is centering on some means to provide for soaring health costs through contributions by citizens and their employers.

No doubt this tack must be pursued, but the politicians must also consider the contribution to the problem by the health care industry. Hopefully, out of the discussions that will follow over the next several years, there will be the acceptance that paying for care *after* the fact of illness is much more expensive than providing means of prevention *against* illness in the first place. This returns us to a prime need for research on dementia—finding the causes and providing prevention against their ravage. By no means should research efforts to improve the status and quality of life for dementia patients and caregivers be relegated to a secondary status, though. Increased efforts must be encouraged here as well.

Meantime, an attempt to forecast the future seems most likely to proceed in the following general directions.

More of the Same

Given the research attitude in various disciplines, a continuation of what is already accepted and followed is the most obvious course to be anticipated. There is much to be gained by the process, though it is not sufficient. The focus of the research, and the techniques employed, differ somewhat from one discipline to another.

Medicine

Much of the medical research has focused on diagnosis in its general sense. Physicians are primarily interested in providing treatment that will cure the ills experienced by the patient. To do so requires knowing what leads to the illness and what treatments are effective for cure. If cure is not possible, the next alternative is to control the condition in order to prevent increases in the illness. If the course is progressive and irreversible, treatment must be provided for ancillary conditions, with an admission that the primary syndrome is untreatable. This last condition is most often found with causes of dementia.

Diagnosis under this circumstance emphasizes making sure that some treatable condition(s) is not responsible for the complaint of the patient. If none can be found, the physician may be left with the necessity to accept the inability to treat in the conventional sense. Medical research, as a result, has emphasized attempts to find some drug or other chemical that can assist the functioning of the patient. In the case of Alzheimer's disease, there is interest in the role of the neurotransmitter acetylcholine (ACh) and the enzyme that produces it, acetyl choline transferase. Though efforts to date have not been successful (using choline, lecithin, and other products to supplant the deficiency in ACh), the search continues in an increasingly sophisticated manner. In time, a means to supply the brain with ACh will be found, and that will give physicians a treatment that will benefit the patient. The disease process may be stopped or, at least, slowed down under these circumstances, even though cure will not be possible.

Physicians are alert to other attempts to develop or use drugs in new ways that may help the Alzheimer's victim. At the same time, many physicians will follow progress in other disciplines as well so that they may inform caregivers and patients of behavioral assists (such as reality orientation, for example).

Though innovative efforts in medicine probably will emerge in the next century, we must expect and encourage the continuation of efforts already underway.

Scientific Research

Although, in special cases, physicians may conduct research into basic issues about dementia, more often this area is attractive to other disciplines such as chemistry, biology, and genetics. The focus of researchers in these areas is on causation—what produces the outcomes that are detrimental to the behavior of a person. To date, research is being conducted on possible chromosomal explanations, neurotransmitter deficiencies, aluminum buildup in cells, mitochondrial inadequacy, immune system decrements, beta amyloid protein involvement, slow-acting viral relationships, and a number of others. None of these appears to be the answer, though more research needs to be done before any can be clearly eliminated as the cause.

There is a basis for the position that the kinds of factors under investigation are not the cause of a syndrome but an accompanying effect. The search needs to be widened, if this is true, and certainly will be as monies are provided to encourage the expansion.

A major effect has come from the invention and refinement of technology. The sophistication resulting from these procedures (particularly the CT, PET, and MRI scans) has increased the accuracy of identification of structural changes in the body and especially of the brain. Eventually, an instrument will be available that will permit examination of structures at the cellular level. At that point, accuracy and precision will be increased not only for diagnosis but for intervention and treatment as well. Cost is a major factor in the use of technology at present, and future inventions probably will be even more expensive. The gains to the potential well-being of patients must override financial considerations alone.

Psychological Research

Psychologists are often involved in the decision-making process through the use of measures designed to assess mental competence of the person. Tests have been developed specific to this purpose, and other measures have been adapted for the determination of competencies in the absence of more direct evidence. The tests used have been studied for their reliability and validity, and the applications by psychologists of the results in decision making have been researched as well. Such studies will continue, both with tests currently available and with new psychometric instruments that will be developed. The data have been used as a part of medical diagnostics but have their role as well in placement decisions (institutionalization, for example) and in program participation (as in reality orientation or reminiscence therapy).

Behavioral changes and effects of dementia will continue to be studied by psychologists as well. Principal emphasis to date has been on the identification and meaning of memory loss, confusion, and disorientation in time and space. In recent years, research has examined more specific factors; for example, memory may be studied in terms of dimensions. In this regard, both semantic and episodic expressions have been investigated. There should be increased sophistication in the models and methods of study. The short-term and long-term effects of dementia will continue to be a major source of research in order to provide patients and caregivers with depth of knowledge and to develop appropriate interventions.

Modes of adjustment adopted both by patient and caregiver are of interest to psychologists as well. There continues to be investigation of burden and stress, with clarification increasing skills in intervention and treatment. Coping methods have been studied in order to identify helpful examples and assist in devising training programs in their use. Supports, including group participation, are an ongoing area of consideration.

These areas of study will continue because they permit applications that are useful and helpful. Beyond these, psychologists should develop models that allow examination of discrete variables at the same time that interactions are more clearly conceived and defined.

Social Research

The dynamics of individual behavior in various settings has been a significant area for study by sociologists and social workers. They have surveyed attitudes of caregivers and patients and used the results both to increase our understanding of specific characteristics and to promote ways of dealing with problems. Institutional qualities have been studied as they impinge on residents and primary caregivers. The roles of aides, paraprofessionals, and professionals have been investigated for their meaning for adaptation in such settings. Group characteristics have been described and assessed for their meaning on individual behavior. Such studies will continue because dynamics are ever-changing while they remain influential.

Recently, there has been an examination of the relationships among the disciplines involved with dementia and the effects these relationships have on the disciplines themselves and the patients and caregivers being served. The medical model has been the preferred one used for intervening with patients and in research. In some recent publications, the effectiveness of the model has been questioned. Increasing efforts in this direction should help clarify what the relationships should be and conditions under which a more effective model may be employed.

Cooperative Efforts

The future should bring an emphasis on multidisciplinary studies that will permit more interaction comparisons. From research done to date, it is clear that univariate approaches do not yield sufficient evidence to understand the scope and influence of dementia. The complexity that has been exposed from such studies does indicate that a comprehensive strategy may disclose dimensions that may be refined for application.

Both patients and caregivers need greater awareness and understanding of the intricate relationship of factors that impinge on their lives. As an example, research indicates that the meaning to the caregiver of the burdens imposed by the caregiving role is more important to adjustment than are the specific burdens themselves. There is the interaction, then, between person and consequences and perceptions that results in an individual who lacks the self-efficacy to feel control over life stresses. The study needs extension to include measures of self-efficacy and feelings of control in order to define the outcomes more explicitly. Essentially, then, there will have been an evolution from, first, the study of burden by person to, second, burden by person by perceptions to, third, burden by person by perceptions by self-efficacy judgments by feelings of control; that is, from two variables to three variables to five variables. The variables chosen must be pertinent and measurable so that the results will add to knowledge and permit extrapolation to further studies. More than one discipline will be involved as well that may bring added strength and increased communication.

Model Building

The need for more coherent investigations requires models that allow systematic testing and consequent modifications. There are a few models within separate disciplines, and these may serve as the base for a more comprehensive structure. Until a multidisciplinary model has been developed, the research efforts are apt to be fragmented and isolated within disciplines. Certainly, some answers result and knowledge accrues, but there will be spotty application. Social workers know and use social work research, gerontologists know and use gerontological research, psychologists know and use psychological research, and so on. One of the major foundations or agencies may need to provide funding to bring representatives in the several disciplines together to develop the essentials that lead to interactive studies.

The Ultimate Goal: Prevention

If there can be a concerted effort to analyze the complex nature of dementia, along with the studies that extend present knowledge and expertise, eventually the day will come when dementing diseases are no longer a source of dread among aging persons. That accomplishment will stand as one of the great achievements in the twenty-first century.

Notes

Chapter 1

1. In some instances, portions of the brain may be "retrained" to take over the functions served by damaged cells. With older persons, this is less likely than with younger ones, however, and the losses resulting from dementia are seldom, if ever, recoverable.
2. When presenting symptoms may result from any of several causes, it is necessary to determine which is the most likely source. The process, based on data that may come from various sources such as family history and occupational setting as well as from medical and psychological signs, is called "differential diagnosis."
3. A "slow virus," in this case, is defined as an infective agent that will pass through filters that bacteria cannot pass through and that takes some period of time (days, months, or years) to bring about adverse effects.
4. The ventricles are the "spaces" or areas between the folds of tissue that make up the brain.

Chapter 2

1. The word *lobe* means nothing more than a generally rounded part that projects from the body to which it is attached, as in "earlobe." In this case, it is a portion of the brain that is separated from other portions by a fissure.
2. In the cortex of the brain, many complex functions are performed that are not yet understood. The term *association area* is used in this text to mean portions of the brain that receive signals from other areas of the cortex and even from structures below the cortex. These signals are analyzed to allow the complicated behaviors that we ascribe to the human "mind."

Chapter 4

1. A cyclotron is an apparatus that furnishes high energy to particles such as protons (a unit always charged with positive electricity). The machine causes the particle to move in a spiral path with increasing energy and, at the proper speed, permits a computer reconstruction of an image.
2. That is, to stimulate production of deficient neurotransmitters and particularly acetylcholine.

Chapter 5

1. Sutherland (1989) defines neuropsychology as the subdiscipline in psychology that studies brain damage in humans in order to infer the brain mechanisms that underlie both normal and impaired behavior. Holden (1988, p. x) describes the field as the study of behavior directly related to functioning of the brain.
2. AD is used for those under age 65, SDAT for those over 65. The distinction is an arbitrary one.

Chapter 6

1. There are physical causes that are expressed as disorders also. Included would be such conditions as organic mood disorder, organic anxiety disorder, organic personality disorder, and so on.
2. This term is used intentionally to distinguish characteristics of the disorders from those of Personality Disorders. The DSM-III-R (1987, p. 335) uses the term *personality disorder* for conditions where personality traits are inflexible or maladaptive, leading to functional impairment or psychological distress. Further, the diagnosis of a Personality Disorder is reserved to long-term functioning. In old age, the disorders interfere in a more discrete fashion. In fact, the expressions are usually situation-specific rather than long-term means of adaptation.
3. Such an acceptance is found for other conditions as well. Psychotics may express themselves in a way that appears rational, and the confabulations of an alcoholic may seem reasonable also.

Chapter 7

1. Today, of course, we would argue that old age does not bring memory inadequacy, confusion, and disorientation. These are anomalies found only in exceptional cases, under unusual circumstances.
2. This possibility may be illustrated by an analogy of physical integrity and recovery. A young adult may hit her or his hand against a desk and feel pain. Usually, the discomfort subsides in a few minutes, and there will be little or no evidences of the blow. An elderly person who strikes his or her hand with the same force is much more likely to feel pain longer, probably develop a bruise, and be days in recovering. The analogy implies that brain cells are more susceptible to damage with increasing age, although there should be no connotation that such cells react as muscles do.
3. In fact, there is no way to prove that intervention for hypertension reduces the number of major strokes, either. It is simply impossible to "prove the absence of" such factors or to demonstrate that an event would have happened except for intervention. We must operate on probability statements, then, without knowing the level of probability that exists in the actual relationship of treatment to stroke reduction.
4. The sample is not representative of the population, so that these figures cannot be presumed to reflect the incidence per year for the country at large.
5. SPECT differs from PET (positron emission tomography) in the fact that it does not require an on-site cyclotron. However, it is less precise in quantifying regional radioactivity in the brain.

Chapter 8

1. Shunting is a surgical procedure where a plastic tube is used to bypass, temporarily, a section of an artery. This permits blood flow that would otherwise be obstructed.
2. In this case, "size" refers to the fact that the infectious agent is left after the fluid that contains it is passed through a filter. This agent remains virulent.
3. The term refers to memory storage that is very brief; say, in hundreths of a second, or tenths of a second.

Chapter 11

1. This approach has already been demonstrated for "normal aging" by the Baltimore Longitudinal Study (Shock, 1984).

References

Adams, R. D., Fisher, C. M., Hakim, S., Ojemann, R. G., & Sweet, W. H. (1965). Symptomatic occult hydrocephalus with normal cerebrospinal fluid pressure. *New England Journal of Medicine, 273,* 117-126.

Alekoumbides, Apostolos, Charter, Richard A., Adkins, Thomas G., & Seacat, George F. (1987). The diagnosis of brain damage by the WAIS, WMS, and Reitan Battery utilizing standardized scores corrected for age and education. *International Journal of Clinical Neuropsychology, 9*(1), 11-28.

Alexianu, Marilena, Tudorache, Bogdana, & Dumitrescu, Alice. (1985). Multi-infarct dementia: Clinical and morphological correlations. *Neurologie et Psychiatrie, 23*(4), 221-229.

Alexopoulos, George S. (1989). Biological abnormalities in late-life depression. *Journal of Geriatric Psychiatry, 22*(1), 25-34.

Alzheimer's Association (1991a). *Newsletter,* 11, 2, p. 5.

Alzheimer's Association (1991b). *Public policy update,* Issue no. 30, July.

Alzheimer's Association (1991c). *Advances in Alzheimer' research.* Winter, 3.

Alzheimer's Association (1987). *Directions in Alzheimer's disease research.* Chicago, ADRDA.

American Psychiatric Association (1987). *The diagnostic and statistical manual of mental disorders* (3rd. ed., rev.). Washington, DC: American Psychiatric Association.

Ames, David, Dolan, Ray, & Mann, Anthony. (1990). The distinction between depression and dementia in the very old. *International Journal of Geriatric Psychiatry, 5*(3), 193-198.

Ancill, Ray J. (1989). Discussion: Cognitive-affective disorders: The co-presentation of depression and dementia in the elderly. *Psychiatric Journal of the University of Ottawa, 14*(2), 370-371.

Andrade, Luis A. (1983). Neurotransmitter disturbances and the proposals of a rational treatment in senile dementia of the Alzheimer type. *Neurobiologia, 46*(2), 125-140.

Aram, D. M., & Ekelman, B. L. (1986). Cognitive profiles of children with early onset unilateral lesions. *Developmental Neuropsychology, 2,* 155-172.

Arie, Tom. (1984). Prevention of mental disorders of old age. *Journal of the American Geriatrics Society, 32*(6), 460-465.

Babins, Leonard (1986). A humanistic approach to Old-Old people: A general model. *Activities, Adaptation and Aging, 8*(3-4), 57-63.

Babins, Leonard (1988). Conceptual analysis of validation therapy. *International Journal of Aging and Human Development, 26*(3), 161-168.

Babins, Leonard H., Dillion, Jackie P., & Merovitz, Steven. (1988). The effects of validation therapy on disoriented elderly. *Activities, Adaptation and Aging, 12*(1-2), 73-86.

273

Baines, Sheila, Saxby, Peter, & Ehlert, Karen. (1987). Reality orientation and reminiscence therapy: A controlled cross-over study of elderly confused people. *British Journal of Psychiatry, 151,* 222-231.

Baker, Nora J. (1985). Reminiscing in group therapy for self-worth. *Journal of Gerontological Nursing, 11*(7), 21-24.

Ban, Thomas A. (1989). Introduction to the diagnosis and treatment of old age dementias. *Modern Problems of Pharmacopsychiatry, 23,* 1-9.

Ban, Thomas A., Conti, L., Morey, L., Lazzerini, F, Cornelli, U., Postiglioni, A., & Grossi, D. (1987). Changes in functioning with glycosaminoglycan polysulfate in primary degeneration and multi-infarct dementia. *Current Therapeutic Research, 42*(4), 614-619.

Bandura, Albert (1977). Self-efficacy: Toward a unifying theory of behavioral change. *Psychological Review, 84,* 191-215.

Bandura, Albert (1982). Self-efficacy mechanisms in human agency. *American Psychologist, 37,* 122-147.

Bandura, Albert (1986a). Fearful expectations and avoidant reactions as coeffects of perceived self-inefficacy. *American Psychologist, 32,* 1389-1391.

Bandura, Albert (1986b). Social foundations of thought and action: A social cognitive theory. Englewood Cliffs, NJ: Prentice Hall.

Barclay, Laurie L., Blass, John P., & Lee, Robert E. (1984). Cerebral metasteses mimicking depression in a "forgetful" attorney. *Journal of the American Geriatrics Society, 32*(11), 866-867.

Barclay, Laurie L., Zemcov, Alexander, Blass, John P., & Sansone, Joseph. (1985). Survival in Alzheimer's disease and vascular dementia. *Neurology, 35*(6), 834-840.

Barker, M. G., & Lawson, J. S. (1968). Nominal dysphasia in dementia. *British Journal of Psychiatry, 114,* 1351-1356.

Bartlett, John G. (1990). Tuberculosis. In William B. Abrams & Robert Berkow (eds.)., *The Merck manual of geriatrics.* Rahway, NJ: Merck Sharp and Dohme Research Laboratories.

Barusch, Amanda S., & Spaid, Wanda M. (1989). Gender differences in caregiving: Why do wives report greater burden? *Gerontologist, 29*(5), 667-676.

Bayles, Kathryn A. (1982). Language function in senile dementia. *Brain and Language, 16,* 265-280.

Bayles, Kathryn A., & Tomoeda, Cheryl K. (1983). Confrontation naming impairment in dementia. *Brain and Language, 19*(1), 98-114.

Belloni-Sonzogni, Amelia, Tissot, Antonella, Tettamanti, Mauro, Frattura, Lucilla, & Spagnoli, Alberto. (1989). Mortality of demented patients in a geriatric institution. *Archives of Gerontology and Geriatrics, 9*(2), 193-197.

Bender, Lauretta (1946). *Bender Visual Motor Gestalt Test.* American Orthopsychiatric Association.

Benjamin, Lisa C., & Spector, John. (1990). The relationship of staff, resident and environmental characteristics to stress experienced by staff caring for the dementing. *International Journal of Geriatric Psychiatry, 5*(1), 25-31.

Benson, D. Frank. (1984). New developments in diagnosis—CAT, PET and NMR. *Psychiatric Annals, 14*(3), 192-197.

Berg, Richard, Franzen, Michael, & Wedding, Danny. (1987). *Screening for brain impairment: A manual for mental health practice.* New York: Springer.

Besson, J. A., Mutch, W. J., Smith, F. W., & Corrigan, F. M. (1985).The relationship between Parkinson's disease and dementia: A study using proton NMR imaging parameters. *British Journal of Psychiatry, 147,* 380-382.

Besson, J. A, Corrigan, F. M., Foreman, E. Iljon, Eastwood, L. M., Smith, F. W., & Ashcroft, G. W. (1985). Nuclear magnetic resonance (NMR); II. Imaging in dementia. *British Journal of Psychiatry, 146,* 31-35.

Besson, J.A., Crawford, J. R., Parker, D.M., & Smith, F. W. (1989). Magnetic resonance imaging in Alzheimer's disease, multi-infarct dementia, alcoholic dementia and Korsakoff's psychosis. *Acta Psychiatrica Scandinavica, 80* (5), 451-458.

Birkel, Richard C., & Jones, Constance J. (1989). A comparison of the caregiving networks of dependent elderly individuals who are lucid and those who are demented. *Gerontologist, 29* (1), 114-119.

Birkett, D. Peter (1989). Advising families about inheritance of dementia. *Loss, Grief and Care, 3* (3-4), 105-109.

Blazer, Dan G. II (1982). *Depression in late life.* St. Louis: C. V. Mosby.

Blazer, Dan G. II. (1990). Anxiety disorders. In William B. Abrams & Robert Berkow (eds.), *The Merck manual of geriatrics.* Rahway, NJ: Merck Sharp and Dohme Research Laboratories.

Bledsoe, Nancy, & Lutz-Ponder, Patricia. (1986). Group counseling with nursing home residents. *Journal of Specialists in Group Work, 11* (1), 37-41.

Boller, Francois, Lopez, Oscar L., & Moossy, John. (1989). Diagnosis of dementia: Clinicopathologic correlations. *Neurology, 39* (1), 76-79.

Bowen, D. M., Davison, A. N., Francis, P. T., Palmer, A. M., & Pearce, B. R. (1985). Neurotransmitter and metabolic dysfunction in Alzheimer's dementia: Relationship to histopathological features. In F. Clifford Rose (ed.), *Modern approaches to the dementias. Part I: Etiology and pathophysiology.* New York: Karger.

Bowlby, John. (1990). *Charles Darwin: A new life.* New York: Norton.

Brandt, Jason. (1985). Access to knowledge in the dementia of Huntington's disease. *Developmental Neuropsychology, 1* (4), 335-348.

Brandt, Jason, & Butters, Nelson. (1986). The neuropsychology of Huntington's disease. *Trends in Neurosciences, 9* (3), 118-120.

Brenner, Richard P., Reynolds, Charles F., & Ulrich, Richard F. (1989). EEG findings in depressive pseudodementia and dementia with secondary depression. *Electroencephalography and Clinical Neurophysiology, 72* (4), 298-304.

Brink, T. L., Carter, Mary Ann, Janson, Eleanor, Love, Donna, Menn, Mary Ellen, and Peratis, Tina. (1985). Paranoid performance on the SRT. *Clinical Gerontologist, 3* (3), 52-55.

Brink, T. L., Yesavage, J. A., Lum, O., Heersema, P., Adey, M., & Rose, T. L. (1982). Screening tests for geriatric depression. *Clinical Gerontologist, 1* (1), 37-43.

Brinkman, Samuel D., & Braun, Paul. (1984). Classification of dementia patients by a WAIS profile related to central cholinergic deficiencies. *Journal of Clinical Neuropsychology, 6* (4), 393-400.

Brodsky, Patricia, Brodsky, Marvin, Lee, Henry, & Sever, Joy. (1986). Two evaluation studies of Reitan's REHABIT program for the retraining of brain dysfunctions. *Perceptual and Motor Skills, 63* (2), 501-502.

Brown, Lisa J., Potter, Jane F., & Foster, Betty G. (1990). Care-giver burden should be evaluated during geriatric assessment. *Journal of the American Geriatrics Society, 38* (4), 455-460.

Brun, Anne. (1987). Frontal lobe degeneration of non-Alzheimer type:I. Neuropathology. *Archives of Gerontology and Geriatrics, 6* (3), 193-208.

Buckholdt, David R., & Gubrium, Jaber F. (1983). Therapeutic pretense in reality orientation. *International Journal of Aging and Human Development, 16* (3), 167-181.

Buechel, Heidi (1986). Reminiscence: A review and prospectus. *Physical and Occupational Therapy in Geriatrics, 5* (2), 25-37.

Burdz, Michael P., Eaton, Warren O., & Bond, John B. (1988).Effects of respite care on dementia and nondementia patients and their caregivers. *Psychology and Aging, 3* (1), 38-42.

Burnside, Irene. (1990). Reminiscence: An independent nursing intervention for the elderly. *Issues in Mental Health Nursing, 11* (1), 33-48.

Busch, Charles D. (1984). Common themes in group psychotherapy with older adult nursing home residents: A review of selected literature. *Clinical Gerontologist, 2* (3), 25-38.

Butler, Robert N. (1963). The life review: An interpretation of reminiscence in the aged. *Psychiatry, 26,* 65-75.

Butler, Robert N. (1990). Senile dementia of the Alzheimer type (SDAT). In William B. Abrams and Robert Berkow (eds.), *The Merck manual of geriatrics.* (pp. 933-938). Rahway, NJ: Merck Sharp and Dohme Research Laboratories.

Butters, Nelson. (1984). The clinical aspects of memory disorders:Contributions from experimental studies of amnesia and dementia. *Journal of Clinical Neuropsychology, 6* (1), 17-36.

Caird, F. I. (1985). Recent advances in the diagnosis of dementia in old age. In F. Clifford Rose (Ed.), *Modern approaches to the dementias. Part II: Clinical and therapeutic aspects* (pp. 58-62). New York: Karger.

Calne, Donald B. (1989). Is "Parkinson's disease" one disease? *Journal of Neurology, Neurosurgery and Psychiatry,* June Special Supplement, 18-21.

Caltagirone, Carlo, Carlesimo, Augusto, Nocentini, Ugo, & Vicari, Stefano. (1989). Defective concept formation in Parkinsonians is independent from mental deterioration. *Journal of Neurology, Neurosurgery and Psychiatry, 52* (3), 334-337.

Caplan, Louis R. (1990). Cerebrovascular disease. In William B. Abrams & Robert Berkow (eds.), *The Merck manual of geriatrics.* Rahway, NJ: Merck Sharp and Dohme Research Laboratories.

Capuzzi, Dave, Gross, Doug, & Friel, Susan E. (1990). Recent trends in group work with elders. *Generations, 14* (1), 43-48.

Catala, I., Ferrer, I., Galofre, E., & Fabregues, I. (1988). Decreased numbers of dendritic spines on cortical pyramidal neurons in dementia: A quantitative Golgi study on biopsy samples. *Human Neurobiology, 6* (4), 255-259.

Charatan, Fred B. (1985). Depression and the elderly: Diagnosis and treatment. *Psychiatric Annals, 15* (5), 313-316.

Charter, Richard A., & Alekoumbides, Apostolos. (1988). An abbreviated version of a psychometric battery for the diagnosis of brain damage utilizing standardized scores corrected for age and education. *International Journal of Clinical Neuropsychology, 10* (3), 123-129.

Chenoweth, Barbara, & Spencer, Beth. (1986). Dementia: The experience of family caregivers. *Gerontologist, 26* (3), 267-272.

Christie, J. E., Kean, D. M., Douglas, R. H., Engleman, H. M., St. Clair, D. and Blackburn, I.M. (1988). Magnetic resonance imaging in pre-senile dementia of the Alzheimer type, multi-infarct dementia and Korsakoff's syndrome. *Psychological Medicine, 18* (2), 319-329.

Chui, Helena C. (1989). Dementia: A review emphasizing clinico-pathologic correlation and brain-behavior relationships. *Archives of Neurology, 46* (7), 806-814.

Coben, Lawrence A., Danziger, Warren L., and Berg, Leonard. (1983). Frequency analysis of the resting awake EEG in mild senile dementia of Alzheimer type. *Electroencephalography and Clinical Neurophysiology, 55* (4), 372-380.

Coben, Lawrence A., Danziger, Warren, & Storandt, Martha. (1985). A longitudinal EEG study of mild senile dementia of Alzheimer type: Changes at 1 year and 2.5 years. *Electroencephalography and Clinical Neurophysiology, 61* (2), 101-112.

Cohen, Gene D. (1988). *The brain in human aging.* New York: Springer.

Cole, Martin G. (1988). The course of multi-infarct dementia: An uncontrolled longitudinal study. *Journal of Clinical and Experimental Gerontology, 10* (1-2), 13-22.

Colgan, John. (1985). Regional density and survival in senile dementia: An interim report on a prospective computed tomographic study. *British Journal of Psychiatry, 147,* 63-66.

Colerick, Elizabeth J., & George, Linda K. (1986). Predictors of institutionalization among caregivers of patients with Alzheimer's Disease. *Journal of the American Geriatrics Society, 34* (7), 493-498.

Comfort, Alex. (1984). Alzheimer's disease or "Alzheimerism"? *Psychiatric Annals, 14* (2), 130-132.

Constantinidis, Jean. (1985). Pick dementia: Anatomoclinical correlations and pathophysiological considerations. In F. Clifford Rose (ed.), *Modern approaches to the dementias. Part I: Etiology and pathophysiology* (pp. 72-97). New York: Karger.

Corona, G. L., Cucchi, M. L., Frattini, P., Santogostino, G., Schinelli, S., Romani, A., Pola, A., Zerbi, F., & Savoldi, F.(1989). Clinical and biochemical responses to therapy in Alzheimer's disease and multi-infarct dementia. *European Archives of Psychiatry and Neurological Sciences, 239* (2), 79-86.

Corthesy, D., Hungerbuhler, J. P., Assar, G., & Regli, F. (1985). Atrophie cerebrale et demense dans la maladie de Parkinson. *Schweizer Archiv fur Neurologie, Neurochirugie und Psychiatrie, 136* (10), 75-85.

Crawford, John R. (1989). Estimation of premorbid intelligence: A review of recent developments. In John R. Crawford & Denis M. Parker (eds.), *Developments in clinical and experimental neuropsychology* (pp. 55-74). New York: Plenum Press.

Cummings, Jeffrey L. (1988). Intellectual impairment in Parkinson's disease: Clinical, pathologic, and biochemical correlates. *Journal of Geriatric Psychiatry and Neurology, 1* (1), 24-36.

Cummings, Jeffrey L., & Benson, Frank. (1988). Psychological dysfunction accompanying subcortical dementias. *Annual Review of Medicine, 39,* 53-61.

Cunliffe, Penny. (1984). Reality orientation with psychogeriatric patients: An initial two-month programme. *British Journal of Occupational Therapy, 47* (11), 341-344.

DeBettignies, Barbara H., Mahurin, Roderick K., & Pirozzolo, Francis J. (1990). Insight for impairment in independent living skills in Alzheimer's disease and multi-infarct dementia. *Journal of Clinical and Experimental Neuropsychology, 12* (2), 355-363.

Degrell, Istvan, & Niklasson, Frank. (1988). Purine metabolites in the CSF in presenile and senile dementia of the Alzheimer type, and in multi-infarct dementia. *Archives of Gerontology and Geriatrics, 7* (2), 173-178.

Degrell, Istvan, Hellsing, Kristoffer, Nagy, Erzsebett, & Niklasson, Frank. (1989). Amino acid concentrates in cerebrospinal fluid in presenile and senile dementia of Alzheimer type and multi-infarct dementia. *Archives of Gerontology and Geriatrics, 9* (2), 123-135.

Deisenhammer, E., Reisecker, F., Leblhuber, Friedrick, Markut, H., Hoell, K., Trenkler, J., & Steinheusel, H. (1989). Single photon emission computed tomography (SPECT) and X-ray CT in patients with dementia. *Psychiatry Research, 29* (3), 443-445.

de la Monte, Suzanne M., Hutchins, Grover M., & Moore, G. William. (1989). Racial differences in the etiology of dementia and frequency of Alzheimer lesions in the brain. *Journal of the National Medical Association, 81* (6), 644-652.

Delaney, Richard C. (1982). Screening for organicity: The problem of subtle neuropsychological deficit and diagnosis. *Journal of Clinical Psychology, 38* (4), 843-846.

de Ruiter, J. P., & Uylings, H. B. (1987). Morphometric and dendritic analysis of fascia dentata granule cells in human aging and senile dementia. *Brain Research, 402* (2), 217-229.

de Smet, Yves, Ruberg, Merle, Sedaru, Michel, Dubois, Bruno, Lhermitti, Francois, & Agid, Yves. (1982). Confusion, dementia and anticholinergics in Parkinson's disease. *Journal of Neurology, Neurosurgery and Psychiatry, 45*(12), 1161-1164.

Deutsch, Georg, & Tweedy, James R. (1987). Cerebral blood flow in severity-matched Alzheimer and multi-infarct patients. *Neurology, 37*(3), 431-438.

Dewan, Mantosh J., & Bick, Peter A. (1985). Normal pressure hydrocephalus and psychiatric patients. *Biological Psychiatry, 20*(10), 1127-1131.

Dietch, James T., Hewett, Linda J., & Jones, Sue. (1989). Adverse effects of reality orientation. *Journal of the American Geriatrics Society, 37*(10), 974-976.

Dieudonne, L. (1984). Maladie de Parkinson et troubles psychiques. *Feuillets Psychiatriques de Liege, 17*(1-2), 124-128.

Direnfeld, Lorne K., Albert, Martin L., Volicer, Ladislav, Langlais, Philip J., Marquis, Judith, & Kaplan, Edith. (1984). Parkinson's disease: The possible relationship of laterality to dementia and neurochemical findings. *Archives of Neurology, 41*(9), 935-941.

Doebler, Jeffrey A. Rhoads, Robert E., Anthony, Adam, and Markesbery, William R. (1989). Neuronal RNA in Pick's and Alzheimer's diseases: Comparison of disease-susceptible and disease-resistant cortical areas. *Archives of Neurology, 46*(2), 134-137.

Drinka, Theresa J. Smith, Jane C., & Drinka, Paul J. (1987). Correlates of depression and burden for informal caregivers of patients in a geriatric referral clinic. *Journal of the American Geriatrics Society, 35*(6), 522-525.

Dunkle, Ruth E., & Nevin, Michael (1987). Stress of the caregiver: Effective management of dementia patients in hospital and community settings. *Journal of Sociology and Social Welfare, 14*(1), 73-84.

Dura, Jason R., Haywood-Niler, Elizabeth, & Kiecolt-Glaser, Janice K. (1990). Spousal caregivers of persons with Alzheimer's and Parkinson's disease dementia: A preliminary comparison. *Gerontologist, 30*(3), 332-336.

Eastman, Peggy. (1991). Finding the key: Scientists gaining on Alzheimer's. *AARP Bulletin, 32*(1), 17.

Edwards, Allen Jack. (1974). Introduction. In David Wechsler, *The selected papers of David Wechsler*. New York: Academic Press.

Emery, Olga B., & Breslau, Lawrence D. (1989). Language deficits in depression: Comparisons with SDAT and normal aging. *Journals of Gerontology, 44*(3), M85-M92.

Erkinjuntti, Timo. (1987a). Differential diagnosis between Alzheimer's disease and vascular dementia: Evaluation of common clinical methods. *Acta Neurologica Scandinavica, 76*(6), 433-442.

Erkinjuntti, Timo. (1987b). Types of multi-infarct dementia. *Acta Neurologica Scandinavica, 75*(6), 391-399.

Erkinjuntti, Timo, Ketonen, L., Sulkava, R., Vuorialho, M., & Palo, J. (1987). CT in the differential diagnosis between Alzheimer's disease and vascular dementia. *Acta Neurologica Scandinavica, 75*(4), 262-270.

Ettlin, Thierry M., Staehelin, Hannes B., Kischka, Udo, Ulrich, Jurg, Scollo-Lavizzari, Giuseppe, Wiggli, Urs, & Seiler, Walter O. (1989). Computed tomography, electroencephalography,and clinical features in the differential diagnosis of senile dementia: A prospective clinicopathologic study. *Archives of Neurology, 46*(11), 1217-1220.

Feil, Naomi (1985). Resolution: The final life task. *Journal of Humanistic Psychology, 25*(2), 91-105.

Feil, Naomi (1982). *VF validation: The Feil method*. Cleveland, Edward Feil Productions.

Fields, W. S. (1985). Vascular disease and dementia. In F. Clifford Rose (ed.), *Modern approaches to the dementias. Part I: Etiology and pathophysiology* (pp. 12-17). New York: Karger.

Fischer, Peter, Gatterer, Gerald, Marterer, Alice, & Danielczyk, Walter (1988). Non-specificity of semantic impairment in dementia of Alzheimer's type. *Archives of Neurology, 45*(12), 1341-1343.

Fisk, Albert A. (1981). *A new look at senility: Its causes, diagnosis, treatment and management.* Springfield, IL: Charles C Thomas.

Fogel, Barry S., & Faust, David. (1987). Neurologic assessment, neurodiagnostic tests and neuropsychology in medical psychiatry. In Alan Stoudemire & Barry S. Fogel (eds.), *Principles of medical psychiatry.* Orlando, FL.: Grune & Stratton.

Folsom, Geneva S. (1986). "Worth repeating" reality orientation: Full circle. *Activities, Adaptation and Aging, 8*(3-4), 65-73.

Folstein, M. F., Folstein, S. E., & McHugh, P. R. (1975). "Mini-mental state": A practical method for grading the cognitive state of patients for the clinician. *Journal of Psychiatric Research, 12,* 189-198.

Forsythe, Emma. (1988-1989). One-to-one therapeutic recreation activities for the bed and/or room bound. *Activities, Adaptation and Aging, 13*(1-2), 63-76.

Franzen, Michael D. (1989). *Reliability and validity in neuropsychological assessment.* New York: Plenum Press.

Franzen, Michael D., & Robbins, Douglas E. (1989). The Halstead-Reitan Neuropsychological Battery. In Michael D. Franzen, (Ed.), pp. 91-107). *Reliability and validity in neuropsychological assessment.* New York: Plenum Press.

Freedman, Morris, & Oscar-Berman, Marlene. (1989). Spatial and visual learning deficits in Alzheimer's and Parkinson's disease. *Brain and Cognition, 11*(1), 114-126.

Fuld, Paula A. (1984). Test profile of cholinergic dysfunction and of Alzheimer-type dementia. *Journal of Clinical Neuropsychology, 6*(4), 380-392.

Galvez, Sergio, & Cartier, Luis. (1984). Computed tomography findings in 15 cases of Creutzfeldt-Jakob disease with histological verification. *Journal of Neurology, Neurosurgery and Psychiatry, 47*(11), 1244-1246.

Garland, Jeffrey. (1985). Adaptation skills in the elderly, their supporters and carers. *British Journal of Medical Psychology, 58*(3), 267-274.

Gemmell, Howard G., Sharp, P. F., Smith, F. W., Besson, J. A. O., Ebmier, K. P., Davidson, J., Evans, N. T. S., Roeda, D., Newton, R., & Mallard, J.R. (1989). Cerebral blood flow measured by SPECT as a diagnostic tool in the study of dementia. *Psychiatric Research, 29*(3), 327-329.

George, Linda K., & Gwyther, Lisa P. (1986). Caregiver well-being: A multidimensional examination of family caregivers of demented adults. *Gerontologist, 26*(3), 253-259.

Gerner, Robert H. (1987). Geriatric depression and treatment with trazodone. *Psychopathology, 20*(suppl. 1), 82-91.

Gershon, Samuel & Herman, Stephen P. (1982). The differential diagnosis of dementia. *Journal of the American Geriatrics Society, 30*(11), 58-66.

Gibbs, C. J., & Gadjusek, M. (1978). Subacute spongiform virus encephalopathies: The transmissable virus dementia. In R. Katzman, R. D. Terry, & K. L. Bick (eds.), *Alzheimer's disease: Senile dementia and related disorders.* New York: Raven.

Gibbs, Clarence J., Jr., Gadjusek, D. Carleton, & Masters, Colin L. (1978). Considerations of transmissable subacute and chronic infections, with a summary of the clinical, pathological and virological characteristics of Kuru, Creutzfeldt-Jakob disease and scrapie. In Kalidas Nandy (ed.), *Senile dementia: A biomedical approach* (pp. 115-129). New York: Elsevier.

Gilhooly, Mary L., & Whittick, Janice E. (1989). Expressed emotion in caregivers of the dementing elderly. *British Journal of Medical Psychology, 62*(3), 265-272.

Gilles, Christian, Ryckaert, Pierre, deMol, Jacques, deMaertelaere, Viviane, & Mendlewicz, Julien. (1989). Clonidine-induced growth hormone secretion in elderly patients with senile dementia of the Alzheimer type and major depressive disorder. *Psychiatric Research, 27*(3), 277-286.

Girotti, F., Soliveri, P., Carella, F., Piccolo, I., Caffarra, P., & Musicco, M. (1988). Dementia and cognitive impairment in Parkinson's disease. *Journal of Neurology, Neurosurgery and Psychiatry, 51*(12), 1498-1502.

Globus, Mordecai, Mildworf, Bracha, & Melamed, Eldad. (1985). Cerebral blood flow and cognitive impairment in Parkinson's disease. *Neurology, 35*(8), 1135-1139.

Godfrey, Hamish P., & Knight, Robert G. (1987). Interventions for amnesiacs: A review. *British Journal of Clinical Psychology, 26*(2), 83-91.

Golden, C. J., Hammeke, T.A., & Purisch, A. D. (1985). *The Luria-Nebraska Neuropsychological Battery.* Los Angeles, Western Psychological Services.

Goldwasser, A. Norman, Auerbach, Stephen M., and Harkins, Stephen W. (1987). Cognitive, affective, and behavioral effects of reminiscence group therapy on demented elderly. *International Journal of Aging and Human Development, 25*(3), 209-222.

Goodnick, P., & Gershon, S. (1984). Chemotherapy of cognitive disorders in geriatric subjects. *Journal of Clinical Psychiatry, 45*(5), 196-209.

Gotestam, K. Gunnar. (1987). Learning versus environmental support for increasing reality orientation in senile demented patients. *European Journal of Psychiatry, 1*(3), 7-12.

Gottfries, C. G. (1985). Alzheimer's disease and senile dementia:Biochemical characteristics and aspects of treatment. *Psychopharmacology, 86*(3), 245-252.

Graff-Radford, Neill R., & Godersky, John C. (1986). Normal pressure hydrocephalus: Onset of gait abnormality before dementia predicts good surgical outcome. *Archives of Neurology, 43*(9),940-942.

Granholm, Eric, & Butters, Nelson. (1988). Associative encoding and retrieval in Alzheimer's and Huntington's disease. *Brain and Cognition, 7*(3), 335-347.

Granholm, Eric, Wolfe, Jessica, & Butters, Nelson. (1985). Affective-arousal factors in the recall of thematic stories by amnesic and demented patients. *Developmental Neuropsychology, 1*(4), 317-333.

Gray, Jeffrey W., Rattan, Arlene I., & Dean, Raymond S. (1986). Differential diagnosis of dementia and depression in the elderly using neuropsychological methods. *Archives of Clinical Neuropsychology, 1*(4), 341-349.

Greene, Vernon L., & Monahan, Deborah J. (1989). The effect of a support and education program on stress and burden among family caregivers to frail elderly persons. *Gerontologist, 29*(4), 472-477.

Gregory, David M., Peters, Nettie, & Cameron, Cynthia F. (1990). Elderly male spouses as caregivers: Toward an understanding of their experience. *Journal of Gerontological Nursing, 16*(3), 20-24.

Griffiths, R. A., Good, W. R., Watson, N. P., O'Donnell, H. F., Fell, P. J., & Shakespeare, J. M. (1987). Depression, dementia and disability in the elderly. *British Journal of Psychiatry, 150,* 482-493.

Gropper-Katz, Elise I. (1987). Reality orientation research. *Journal of Gerontological Nursing, 13*(8), 13-18.

Groth-Marnat, Gary (1990). *Handbook of psychological assessment* (2nd. ed.). New York: Wiley.

Gruetzner, Howard. (1988). *Alzheimer's: A caregiver's guide and sourcebook.* New York: Wiley.

Guilford, J. P. (1959). Three faces of intellect. *American Psychologist, 14,* 469-479.

Gurland, Barry J., & Cross, Peter S. (1982). Epidemiology of psychopathology in old age: Some implications for clinical services. *Psychiatric Clinics of North America, 5*(1), 11-26.

Gurland, Barry J., Copeland, J., Kuriansky, J., Kelleher, M., Sharpe, L., & Dean, L. L. (1983). *The mind and mood of aging: Mental health problems of the elderly in New York and London.* New York: Hawthorne Press.

Gustafson, Lars. (1987). Frontal lobe degeneration of non-Alzheimer type: II. Clinical picture and differential diagnosis. *Archives of Gerontology and Geriatrics, 6*(3), 209-223.

Guyton, Arthur C. (1991). *Textbook of medical physiology,* (8th ed.). Philadelphia: W. B. Saunders.

Habegger, Catherine E., & Blieszner, Rosemary. (1990). Personal and social aspects of reminiscence: An exploratory study of neglected dimensions. *Activities, Adaptation and Aging, 14*(4), 21-38.

Haber, Paul A. L. (1990). Diagnostic and therapeutic technology. In William B. Abrams & Robert Berkow (eds.), *The Merck manual of geriatrics* (pp. 212-225). Rahway, NJ: Merck Sharp and Dohme Research Laboratories.

Hachinski, V. C., Iliff, L. D., Zhilka, D., Du Boulay, G. H. D., McAllister, V. L., Marshall, J., Russell, R. W. R., & Symon, L. (1975). Cerebral blood flow in dementia. *Archives of Neurology, 32,* 632-637.

Hagberg, Bo, & Gustafson, Lars (1985). On diagnosis of dementia:Psychometric investigation and clinical psychiatric evaluation in relation to verified diagnosis. *Archives of Gerontology and Geriatrics, 4*(4), 321-332.

Hagstadius, Stefan, Gustafson, Lars, & Risberg, Jarl. (1984). The effects of bromvincamine and vincamine on regional cerebral blood flow and mental functions in patients with multi-infarct dementia. *Psychopharmacology, 83*(4), 321-326.

Haley, William E., & Pardo, Kinta M. (1989). Relationship of severity of dementia to caregiving stressors. *Psychology and Aging, 4*(4), 389-392.

Haley, William E., Brown, S. Lane, & Levine, Ellen G. (1987a). Experimental evaluation of the effectiveness of group intervention for dementia caregivers. *Gerontologist, 27*(3), 376-382.

Haley, William E., Brown, S. Lane, & Levine, Ellen G. (1987b). Family caregiver appraisals of patient behavioral disturbance in senile dementia. *Clinical Gerontologist, 6*(4), 25-34.

Haley, William E., Levine, Ellen G., Brown, S. Lane, & Bartolucci, Alfred A. (1987). Stress appraisal, coping, and social support as predictors of adaptational outcome among dementia care-givers. *Psychology and Aging, 2*(4), 323-330.

Haley, William E., Levine, Ellen G., Brown, S. Lane, Berry, Jack W., and Hughes, Glenn H. (1987). Psychological, social, and health consequences of caring for a relative with senile dementia. *Journal of the American Geriatrics Society, 35,* 405-411.

Hamlet, Elizabeth & Reed, Sharon. (1990). Caregiver education and support group: A hospital based group experience. *Journal of Gerontological Social Work, 15*(1-2), 75-88.

Harrell, Lindy E., Callaway, Ross, & Sekar, B. Chandra (1987). Magnetic resonance imaging and the diagnosis of dementia. *Neurology, 37*(3), 540-543.

Harries-Jones, R., Knight, R., Will, R. G., Cousens, S., Smith, P. G., & Matthews, W. B. (1988). Creutzfeldt-Jacob disease in England and Wales, 1980-1984: A case-control study of potential risk factors. *Journal of Neurology, Neurosurgery and Psychiatry, 51*(9), 1113-1119.

Hart, Joanna, and Fleming, Richard, (1985). An experimental evaluation of a modified reality orientation therapy. *Clinical Gerontologist, 3*(4), 35-44.

Hart, Robert P., Kwentus, Joseph A., Wade, James B., & Hamer, Robert M. (1987). Digit symbol performance in mild dementia and depression. *Journal of Consulting and Clinical Psychology, 55*(2), 236-238.

Hartwig, William. (1983). Neuropsychological assessment of normal pressure hydrocephalus. *Clinical Neuropsychology, 5*(2), 88-92.

Heinricks, R. Walter and Celinski, Marek J. (1987). Frequency of occurrence of a WAIS dementia profile in male head trauma patients. *Journal of Clinical and Experimental Neuropsychology, 9*(2), 187-190.

Helkala, Eeva Liisa, Laulumaa, Veikko, Soinenen, Hilka, and Riekkinen, Paava J. (1989). Different error pattern of episodic and semantic memory in Alzheimer's disease and Parkinson's disease with dementia. *Neuropsychologia, 27*(10), 1241-1248.

Henderson, A. S. (1990). The social psychiatry of later life. *British Journal of Psychiatry, 156,* 645-653.

Henderson, A. S. (1989). Psychiatric epidemiology and the elderly. *International Journal of Geriatric Psychiatry, 4*(5), 249-253.

Hess, Noel. (1987). King Lear and some anxieties of old age. *British Journal of Medical Psychology, 60*(3), 209-215.

Heston, Leonard L., & White, June A. (1991). *The vanishing mind: A practical guide to Alzheimer's disease and other dementias.* New York: Freeman.

Heston, Leonard L., White, June A., & Mastri, Angeline R. (1987). Pick's disease: Clinical genetics and natural history. *Archives of General Psychiatry, 44*(5), 409-411.

Hier, Daniel B., Warach, Joshua D., Gorelick, Philip B., & Thomas, Joseph. (1989). Predictors of survival in clinically diagnosed Alzheimer's disease and multi-infarct dementia. *Archives of Neurology, 46*(11), 1213-1216.

Hietanen, Marja, & Teravainen, Heikki (1988). The effect of age of disease onset on neuropsychological performance in Parkinson's disease. *Journal of Neurology, Neurosurgery and Psychiatry, 51*(2), 244-249.

Hoch, Carolyn C., Reynolds, Charles F., Kupfer, David J., Houck, Patricia R., Berman, Susan R., & Stack, Jacqueline A. (1986). Sleep-disordered breathing in normal and pathologic aging. *Journal of Clinical Psychiatry, 47*(10), 499-503.

Hofman, A., Schulte, W., Tanja, T. A., Van Duijn, C. M., Haaxma, R., Lameris, A. J., Otten, V. M., & Saan, R. J. (1989). History of dementia and Parkinson's disease in 1st-degree relatives of patients with Alzheimer's disease. *Neurology, 39*(12), 1589-1592.

Hogan, Sharon. (1990). Care for the caregiver: Social policies to ease their burden. *Journal of Gerontological Nursing, 16*(5),12-17.

Holden, Una. (Ed.). (1988). *Neuropsychology and aging.* New York: New York University Press.

Holland, Audrey L., McBurney, Donald H., Moossy, John, & Reinmuth, O. M. (1985). The dissolution of language in Pick's disease with neurofibrillary tangles: A case study. *Brain and Language, 24*(1), 36-58.

Holland, Lynn. (1987). Life review and communication therapy for dementia patients. *Clinical Gerontologist, 6*(3), 62-65.

Horn, J. L. (1968). Organization abilities and the development of intelligence. *Psychological Review, 75,* 242-259.

Houlihan, John P. (1987). Families caring for frail and demented elderly: A review of selected findings. *Family Systems Medicine, 5*(3), 344-356.

Hovestadt, A., van Woerkom, T. C., & Hekster, R. E. (1986). The use of CT-scanning in psychiatric illness: A retrospective study of 226 patients. *Tijdschrift voor Psychiatrie, 28*(3), 178-187.

Huber, Steven J., & Paulson, George W. (1987). Memory impairment associated with progression of Huntington's disease. *Cortex, 23*(2), 275-283.

Huber, Steven J., & Paulson, George W. (1985). The concept of sub-cortical dementia. *American Journal of Psychiatry, 142*(11), 1312-1317.

Huber, Steven J., Shuttleworth, Edwin C., & Paulson, George W. (1986). Dementia in Parkinson's disease. *Archives of Neurology, 43* (10), 987-990.

Huber, Steven J., Shuttleworth, Edwin C., & Freidenberg, Donald L.(1989). Neuropsychological differences between the dementias of Alzheimer's and Parkinson's diseases. *Archives of Neurology, 46* (12), 1287-1291.

Huber, Steven J., Shuttleworth, Edwin C., Christy, Jeffrey A., Chakeres, Donald W., Curtin, Andrew, & Paulson, George W. (1989). Magnetic resonance imaging in dementia of Parkinson's disease. *Journal of Neurology, Neurosurgery and Psychiatry, 52* (11), 1221-1227.

Hughes, Charles P. (1978). The differential diagnosis of dementia in the senium. In Kalidas Nandy (Ed.), *Senile dementia: A biomedical approach* (pp. 201-208). New York: Elsevier.

Hughston, George A., & Cooledge, Nancy J. (1989). The life review: An underutilized strategy for systemic family intervention. *Journal of Psychotherapy and the Family, 5* (1-2), 47-55.

Ihl, Ralf, Eilles, C., Frlich, Lutz, Maurer, Konrad, Dierks, T., & Perisic, I. (1989). Electrical brain activity and cerebral blood flow in dementia of the Alzheimer type. *Psychiatry Research, 29* (3), 449-452.

Iqbal, K., Grundke-Iqbal, I., & Wisniewski, H. M. (1985). Alzheimer neurofibrillary tangles: Biochemical properties. In F. Clifford Rose (Ed.), *Modern approaches to the dementias. Part I: Etiology and pathophysiology* (pp. 98-105). New York: Karger.

Jacobs, Diane, Salmon, David P., Troster, Alexander I., & Butters, Nelson (1990). Intrusion errors in the figural memory of patients with Alzheimer's and Huntington's disease. *Archives of Clinical Neuropsychology, 5* (1), 49-57.

Jagust, William J., Budinger, Thomas F., & Reed, Bruce R. (1987). The diagnosis of dementia with single photon emission computed tomography. *Archives of Neurology, 44* (3), 258-262.

Jagust, William J., Friedland, Robert P., & Budinger, Thomas F.(1985). Positron emission tomography with (-sup-1-sup-8F) Fluorodeoxyglucose differentiates normal pressure hydrocephalus from Alzheimer-type dementia. *Journal of Neurology, Neurosurgery and Psychiatry, 48* (11), 1091-1096.

Jarvik, Lissy F. (1988). Aging of the brain: How can we permit it? *Gerontologist, 28* (5), 739-746.

Jayakumar, P. N., Taly, A. B., Shanmugam, V., Nagaraja, D., & Arya, B. Y. T. (1989). Multi-infarct dementia: A computed tomographic study. *Acta Neurologica Scandinavica, 79* (4), 292-295.

Jenkins, Terry S., Parham, Iris A., & Jenkins, Larry R. (1985). Alzheimer's disease: Caregivers' perceptions of burden. *Journal of Applied Gerontology, 4* (2), 40-57.

Jerison, Harry J. (1985). On the evaluation of mind. In David A. Oakley (ed.), *Brain and mind.* London: Methuen.

Johanson, Aki, & Hagberg, Bo. (1989). Psychometric characteristics in patients with frontal lobe degeneration of non-Alzheimer type. *Archives of Gerontology and Geriatrics, 8* (2), 129-137.

Johnson, Richard P., & Frederiksen, Lee W. (1983). Process vs. outcome feedback and goal setting in a human service organization. *Journal of Organizational Behavior Management, 5* (3-4),37-56.

Jorm, A. F., Korten, A. E., & Henderson, A. S. (1987). The prevalence of dementia: A quantitative integration of the literature. *Acta Psychiatrica Scandinavica, 76* (5), 465-479.

Joynt, Robert J. (1990). Normal aging and patterns of neurologic disease. In William B. Abrams & Robert Berkow (Eds.), *The Merck manual of geriatrics* (pp. 926-929). Rahway, NJ: Merck Sharp and Dohme Research Laboratories.

Judd, Brian W., Meyer, John S., Rogers, Robert L., Gandhi, Sumil, Tanahashi, Norio, Mortel, Karl F., & Tawaklma, Talat. (1986). Cognitive performance correlates with cerebrovascular impairments in multi-infarct dementia. *Journal of the American Geriatrics Society, 34*(5), 355-360.

Kahan, Jason, Kemp, Bryan, Staples, Fred R., & Brummel-Smith, Kenneth (1985). Decreasing the burden in families caring for a relative with a dementing illness. *Journal of the American Geriatrics Society, 33*(10), 664-670.

Kahn, R.L., Goldfarb, A. I., Pollack, M., & Peck, R. (1960). Brief objective measures for the determination of mental status in the aged. *American Journal of Psychiatry, 117,* 326-328.

Kamo, H. McGeer, P. L., Harrop, R., McGeer, E. G, Kalne, D. B., Martin, W. R. W. and Pate, B. D. (1987). Positron emission tomography and histopathology in Pick's disease. *Neurology, 37*(3),439-445.

Kamp, P. E., den Hartog-Jager, W. A., Maathuis, J., de Groot, P. A., de Jong, J. M. B. V., & Bolhuis, P. A. (1986). Brain gangliosides in the presenile dementia of Pick. *Journal of Neurology, Neurosurgery and Psychiatry, 49*(8), 881-885.

Kase, Carlos S. (1986). "Multi-infarct" dementia: A real entity? *Journal of the American Geriatrics Society, 34*(6), 482-484.

Kato, Hiroyuki, Sugawara, Y., Ito, H., & Kogure, K. (1990). White matter lucencies in multi-infarct dementia: A somatosensory evoked potentials and CT study. *Acta Neurologica Scandinavica, 81*(2), 181-183.

Katzman, R. (1985). Clinical presentation of the course of Alzheimer's disease: The atypical patient. In F. Clifford Rose (ed.), *Modern approaches to the dementias. Part II: Clinical and therapeutic aspects.* (pp. 12-18). New York: Karger.

Kermis, Marguerite D. (1986). *Mental health in late life.* Boston: Jones & Bartlett.

Kidd, M., Allsop, D., & Landon, M. (1985). Senile plaque amyloid. In F. Clifford Rose (ed.), *Modern approaches to the dementias. Part I: Etiology and pathophysiology* (pp. 114-126). New York: Karger.

Killeen, Mary. (1990). The influence of stress and coping on family caregivers' perceptions of health. *International Journal of Aging and Human Development, 30*(3), 197-211.

Kim, Kye Y., & Hershey, Linda A. (1988). Diagnosis and treatment of depression in the elderly. *International Journal of Psychiatry in Medicine, 18*(3), 211-221.

Knesevich, John W., Martin, Ronald L., Berg, Leonard & Danziger, Warren. (1983). Preliminary report on affective symptoms in the early stages of senile dementia of the Alzheimer type. *American Journal of Psychiatry, 140*(2), 233-235.

Knight, Robert G., Godfrey, Hamish P., & Shelton, Eric J. (1988). The psychological deficits associated with Parkinson's disease. *Clinical Psychology Review, 8*(4), 391-410.

Knopman, D. S., Christensen, K. J., Schut, L. J., Harbaugh, R. E., Reeder, T., Ngo, T., & Frey, W. (1989). The spectrum of imaging and neuropsychological findings in Pick's disease. *Neurology, 39*(3), 362-368.

Kohut, Sylvester, Jr., Kohut, Jeraldine J., & Fleishman, Joseph J.(1983). *Reality orientation for the elderly* (2nd. ed.). Oradell, NJ: Medical Economics Books.

Kontiola, Paivi, Laaksonen, Ritva, Sulkava, Raimo, & Erkinjuntti, Timo (1990). Pattern of language impairment is different in Alzheimer's disease and multi-infarct dementia. *Brain and Language, 38*(3), 364-383.

Kosberg, Jordan I., Cairl, Richard E., & Keller, Donald M. (1990). Components of burden: Interventive implications. *Gerontologist, 30*(2), 236-242.

Kral, Vojtech A., & Emery, Olga B. (1989). Long-term follow-up of depressed pseudodementia of the aged. *Canadian Journal of Psychiatry, 34*(5), 445-446.

Kunz, Ulrich, Heintz, P., Ehrenheim, Ch., Stolke, D., Dietz, H., & Hundeshagen, H. (1989). MRI as the primary diagnostic instrument in normal pressure hydrocephalus? *Psychiatry Research, 29*(3), 287-288.

Lader, Malcolm. (1982). Differential diagnosis of anxiety in the elderly. *Journal of Clinical Psychiatry, 43*(9, sect. 2), 4-7.

Lappe, Joan M. (1987). Reminiscing: The life review therapy. *Journal of Gerontological Nursing, 13*(4), 12-16.

Larrabee, Glenn J. Largen, John W., & Levin, Harvey S. (1985). Sensitivity of age-decline resistant ("hold") WAIS subtests to Alzheimer's disease. *Journal of Clinical and Experimental Neuropsychology, 7*(5), 497-504.

la Rue, Asenath. (1986). Neuropsychological assessment of older adults. *Clinical Psychologist, 39*(4), 96-98.

Lawton, M. Powell, Brody, Elaine M., & Saperstein, Avalie R.(1989). A controlled study of respite service for caregivers of Alzheimer's patients. *Gerontologist, 29*(1), 8-16.

Lazarus, Lawrence W., Newton, Nancy, Cohler, Bertram, Lesser, Jary, & Schweon, Craig. (1987). Frequency and presentation of depressive symptoms in patients with primary degenerative dementia. *American Journal of Psychiatry, 144*(1), 41-45.

Le Doux, Joseph E. (1985). Brain, mind and language. In David A. Oakley (Ed.), *Brain and mind.* London: Methuen.

Leuchter, Andrew F., Spar, James E., Walter, Donald O., & Weiner, Herbert. (1987). Electroencephalographic spectra and coherence in the diagnosis of Alzheimer's type and multi-infarct dementia: A pilot study. *Archives of General Psychiatry, 44*(11), 993-998.

Levi, Joseph, Oppenheim, Sadi, & Wechsler, David. (1945). Clinical use of the mental deterioration index of the Bellevue-Wechsler Scale. *Journal of Abnormal and Social Psychology, 40,* 405-407.

Levine, Norman B., Dastoor, Dolly P., & Gendron, Carole E. (1983).Coping with dementia: A pilot study. *Journal of the American Geriatrics Society, 31*(1), 12-18.

Levy, Linda L. (1987). Psychosocial intervention and dementia: I. State of the art, future directions. *Occupational Therapy in Mental Health, 7*(1), 69-107.

Lezak, M. (1983). *Neuropsychological assessment* (2nd. ed.). New York: Oxford University Press.

Lichtenberg, Peter A., & Barth, Jeffrey T. (1989). The dynamic process of caregiving in elderly spouses: A look at longitudinal case reports. *Clinical Gerontologist, 9*(1), 31-44.

Lindsey, James, & Murphy, Elaine. (1989). Dementia, depression and subsequent institutionalization: The effect of home support.*International Journal of Geriatric Psychiatry, 4*(1), 3-9.

Liston, Edward H., & la Rue, Asenath (1983). Clinical differentiation of primary degenerative and multi-infarct dementia: A critical review of the evidence: I. Clinical studies. *Biological Psychiatry, 18*(12), 1451-1465.

Lloyd, Chris. (1985). Reality orientation: Its application as a ward based program for the institutionalized elderly. *Activities, Adaptation and Aging, 7*(2), 91-97.

London, Eric, deLeon, Mony J., George, Ajax E., Englund, Elisabet, Ferris, Steven, Gentes, Cynthia, & Reisberg, Barry. (1986). Periventricular lucencies in the CT scan of aged and demented patients. *Biological Psychiatry, 21*(10), 960-962.

Loring, David W., & Largen, John W. (1985). Neuropsychological patterns of presenile and senile dementia of the Alzheimer type. *Neuropsychologia, 23*(3), 351-357.

Loring, David W., Sheer, Daniel E., & Largen, John W. (1985). Forty hertz EEG activity in dementia of the Alzheimer type and multi-infarct dementia. *Psychophysiology, 22*(1), 116-121.

Loring, David W., Meador, K.J., Mahurin, Roderick K., & Largen, John W. (1986). Neuro-psychological performance in dementia of the Alzheimer type and multi-infarct dementia. *Archives of Clinical Neuropsychology, 1* (4), 335-340.

Lucas-Blaustein, Mary J., Filipp, Laura, Dungan, Cheryl, & Tune, Larry. (1988). Driving in patients with dementia. *Journal of the American Geriatrics Society, 36* (12), 1087-1091.

Lund, Dale A. Pett, Marjorie A. and Caserta, Michael S. (1987). Institutionalizing dementia victims: Some caregiver considerations. *Journal of Gerontological Social Work, 11* (1-2), 119-135.

Lundervold, Duane, & Lewin, Lewis M. (1987). Effects of in-home respite care on caregivers of family members with Alzheimer's disease. *Journal of Clinical and Experimental Gerontology, 9* (3), 201-214.

Lyman, Karen A. (1989). Bringing the social back in: A critique of the biomedicalization of dementia. *Gerontologist, 29* (5), 597-605.

Mace, Nancy.(1986). Home and community services for Alzheimer's disease. *Physical and Occupational Therapy in Geriatrics, 4* (3), 5-13.

Maletta, Gabe J. (1990). The concept of "reversible" dementia: How nonreliable terminology may impair effective treatment. *Journal of the American Geriatrics Society, 38* (2), 136-140.

Maloney, Charlotte C., & Daily, Terran (1986). An eclectic group program for nursing home residents with dementia. *Physical and Occupational Therapy in Geriatrics, 4* (3), 55-80.

Marples, Margot. (1986). Helping family members cope with a senile relative. *Social Casework, 67* (8), 490-498.

Martin, David C., Miller, Judson K., Kapoor, Wishwa, Arena, Vincent C., & Boller, Francois. (1987). A controlled study of survival with dementia. *Archives of Neurology, 44* (11), 1122-1126.

Martin, Joseph B. (1984). Huntington's disease: New approaches to an old problem. *Neurology, 34* (8), 1059-1072.

Martin, Joseph B., & Gusella, James F. (1986). Huntington's disease: Pathogenesis and management. *New England Journal of Medicine, 315* (20), 1267-1276.

Martone, Maryann, Butters, Nelson, Payne, Melanie, Becker, James T, & Sax, Daniel S. (1984). Dissociations between skill learning and verbal recognition in amnesia and dementia. *Archives of Neurology, 41* (9), 965-970.

Mayeux, Richard. (1987). The psychiatric and sexual complications of Parkinson's disease. *Medical Aspects of Human Sexuality, 21* (3), 68-72.

Mayeux, Richard, Stern, Yaakov, Rosenstein, Ruth, Marder, Karen, Hauser, Allen, Cote, Lucien, & Fahn, Stanley. (1988). An estimate of the prevalence of dementia in idiopathic Parkinson's disease. *Archives of Neurology, 45* (3), 260-262.

McCue, Michael, Goldstein, Gerald, & Shelly, Carolyn. (1989). The application of a short form of the Luria-Nebraska Neuropsychological Battery to discriminate between dementia and depression in the elderly. *International Journal of Clinical Neuropsychology, 11* (1), 21-29.

McHugh, Paul R. (1989). The neuropsychiatry of basal ganglia disorders: A triadic syndrome and its explanation. *Neuropsychiatry, Neuropsychology and Behavioral Neurology, 2* (4), 239-247.

McNew, Judith A. (1987). Alzheimer's disease: Conceptualizing care-giver competence and practice implications. *Journal of Applied Social Sciences, 11* (2), 167-190.

Meyer, John S., McClintic, Karen L., Rogers, Robert L., Sims, Penne, and Mortel, Karl F. (1988). Aetiological considerations and risk factors for multi-infarct dementia. *Journal of Neurology, Neurosurgery and Psychiatry, 51* (12), 1489-1497.

Meyer, John S., Rogers, Robert L., McClintic, Karen, Mortel, Karl F., & Lotfi, Jamshid. (1989). Randomized clinical trial of daily aspirin therapy in multi-infarct dementia: A pilot study. *Journal of the American Geriatrics Society, 37*(6), 549-555.

Miller, Edgar. (1977). *Abnormal ageing: The psychology of senile and presenile dementia.* London: Wiley.

Miller, Edgar. (1983). A note on the interpretation of data derived from neuropsychological tests. *Cortex, 19*(1), 131-132.

Mindham, R. H., Ahmed, S. W., & Clough, C. G. (1982). A controlled study of dementia in Parkinson's disease. *Journal of Neurology, Neurosurgery and Psychiatry, 45*(11), 969-974.

Mindham, R. H., Steele, Cynthia, Folstein, Michael F., & Lucas, Jane (1985). A comparison of the frequency of major affective disorders in Huntington's disease and Alzheimer's disease. *Journal of Neurology, Neurosurgery and Psychiatry, 48*(11), 1172-1174.

Mitsuyama, Yoshia. (1984). Presenile dementia with motor neuron disease in Japan: Clinicopathological review of 26 cases. *Journal of Neurology, Neurosurgery and Psychiatry, 47*(9), 953-959.

Moak, Gary S. (1990). Characteristics of demented and nondemented geriatric admissions to a state hospital. *Hospital and Community Psychiatry, 41*(7), 799-801.

Mobily, Kenneth E., & Hoeft, Thea M. (1985). The family's dilemma: Alzheimer's disease. *Activities, Adaptation and Aging, 6*(4), 63-71.

Molsa, Pekka K., Marttila, R. J., and Rinne, U. K. (1986). Survival and cause of death in Alzheimer's disease and multi-infarct dementia. *Acta Neurologica Scandinavica, 74*(2), 103-107.

Molsa, Pekka K., Poljarvi, Leo, Rinne, Juha O., Rinne, Urpo K., & Sako, Erkki (1985). Validity of clinical diagnosis in dementia: A prospective clinicopathological study. *Journal of Neurology, Neurosurgery and Psychiatry, 48*(11), 1085-1090.

Montgomery, Rhonda J., & Borgatta, Joseph F. (1989). The effects of alternative support strategies on family caregiving. *Gerontologist, 29*(4), 457-464.

Montgomery, Rhonda J., Gonyea, J. G., & Hooyman, N. R. (1985). Caregiving and the experience of subjective and objective burden. *Family Relations: Journal of Applied Family and Child Studies, 34*(1), 19-26.

Moody, Harry R. (1988). Twenty-five years of the life review: Where did we come from? Where are we going? *Journal of Gerontological Social Work, 12*(3-4), 7-21.

Moritz, Deborah J., Kasl, Stanislav V., & Berkman, Lisa F. (1989).The health impact of living with a cognitively impaired elderly spouse: Depressive syndromes and social functioning. *Journal of Gerontology, 44*(1), S17-S27.

Morris, Lorna W., Morris, Robin G., & Britton, Peter G. (1988).The relationship between marital intimacy, perceived strain and depression in spouse caregivers of dementia sufferers. *British Journal of Medical Psychology, 61*(3), 231-236.

Morris, Lorna W. Morris, Robin G., & Britton, Peter G. (1989). Cognitive style and perceived control in spouse caregivers of dementia sufferers. *British Journal of Medical Psychology, 62*(2), 173-179.

Morycz, Richard K. (1985). Caregiving strain and the desire to institutionalize family members with Alzheimer's disease: Possible predictors and model development. *Research on Aging, 7*(3), 329-361.

Motenko, Aluma K. (1989). The frustrations, gratifications, and well-being of dementia caregivers. *Gerontologist, 29*(2), 166-172.

Nebes, Robert D. (1989). Semantic memory in Alzheimer's disease. *Psychological Bulletin, 106*(3), 377-394.

Nelson, Aaron, Fogel, Barry S., & Faust, David. (1986). Bedside cognitive screening instruments: A critical assessment. *Journal of Nervous and Mental Diseases, 174*(2), 73-83.

Nelson, H. E., & O'Connell, A. (1978). Dementia: The estimation of pre-morbid intelligence levels using the new adult reading test. *Cortex, 14,* 234-244.

Neufeld, M. Y., Inzelberg, R., & Korczyn, A. D. (1988). EEG in demented and non-demented parkinsonian patients. *Acta Neurologica Scandinavica, 78*(1), 1-5.

Newton, H., Pickard, J. D., & Weller, R. O. (1989). Normal pressure hydrocephalus and cerebrovascular disease: Findings of post-mortem. *Journal of Neurology, Neurosurgery and Psychiatry, 52*(6), 804.

Novak, Mark, & Guest, Carol. (1989). Caregiver response to Alzheimer's disease. *International Journal of Aging and Human Development, 28*(1), 67-79.

Oakley, David A., & Eames, Lesley C. (1985). The plurality of consciousness. In David A. Oakley (Ed.), *Brain and mind.* London: Methuen.

O'Boyle, Michael, & Amadeo, Marco. (1989). "Don't know" responses in elderly demented and depressed patients. *Journal of Geriatric Psychiatry and Neurology, 2*(2), 83-86.

O'Connor, Daniel W., Pollitt, Penelope A., Roth, Martin, Brook, Peter B., & Reiss, Bernard B. (1990). Memory complaints and impairment in normal, depressed, and demented elderly persons identified in a community survey. *Archives of General Psychiatry, 47*(3), 224-227.

Orr-Rainey, Nancy. (1991). Today's goals/tomorrow's fact: Special care units. Workshop, Southwestern Missouri Chapter of the Alzheimer's Association, October 24.

Orten, James D., Allen, Mary, & Cook, Jacque. (1989). Reminiscence groups with confused nursing center residents: An experimental study. *Social Work in Health Care, 14*(1), 73-86.

Oyebode, J. R., Barker, W. A., Blessed, G., Dick, D. J., & Britton, P.G. (1986). Cognitive functioning in Parkinson's disease: In relation to prevalence of dementia and psychiatric diagnosis. *British Journal of Psychiatry, 149,* 720-725.

Paire, Jane A., & Karney, Ronald J. (1984). The effectiveness of sensory stimulation for geropsychiatric inpatients. *American Journal of Occupational Therapy, 38*(8), 505-509.

Panella, John J., Lilliston, Barbara A., Brush, Dorothea & McDowell, Fletcher H. (1984). Day care for dementia patients: An analysis of a four-year program. *Journal of the American Geriatrics Society, 32*(12), 883-886.

Parker, Cynthia, & Somers, Carole. (1983). Reality orientation on a geropsychiatric unit. *Geriatric Nursing, 4*(3), 163-165.

Parlato, V., Carlomagno, Sergio, Merla, F., & Bonavita, V. (1988). Patterns of verbal memory impairment in dementia: Alzheimer disease vs. multi-infarctual dementia. *Acta Neurologica, 10*(6), 343-351.

Passafiume, Domenico & Boller, Francois (1984). Neuropsychological impairments of patients with Parkinson's Disease. *Archivio di Neurologia e Psichiatria, 45*(2), 211-224.

Passeri, M., & Cucinotta, D. (1989). Ateroid in the clinical treatment of multi-infarct dementia. *Modern Problems of Pharmacopsychiatry, 23,* 85-94.

Pearce, J. M. S., & Flowers, K. (1985). Dementia: A syndrome or an entity? In F. Clifford Rose (ed.), *Modern approaches to the dementias. Part II: Clinical and therapeutic aspects* (pp. 19-23). New York: Karger.

Pearlson, Godfrey D., Rabins, Peter V., Kim, Won S., Speedie, Lynn J., Moberg, Paul J., Burns, Alistair, & Bascom, Mary J. (1989). Structural brain CT changes and cognitive deficits in elderly depressives with and without reversible dementia. *Psychological Medicine, 19*(3), 573-584.

Pearson, Jane L., Teri, Linda, Reifler, Burton V., & Raskind, Murray A. (1989). Functional status and cognitive impairment in Alzheimer's patients with and without depression. *Journal of the American Geriatrics Society, 37*(12), 1117-1121.

Pfeiffer, Eric. (1978). Clinical manifestations of senile dementia.In Kalidas Nandy (ed.), *Senile dementia: A biomedical approach* (pp. 171-182). New York: Elsevier.

Pierce, David. (1987). Deliberate self-harm in the elderly. *International Journal of Geriatric Psychiatry, 2*(2), 105-110.

Pilisuk, Marc, & Parks, Susan H. (1988). Caregiving: Where families need help. *Social Work, 33*(5), 436-440.

Poulton, James L., & Strassberg, Donald S. (1986). The therapeutic use of reminiscence. *International Journal of Group Psychotherapy, 36*(3), 381-398.

Powell, Artiss L., Cummings, Jeffrey L., Hill, Mary A., & Benson, D. Frank. (1988). Speech and language alterations in multi-infarct dementia. *Neurology, 38*(5), 717-719.

Pratt, Clara C., Schmall, Vicki L., Wright, Scott, & Cleland, Marilyn. (1985). Burden and coping strategies of caregivers to Alzheimer's patients. *Family Relations Journal of Applied Family and Child Studies, 34*(1), 27-33.

Pratt, Clara C., Schmall, Vicki L., & Wright, Scott. (1986). Family caregivers and dementia. *Social Casework, 67*(2), 119-124.

Pratt, Clara C., Wright, Scott, & Schmall, Vicki (1987). Burden, coping and health status: A comparison of family caregivers to community dwelling and institutionalized Alzheimer's patients. *Journal of Gerontological Social Work, 10*(1-2), 99-112.

Predescu, V., Alexianu, Marilene, Tudorache, Bogdana, & Tudor, Sanda. (1983). Psychopathological correlations in multi-infarct dementia. *Neurologie et Psychiatrie, 21*(3), 231-233.

Proulx, Guy B., & Campbell, Kenneth B. (1986). The management of apparent "paranoid" behaviour in a patient with multi-infarct dementia. *Clinical Gerontologist, 6*(2), 121-128.

Pruchno, Rachel A., & Resch, Nancy L. (1989). Aberrant behaviors and Alzheimer' disease: Mental health effects on spouse care-givers. *Journal of Gerontology, 44*(5), S177-S182.

Quarrell, O. W., & Harper, Peter S. (1986). Huntington's chorea without dementia. *British Journal of Psychiatry, 148,* 612-613.

Quattrochi-Turbin, Susan J., & Jason, Leonard A. (1987-1988). The effects of cognitive and behavioral strategies in enhancing behavioral functioning among residents of a nursing home. *Gerontology and Geriatric Education, 8*(1-2), 133-148.

Quayhagen, Mary P., & Quayhagen, Margaret (1989). Differential effects of family-based strategies on Alzheimer's disease. *Gerontologist, 29*(2), 150-155.

Rabins, Peter V. (1982). Psychopathology of Parkinson's disease. *Comprehensive Psychiatry, 23*(5), 421-429.

Rai, G. S., Scott, L., & Beston, B. (1989). Assessment of the objective value of Mini-Mental State Examination. *Journal of Clinical and Experimental Gerontology, 11*(1-2), 41-46.

Raichle, Marcus E., Grubb, Robert L., Gado, Mokhtar H., Eichling, John O., & Hughes, Charles P. (1978). Cerebral hemodynamics and metabolism in dementia: Features distinguishing normal pressure hydrocephalus from atrophy. In Kalidas Nandy (ed.), *Senile dementia: A biomedical approach* (pp. 131-138). New York: Elsevier.

Reding, Michael J., Haycox, James, Wigforss, Karen, Brush, Dorothea and Blass, John P. (1984). Follow-up of patients referred to a dementia service. *Journal of the American Geriatrics Society, 32*(4), 265-268.

Reed, Bruce R., Stone, Arthur A., & Neale, John M. (1990). Effects of caring for a demented relative on elders' life events and appraisals. *Gerontologist, 30*(2), 200-205.

Reifler, Burton V. (1986). Mixed cognitive-affective disturbances in the elderly: A new classification. *Journal of Clinical Psychiatry, 47*(7), 354-356.

Reifler, Burton V., & Larson, Eric B. (1985). Alzheimer's disease and long-term care: The assessment of the patient. *Journal of Geriatric Psychiatry, 46,* 9-26.

Reinikainen, K., Soininen, H., Kosma, V-M., Halonen, T., Jolkkonen, J., & Riekkinen, P. J. (1985). Neurotransmitters in senile dementia of Alzheimer type and in vascular dementia. In F. Clifford Rose (Ed.), *Modern approaches to the dementias. Part I: Etiology and pathophysiology* (pp. 184-197). New York: Karger.

Reynolds, Charles F., Kupfer, David J., Houck, Patricia R., Hoch, Carolyn C., Stark, Jacqueline A., Berman, Susan R., & Zimmer, Ben. (1988). Reliable discrimination of elderly depressed and demented patients by electroencephalographic sleep data. *Archives of General Psychiatry, 45* (3), 258-264.

Rinn, William E. (1988). Mental decline in normal aging: A review. *Journal of Geriatric Psychiatry and Neurology, 1* (3), 144-158.

Rinne, U.K. (1983). Problems associated with long-term levodopa treatment of Parkinson's disease. *Acta Neurologica Scandinavica, 68* (Suppl. 95), 19-26.

Rinne, John O., Rummukainen, Jaana, Paljarvi, Leo, & Rinne, Urpo K. (1989). Dementia in Parkinson's disease is related to neuronal loss in the medial substantia nigra. *Annals of Neurology, 26* (1), 47-50.

Risberg, Jarl. (1987). Frontal lobe degeneration of non-Alzheimer type: III. Regional cerebral blood flow. *Archives of Gerontology and Geriatrics, 6* (3), 225-233.

Robb, Susanne S., Stegman, Charles E. and Wolanin, Mary O. (1986). No research vs. research with compromised results: A study of validation therapy. *Nursing Research, 35* (2), 113-118.

Robertson, Duncan, Rockwood, Kenneth, & Stolee, Paul (1982). A short mental status questionnaire. *Canadian Journal on Aging, 1* (1-2), 16-20.

Rogers, Daniel. (1986). Bradyphrenia in parkinsonism: A historical review. *Psychological Medicine, 16* (2), 257-265.

Rogers, Robert L., Meyer, John S., Mortel, Karl F., Mahurin, Roderick K. and Judd, Brian W. (1986). Decreased cerebral blood flow precedes multi-infarct dementia, but follows senile dementia of Alzheimer type. *Neurology, 36* (1), 1-6.

Rorsman, Birgitta, Hagnell, Olle, & Lanke, Jan. (1985). Mortality and age psychosis in the Lundby study: Death risk of senile and multi-infarct dementia: Changes over time in a prospective study of a total population followed over 25 or 15 years. *Neuropsychobiology, 14* (1), 13-16.

Rorsman, Birgitta, Hagnell, Olle, & Lanke, Jan. (1986). Prevalence and incidence of senile and multi-infarct dementia in the Lundby study: A comparison between the time periods 1947-1957 and 1957-1972. *Neuropsychobiology, 15* (3-4), 122-129.

Rosin, A. J., Abramowitz, L., Diamond, J. and Jesselson, P. (1985). Environmental management of senile dementia. *Social Work in Health Care, 11* (1), 33-43.

Rosser, M. N., Mountjoy, C. Q., Roth, M. and Reynolds, G. P. (1985). Ascending systems in Alzheimer's disease. In F. Clifford Rose (Ed.), *Modern approaches to the dementias. Part I: Etiology and pathophysiology* (pp. 198-212). New York: Karger.

Russell, E. W. (1975). A multiple scoring method for the assessment of complex memory functions. *Journal of Consulting and Clinical Psychology, 43,* 800-809.

Satz, P., & Mogel, S. (1962). An abbreviation of the WAIS for clinical use. *Journal of Clinical Psychology, 18,* 77-79.

Satz, Paul, Van Gorp, Wilfred G., Soper, Henry V., & Mitrushina, Maura (1987). WAIS-R marker for dementia of the Alzheimer type? An empirical and statistical induction study. *Journal of Clinical and Experimental Neuropsychology, 9* (6), 767-774.

Scheltens, Ph., Hazenberg, G.J., Lindeboom, J., Valk, J., & Wolters, E. Ch. (1990). A case of progressive aphasia without dementia: "Temporal" Pick's disease? *Journal of Neurology, Neurosurgery and Psychiatry, 53* (1), 79-80.

Schmidt, Gregory. (1986). Psychiatric symptoms caused by medical illness in the chronically mentally ill elderly. *New Directions for Mental Health Services, 29,* 59-70.

Schmidt, Gregory L. (1989). Reversible mental illness: The role of the family in therapeutic context. *Journal of Psychotherapy and the Family, 5*(1-2), 89-96.

Schroth, Gerhard, & Klosa, U. (1989). MRI of CSF flow in normal pressure hydrocephalus. *Psychiatry Research, 29*(3), 289-290.

Schultz, Katheryn A., Schmitt, Frederick A., Logue, Partick E. and Rubin, David C. (1986). Unit analysis of prose memory in clinical and elderly populations. *Developmental Neuropsychology, 2*(2), 77-87.

Schwab, Marilyn, Rader, Joanne, & Doan, Judy. (1985). Relieving the anxiety and fear in dementia. *Journal of Gerontological Nursing, 11*(5), 8-15.

Schwarb, Susanne, Koberle, Suse, & Spiegel, R. (1988). The Alzheimer's Disease Assessment Scale (ADAS): An instrument for early diagnosis of dementia? *International Journal of Geriatric Psychiatry, 3*(1), 45-53.

Scott, Jean Pearson, Roberto, Karen A., & Hutton, J. Thomas. (1986). Families of Alzheimer's victims: Family support to the caregivers. *Journal of the American Geriatrics Society, 34,* 348-354.

Segall, Mary, & Wykle, May. (1988-1989). The Black family's experience with dementia. *Journal of Applied Social Sciences, 13*(1), 170-191.

Shamoian, Charles A. (1985). Assessing depression in elderly patients. *Hospital and Community Psychiatry, 36*(4), 338-339, 345.

Shefer, V. F. (1985). Multiinfarction dementia. *Zhurnal Nevropatologii i Psikhiatrii, 85*(7), 976-979.

Sherman, Edmund. (1985). A phenomenological approach to reminiscence and life review. *Clinical Gerontologist, 3*(4), 3-16.

Shibayama, Hiroto, Kasahara, Y., & Kobayashi, H. (1986). Prevalence of dementia in a Japanese elderly population. *Acta Psychiatrica Scandinavica, 74*(2), 144-151.

Shock, Nathan W. (1984). *Normal human aging: The Baltimore longitudinal study of aging.* Washington, DC: U.S. Government Printing Office.

Shoulson, Ira. (1978). Dementia in Huntington's disease and cognition effects of muscimol therapy. In Kalidas Nandy (ed.), *Senile dementia: A biomedical approach* (pp. 251-258). New York: Elsevier.

Shoulson, Ira. (1990). Huntington's disease: Cognitive and psychiatric features. *Neuropsychiatry, Neuropsychology and Behavioral Neurology, 3*(1), 15-22.

Simank, Margaret H., & Strickland, Kenny J. (1985–1986). Assisting families in coping with Alzheimer's disease and other related dementias with the establishment of a mutual support group. *Journal of Gerontological Social Work, 9*(2), 49-58.

Sims, N. R., Finnegan, J. M., Blass, John P., Bowen, D. M., & Neary, D. (1987). Mitochondrial function in brain tissue in primary degenerative dementia. *Brain Research, 436*(1), 30-38.

Sistler, Audrey. (1989). Adaptive coping of older caregiving spouses. *Social Work, 34*(5), 415-420.

Skelton-Robinson, M., & Jones, S. (1984). Nominal dysphasia and the severity of senile dementia. *British Journal of Psychiatry, 145,* 168-171.

Slaby, Andrew E., & Cullen, Leah Oscar (1987). Dementia and delirium. In Alan Stoudemire and Barry S. Fogel (eds.), *Principles of medical psychiatry.* Orlando, Grune & Stratton.

Smith, D. A., & Lantos, P. L. (1983). A case of combined Pick's disease and Alzheimer's disease. *Journal of Neurology, Neurosurgery and Psychiatry, 46*(7), 675-677.

Smith, Georgia H. (1986). A comparison of the effects of three treatment interventions on cognitive functioning of Alzheimer patients. *Music Therapy, 6A*(1), 41-56.

Smith, Stan, Butters, Nelson, White, Roberta, Lyon, Lauren, & Granholm, Eric. (1988). Priming semantic relations in patients with Huntington's disease. *Brain and Language, 33*(1), 27-40.

Soininen, H., Partenen, V. J., Helkala, Eeva Liisa, & Riekkinen, Paavo J. (1982). EEG findings in senile dementia and normal aging. *Acta Neurologica Scandinavica, 65*(1), 59-70.

Soloman, Kenneth. (1990). Mental health and the elderly. In Abraham Monk (Ed.), *Handbook of gerontological services* (pp. 228-267). New York: Columbia University Press.

Spar, James E. (1982). *Dementia in the aged.* Psychiatric Clinics of North America, 5(1), 67-86.

Speedie, Lynn, Rabins, Peter V., Pearlson, Godfrey D., & Moberg, Paul J. (1990). Confrontation naming deficit in dementia and depression. *Journal of Neuropsychiatry and Clinical Neurosciences, 2*(1), 59-63.

Staight, Paula R., & Harvey, S. Marie (1990). Caregiver burden: A comparison between elderly women as primary and secondary caregivers for their spouses. *Journal of Gerontological Social Work, 15*(1-2), 89-104.

Starr, Cynthia. (1990). Alzheimer's: The stranger among us. *Drug Topics,* Sept. 3, 34-36, 41-42, 44.

St. Clair, D., & Whalley, L. J. (1983). Hypertension, multi-infarct dementia and Alzheimer's disease. *British Journal of Psychiatry, 143,* 274-276.

Stern, Matthew B., Gur, Ruben C., Saykin, Andrew J., & Hurtig, Howard I. (1986). Dementia of Parkinson's disease and Alzheimer's disease: Is there a difference? *Journal of the American Geriatrics Society, 34*(6), 475-478.

Steuer, Joanne L., & Clark, Elizabeth O. (1982). Family support groups within a research project on dementia. *Clinical Gerontologist, 1*(1), 87-95.

Stigsby, Bent. (1988). Dementias (Alzheimer's and Pick's disease): Dysfunctional and structural changes. *American Journal of EEG Technology, 28*(2), 83-97.

St. Laurent, Maurice. (1988). Normal pressure hydrocephalus in geriatric medicine: A challenge. *Journal of Geriatric Psychiatry and Neurology, 1*(3), 163-168.

Stoller, Elearnor P., & Pugliesi, Karen L. (1989). Other roles of caregivers: Competing responsibilities or supportive services. *Journals of Gerontology, 44*(6), S231-S238.

Stommel, Manfred, Given, Charles W., & Given, Barbara A. (1990). Depression as an overriding variable explaining caregiver burdens. *Journal of Aging and Health, 2*(1), 81-102.

Storandt, Martha. (1983). Understanding senile dementia: A challenge for the future. *International Journal of Aging and Human Development, 16*(1), 1-6.

Stoudemire, Alan, Hill, Connie, Gulley, Lawrence R., & Morris, Robin G. (1989). Neuropsychological and biomedical assessment of depression-dementia syndromes. *Journal of Neuropsychiatry and Clinical Neurosciences, 1*(4), 347-361.

Striano, S., Meo, R., & Bilo, L. (1988). Conventional EEG in the differential diagnosis of dementia syndromes. *Acta Neurologica, 10*(2), 98-107.

Sturt, Elizabeth. (1986). Application of survival analysis to the inception of dementia. *Psychological Medicine, 16*(3), 583-593.

Sudarsky, Lewis, Morris, James, Romero, Jorge, & Walshe, Thomas M. (1989). Dementia in Parkinson's disease: The problem of clinicopathologic correlation. *Journal of Neuropsychiatry and Clinical Neurosciences, 1*(2), 159-166.

Sulkava, Raimo, & Amberla, Kaarina. (1982). Alzheimer's disease and senile dementia of Alzheimer type: A neuropsychological study. *Acta Neurologica Scandinavica, 65*(6), 651-660.

Sulkava, Raimo, & Erkinjuntti, T. (1987). Vascular dementia due to cardiac arrhythmias and systemic hypotension. *Acta Neurologica Scandinavica, 76*(2), 123-128.

Sulkava, Raimo, Viinikha, Lasse, Erkinjuntti, Timo, & Roine, Risto. (1988). Cerebrospinal fluid neuron-specific enolase is decreased in multi-infarct dementia, but unchanged in Alzheimer's disease. *Journal of Neurology, Neurosurgery and Psychiatry, 51* (4), 549-551.

Sunderland, Trey. (1990). Organic brain disorders: Non-Alzheimer dementias. In William B. Abrams, & Robert Berkow (eds.), *The Merck manual of geriatrics* (pp. 944-948). Rahway, NJ: Merck Sharp and Dohme Research Laboratories.

Sutcliffe, Caroline, & Larner, Stuart (1988). Counseling carers of the elderly at home: A preliminary study. *British Journal of Clinical Psychology, 27* (2), 177-178.

Sutherland, Stuart. (Ed.) (1989). *The international dictionary of psychology.* New York: Continuum.

Swash, M., Smith, C. M., & Hart, S. (1985). The dementia of Alzheimer's disease. In F. Clifford Rose (Ed.), *Modern approaches to the dementias. Part II. Clinical and therapeutic aspects* (pp. 1-11). New York: Karger.

Swearer, Joan M., Drachman, David A., O'Donnell, Brian F., & Mitchell, Ann L. (1988). Troublesome and disruptive behaviors in dementia: Relationships to diagnosis and disease severity. *Journal of the American Geriatrics Society, 36* (9), 784-790.

Taft, Lois B. (1989). Conceptual analysis of agitation in the confused elderly. *Archives of Psychiatric Nursing, 3* (2), 102-107.

Tager, Robert M. (1980). Physical assessment. In Steven H. Zarit, (Ed.), *Aging and mental disorders* (pp. 161-183). New York: Free Press.

Tanahashi, Norio, Meyer, John S., Ishikawa, Yoshiki, Kandula, Prasab, Mortel, Karl F., Rogers, Robert L., Gandhi, Sunil, & Walker, Mary. (1985). Cerebral blood flow and cognitive testing correlate in Huntington's disease. *Archives of Neurology, 42* (12), 1169-1175.

Taulbee, L. A., & Folsom, J. C. (1966). Reality orientation for geriatric patients. *Hospital and Community Psychiatry, 17* (5), 133-135.

Teng, Evelyn Lee, Chui, Helena Chang, Schneider, Lon S., & Metzger, Laura Erickson. (1987). Alzheimer's dementia: Performance on the Mini-Mental State Examination. *Journal of Consulting and Clinical Psychology, 55* (1), 96-100.

Teresi, Jeanne, Toner, John, Bennett, Ruth, & Wilder, David (1988-1989). Caregiver burden and long-term care planning. *Journal of Applied Social Sciences, 13* (1), 192-214.

Terman, Lewis M., & Merrill, Maude A. (1937). *Measuring intelligence.* Cambridge, MA.: Riverside Press.

Terry, Robert D., & Parker, Joseph C. (1990). The pathologic basis for dementia. Unpublished paper presented at Alzheimer' Disease 1990: New Dimensions in Research. Kansas City, KS.

Thompson, Suzanne C., Bundek, Nancy I., & Sobolew-Shubin, Alexandria (1990). The caregivers of stroke patients: An investigation of factors associated with depression. *Journal of Applied Social Psychology, 20* (2), 115-119.

Torack, R. M. (1978). *The pathologic physiology of dementia.* New York: Springer-Verlag.

Tresch, Donald D., Folstein, Marshal F., Rabins, Peter F., & Hazzard, William R. (1985). Prevalence and significance of cardiovascular disease and hypertension in elderly patients with dementia and depression. *Journal of the American Geriatrics Society, 33* (8), 530-537.

Truschke, Edward F. (1991). The FDA/THA debate: The Alzheimer's Association viewpoint. *Newsletter of the Alzheimer's Association, 11,* 2, p. 2.

Tuokko, H., & Crockett, D. (1987). Central cholinergic deficiency WAIS profiles in a non-demented aged sample. *Journal of Clinical and Experimental Neuropsychology, 9* (2), 225-227.

Turner, T. H. (1985). Huntington's chorea without dementia: A problem case. *British Journal of Psychiatry, 146,* 548-550.

Veroff, Amy E., Pearlson, Godfrey D., & Ahn, Hyo S. (1982). CT scan and neuropsychological correlates of Alzheimer's disease and Huntington's disease. *Brain and Cognition, 1* (2), 177-184.

Von Bonin, Gerhardt. (1963). *The evolution of the human brain.* Chicago: University of Chicago Press.

Wallis, Geoffrey G., Baldwin, M., & Higginbotham, P. (1983). Reality orientation therapy: A controlled trial. *British Journal of Medical Psychology, 56* (3), 271-277.

Wands, Kim, Merskey, Harold, Hachinski, Vladimir C., Fishman, Michael, Fox, Hannah, & Boniferro, Mary. (1990). A questionnaire investigation of anxiety and depression in early dementia. *Journal of the American Geriatrics Society, 38* (5) 535-538.

Webb, R. Mark, & Trzepacz, Paula T. (1987). Huntington's disease: Correlates of mental status with chorea. *Biological Psychiatry, 22* (6), 751-761.

Webster's *Medical Desk Dictionary* (1986). Springfield, MA.: Merriam-Webster.

Wechsler, David. (1944). *The measurement of adult intelligence* (3rd ed.). Baltimore, MD: Williams, & Wilkins.

Wechsler, David. (1955). The measurement and evaluation of intelligence in older persons. In Third Congress of the International Association of Gerontology, *Old age in the modern world* (pp. 275-279). London: E. and S. Livingstone.

Wechsler, David. (1961). Intelligence, memory, and the aging process. In Paul S. Hoch and Joseph Zubin (eds.), *Psychopathology of aging* (pp. 152-159). New York: Grune & Stratton.

Wechsler, David (1981). *Manual for the WAIS-R.* New York: Psychological Corporation.

Wechsler, David. (1987). *Wechsler Memory Scale—Revised.* San Antonio, TX.: Psychological Corporation.

Wechsler, David, & Stone, Calvin P. (1973). *Wechsler Memory Scale.* New York: Psychological Corporation.

Weinberger, Daniel R., Berman, Karen F., Iadarola, Mary, Driesen, Naomi, & Zec, Ronald F. (1988). Prefrontal cortical blood flow and cognitive function in Huntington's disease. *Journal of Neurology, Neurosurgery and Psychiatry, 51* (1), 94-104.

Weinstein, Barbara E., & Amsel, Lynn (1986). Hearing loss and senile dementia in the institutionalized elderly. *Clinical Gerontologist, 4* (3), 3-15.

Whall, Ann L. (1986). Identifying the characteristics of pseudo-dementia. *Journal of Gerontological Nursing, 12* (10), 34-35.

Whalley, L. J., Wright, A. F., & St. Clair, D. M. (1985). Genetic factors in Down's syndrome and their possible role in the pathogenesis of Alzheimer's disease. In F. Clifford Rose (Ed.), *Modern approaches to the dementias. Part I: Etiology and pathophysiology* (pp. 18-31). New York: Karger.

Whittick, Janice E. (1988). Dementia and mental handicap: Emotional distress in carers. *British Journal of Clinical Psychology, 27* (2), 167-172.

Wilson, Holly S. (1989). Family caregiving for a relative with Alzheimer's dementia: Coping with negative choices. *Nursing Research, 38* (2), 94-98.

Wilson, Robert S., Fox, Jacob H., Huckman, Michael S., Bacon, Lynd D., & Lobrick, John J. (1982). Computed tomography in dementia. *Neurology, 32* (9), 1054-1057.

Wilson, Robert S., Kaszniak, Alfred W., Bacon, Lynd D., Fox, Jacob H., & Kelly, Mark P. (1982). Facial recognition memory in dementia. *Cortex, 18* (3), 329-336.

Winblad, Bengt, Hardy, John, Backman, Lars, & Nilsson, Lars Goran. (1985). Memory function and brain biochemistry in normal aging and in senile dementia. *Annals of the New York Academy of Sciences, 444,* 255-268.

Winogrond, Iris R., Fisk, Albert A., Kirsling, Robert A., & Keyes, Barbara. (1987). The relationship of caregiver burden and morale to Alzheimer's disease patient function in the therapeutic setting. *Gerontologist, 27* (3), 336-339.

Wisniewski, H. M., Merz, G. S., & Carp, R. I. (1985). Current hypothesis of the etiology and pathogenesis of senile dementia of the Alzheimer type. In F. Clifford Rose (Ed.), *Modern approaches to the dementias.* Part I: Etiology and pathophysiology (pp. 45-53). New York: Karger.

Wolanin, Mary O. (1983). Scope of the problem and its diagnosis. *Geriatric Nursing, 4*(4), 227-230.

Wolfe, Gary R. (1987). Clinical neuropsychology and assessment of brain impairment: An overview. *Cognitive Rehabilitation, 5*(5), 20-25.

Woods, R. T. (1983). Specificity of learning in reality-orientation sessions: A single-case study. *Behaviour Research and Therapy, 21*(2), 173-175.

Wright, Scott D., Pratt, Clara C., & Schmall, Vicki L. (1985). Spiritual support for caregivers of dementia patients. *Journal of Religion and Health, 24*(1), 31-38.

Yahr, Melvin D., & Pang, Stuart W. H. (1990). Movement disorders: Parkinsonian syndrome. In William B. Abrams, & Robert Berkow(eds.), *The Merck manual of geriatrics* (pp. 974-981). Rahway, NJ: Merck Sharp and Dohme Research Laboratories.

Yesavage, J. A., Brink, T. L., Rose, T. L., Lum, O., Huang, V., Adey, M., & Leirer, V. O. (1983). Development and validation of a Geriatric Depression Screening Scale: A preliminary report. *Journal of Psychiatric Research, 17,* 37-49.

Zarit, Steven H. (1980). *Aging and mental disorders.* New York: Free Press.

Zarit, Steven H., & Zarit, Judy M. (1982). Families under stress: Interventions for caregivers of senile dementia patients. *Psychotherapy Theory, Research and Practice, 19*(4), 461-471.

Zarit, Steven H., & Zarit, Judy M. (1986). Dementia and the family: A stress management approach. *Clinical Psychologist, 39*(4), 103-105.

Zarit, Steven H., Anthony, Cheri R., & Boutselis, Mary (1987). Interventions with caregivers of dementia patients: Comparisons of two approaches. *Psychology and Aging, 2*(3), 225-232.

Zarit, Steven H., Orr, Nancy, & Zarit, Judy M. (1985). *The hidden victims of Alzheimer's disease: Families under stress.* New York: New York University Press.

Zimpfer, David G. (1987). Groups for the aging: Do they work? *Journal for Specialists in Group Work, 12*(2), 85-92.

Zubenko, George S. (1990). Progression of illness in the differential diagnosis of primary dementia. *American Journal of Psychiatry, 147*(4), 435-438.

Zubenko, George S., & Moossy, John. (1988). Major depression in primary dementia: Clinical and neuropathologic correlates. *Archives of Neurology, 45*(11), 1182-1186.

Zubenko, George S., Moossy, John, & Kopp, Ursula. (1990). Neurochemical correlates of major depression in primary dementia. *Archives of Neurology, 47*(2), 209-214.

Index